5-HYDROXYTRYPTAMINE
IN PERIPHERAL REACTIONS

5-Hydroxytryptamine
in Peripheral Reactions

Editors

Fred De Clerck, M.Sc.
Laboratory of Haematology
Janssen Pharmaceutica Research
Laboratories
B-2340 Beerse, Belgium

Paul M. Vanhoutte, M.D.
Department of Physiology and Biophysics
Mayo Clinic and Foundation
Rochester, Minnesota

Raven Press ■ New York

Raven Press, 1140 Avenue of the Americas, New York, New York 10036

Made in the United States of America

Library of Congress Cataloging in Publication Data
Main entry under title:

5-hydroxytryptamine in peripheral reactions.

"This volume is the result of a workshop ... held in Beerse, Belgium, in March 1981, under the sponsorship of the Janssen Research Foundation"—Acknowledgement.
Includes bibliographical references and index.
  1. Serotonin—Physiological effect—Congresses.   I. Clerck, Fred de.   II. Vanhoutte, Paul M.   III. Janssen Research Foundation.
[DNLM: 1. Serotonin.   QV 126 Z99]
QP801.S4A16   615.7   82-7585
ISBN 0-89004-772-3   AACR2

Great care has been taken to maintain the accuracy of the information contained in the volume. However, Raven Press cannot be held responsible for errors or for any consequences arising from the use of the information contained herein.

Preface

This volume is a concerted international effort of leading scientists to summarize and discuss present knowledge on the role of 5-hydroxytryptamine in the normal and pathological functioning of peripheral organs.

The first section deals with the sites of production, the storage, and the release of 5-hydroxytryptamine in the intestine, as well as its transport and release in the blood by platelets and its deactivation by endothelial cells.

The second section covers the possible physiological role of 5-hydroxytryptamine in the normal function of the blood vessel wall and the platelets; particular attention is paid not only to the direct effects of 5-hydroxytryptamine on the tissue cells, but also to its potential to markedly amplify the effect of other endogenous neurohumoral mediators. For comparison, the effects of prostacyclin are summarized.

The third section focuses on a number of diseases where 5-hydroxytryptamine could play a role, possibly even in the initiation of the pathological condition. These include: muscular dystrophies, malignant hyperthermia, pulmonary diseases, shock, and hypertension.

Throughout this text, frequent reference is made to the pharmacological and potential therapeutic properties of a new 5-HT_2 (S_2) serotonergic receptor antagonist ketanserin (R41468; 3-{2-[4-(4-fluorobenzoyl)-1-piperidinyl]ethyl}-2,4($1H,3H$)-quinazolinedione). Because this compound is both selective for $5HT_2$-serotonergic receptor sites and devoid of agonistic properties, which so commonly complicate the actions of serotonergic antagonists, it has become a powerful pharmacological tool in unraveling the role of 5-hydroxytryptamine both in health and disease. Its properties are described in more detail in the last section.

This book will be of interest not only to scientists, whether physiologists or pharmacologists, but also to clinical researchers, anesthesiologists, and physicians who manage patients with hypertension, cardiovascular failure, peripheral vascular disease, and muscular dystrophies.

The Editors

Acknowledgments

This volume is the result of a workshop "5-Hydroxytryptamine in Peripheral Reactions" held in Beerse, Belgium, in March 1981, under the sponsorship of the Janssen Research Foundation. The editors are indebted to Dr. P. Janssen for his stimulating interest and criticism during the preparation and performance of this workshop.

Contents

5-Hydroxytryptamine and Pathological Conditions

Pharmacological and Clinical Profiles of Ketanserin

Contributors

H. Ahlman
Department of Surgery III
Sahlgren Hospital
S-41345 Göteborg
Sweden

F. Awouters
Department of Pharmacology
Janssen Pharmaceutica
B-2340 Beerse
Belgium

J. Bach Kolling
Department of Cardiovascular
* Anaesthesia*
Medisch Centrum De Klokkenberg
4800 RA Breda
The Netherlands

T. Barbui
Division of Hematology
Ospedale Riuniti
Bergamo
Italy

S. R. Bloom
Histochemistry Unit
Department of Histopathology
* and Department of Medicine*
Hammersmith Hospital
London W12 OHS, United Kingdom

L. Carreras
Center for Thrombosis
* and Vascular Research*
Department of Medical Research
University of Leuven
Campus Gasthuisberg
Herestraat, 49
B-3000 Leuven
Belgium

L. Ceccatelli
Department of Internal Medicine
School of Medicine
University of Siena
I-53100 Siena
Italy

S. Cortellazzo
Division of Hematology
Ospedale Generale Regionale
Vicenza
Italy

A. Dahlström
Institute of Neurobiology
University of Göteborg
S-41345 Göteborg
Sweden

P. D'Amore
Department of Surgery
Children's Hospital Medical Center
Harvard Medical School
Boston, Massachusetts 02115

J. L. David
Hôpital de Bavière
Université de Liège
Institut de Médecine
B-4200 Liège
Belgium

F. De Clerck
Laboratory of Haematology
Janssen Pharmaceutica
B-2340 Beerse
Belgium

W. De Cock
Clinical Research Unit
St. Bartholomeus
Jan Palfijn ziekenhuis
B-2060 Merksem
Belgium

J. De Cree
Clinical Research Unit
St. Bartholomeus
Jan Palfijn ziekenhuis
B-2060 Merksem
Belgium

G. De Gaetano
Laboratory of Haematosis and
Thrombosis
Istituto "Mario Negri"
I-20157 Milano
Italy

J. De Mey
Laboratory of Oncology
Janssen Pharmaceutica Research
Laboratories
B-2340 Beerse
Belgium

T. Di Perri
Department of Internal Medicine
School of Medicine
University of Siena
I-53100 Siena
Italy

H. Geukens
Clinical Research Unit
St. Bartholomeus
Jan Palfijn ziekenhuis
B-2060 Merksem
Belgium

D. Grahame-Smith
MRC Clinical Pharmacology Unit
University Department of Clinical
Pharmacology
Radcliffe Infirmary
Oxford OX2 6HE
United Kingdom

A. G. Herman
University of Antwerp
Department of Experimental
Pharmacology
B-2610 Wilrijk
Belgium

P. A. J. Janssen
President and Director of Research
Janssen Pharmaceutica
B-2340 Beerse
Belgium

F. Laghi Pasini
Department of Internal Medicine
School of Medicine
University of Siena
I-53100 Siena
Italy

J. Leempoels
Clinical Research Unit
St. Bartholomeus
Jan Palfijn ziekenhuis
B-2060 Merksem
Belgium

D. Lewis
Clinical Research Center
University Hospital
S-58185 Linköping
Sweden

J. Leysen
Department of Biochemical
Pharmacology
Janssen Pharmaceutica
B-2340 Beerse
Belgium

G. L. Makabali
Division of Reproductive Sciences
Department of Obstetrics and Gynecology
The Charles R. Drew Postgraduate
Medical School
Los Angeles, California 90048

A. K. Mandal
Department of Surgery
The Charles R. Drew Postgraduate
Medical School
Los Angeles, California 90048

G. Martelli
Department of Internal Medicine
School of Medicine
University of Siena
I-53100 Siena
Italy

J. A. Morris
Department of Pharmacology, Obstetrics,
and Gynecology
Medical University of South Carolina
Charleston, South Carolina 24425

L. Ooms
Veterinary Department
Janssen Pharmaceutica
B-2340 Beerse
Belgium

J. Polak
Histochemistry Unit
Department of Histopathology and
Department of Medicine
Royal Postgraduate Medical School
Hammersmith Hospital
London W12 OHS, United Kingdom

C. Post
Department of Clinical Pharmacology
University Hospital
S-58185 Linköping
Sweden

R. S. Reneman
Department of Physiology
University of Limburg
6200 MD Maastricht
The Netherlands

H. Scheijgrond
Department of Clinical Research
Janssen Pharmaceutica
B-2340 Beerse
Belgium

D. Shepro
Department of Biology and Surgery
Boston University
Boston, Massachusetts 02115

P. Stoward
Department of Anatomy
The University
Dundee DD1 4HN
Scotland

J. Symoens
Department of Clinical Research
Janssen Pharmaceutica
B-2340 Beerse
Belgium

P. J. A. Van der Starre
Department of Cardiovascular
Anaesthesia
Medisch Centrum "De Klokkenberg"
4800 RA Breda
The Netherlands

P. M. Vanhoutte
Department of Physiology and Biophysics
Mayo Clinic and Foundation
Rochester, Minnesota 55905

J. Van Nueten
Department of Pharmacology
Janssen Pharmaceutica
B-2340 Beerse
Belgium

H. Verhaegen
Clinical Research Unit
St. Bartholomeus
Jan Palfijn ziekenhuis
B-2060 Merksem
Belgium

A. Verheyen
Laboratory of Cell Biology
Janssen Pharmaceutica
Research Laboratories
B-2340 Beerse
Belgium

J. Vermylen
Center for Thrombosis and Vascular
Research
Department of Medical Research
University of Leuven
Campus Gasthuisberg
B-3000 Leuven
Belgium

P. Viero
Division of Hematology
Ospedale Generale Rigionale
Vicenza
Italy

H. Vittoria
Department of Internal Medicine
School of Medicine
University of Siena
I-53100 Siena
Italy

5-Hydroxytryptamine in Peripheral Reactions,
edited by Fred De Clerck and Paul M.
Vanhoutte. Raven Press, New York © 1982.

Storage and Release of 5-Hydroxytryptamine in Enterochromaffin Cells of the Small Intestine

*Håkan Ahlman and **Annica Dahlström

*Department of Surgery III, **Sahlgren Hospital and Institute of Neurobiology,
University of Göteborg, S-413 45 Göteborg, Sweden

In mammals most 5-hydroxytryptamine of the body is located in the enterochromaffin cells of the gastrointestinal tract (23,52). In certain species, e.g., rats and mice, the mast cells also contain large amounts of 5-hydroxytryptamine. Apart from neurons in the central nervous system, enteric intramural nerves also have been suggested to contain and use 5-hydroxytryptamine as transmitter (25,26,59). In the guinea pig, Gershon et al. (25) reported autoradiographic evidence for such 5-hydroxytryptamine-containing enteric neurons, but no objective evidence for the presence of the 5-hydroxytryptamine fluorophore in the myenteric plexus of this species was found spectrocytofluorimetrically (1). However, Gershon (26) reviewed a number of studies, using various methodological approaches, which provide convincing evidence for the existence of such enteric 5-hydroxytryptamine-containing neurons. These neurons normally contain small amounts of 5-hydroxytryptamine and it is, therefore, difficult with present techniques to study their function.

The enterochromaffin cells are part of "the diffuse endocrine system" already recognized by Feyrter (24) in 1938. He found in routine stains of the gut many cells with a very clear cytoplasm ("helle Zellen"). Many of these cells were found to stain brown after fixation in dichromate solutions (cf. ref. 30). Ciaccio (19) had observed as early as 1906 that certain cells of the gut mucosa and adrenal medulla cells stained similarly after dichromate fixation, and had named these cells in the gut "enterochromaffin cells." Many names have been proposed for these cells (e.g., argentaffin cells, basal granulated cells; for review, see ref. 52), but "enterochromaffin cells" is the generally accepted term.

CYTOFLUORIMETRIC METHOD FOR STUDIES OF 5-HYDROXYTRYPTAMINE

The enterochromaffin cells are characterized by numerous, large, irregular and electrondense granules, which contain 5-hydroxytryptamine in addition to various peptides such as motilin and substance P (57) (Fig. 1). We have studied their

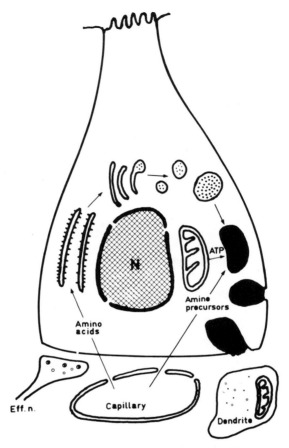

FIG. 1a. Schematic drawing of an epithelial enterochromaffin cell in close contact with nerve terminals, dendrites, and capillaries. Synthesis of 5-hydroxytryptamine and polypeptide hormones from amine precursors and amino acids; both compounds are probably stored together in individual granules.

5-hydroxytryptamine content by using a cytofluorimetric technique, where the intensity of the formaldehyde-induced fluorescence is recorded and quantified in individual cells.

The gut specimens studied were cut into small pieces (3 × 4 × 4 mm), of the whole intestinal wall, which were placed on coded paper strips. The specimens were then quickly frozen in liquid propane, cooled by liquid nitrogen. After freeze-drying at −50°C for 2 to 3 days, the specimens were warmed up to room temperature while exposed to air, and allowed to react in a closed vessel with paraformaldehyde gas, generated from paraformaldehyde powder at the bottom of the vessel, at +80°C for 1 hr. Following embedding in paraffin *in vacuo*, thin sections (8–10 μm)were cut, placed on a clean glass slide, and mounted, without previous deparaffination, in a mixture of Entellane® and xylene. The sections were examined in a fluorescence

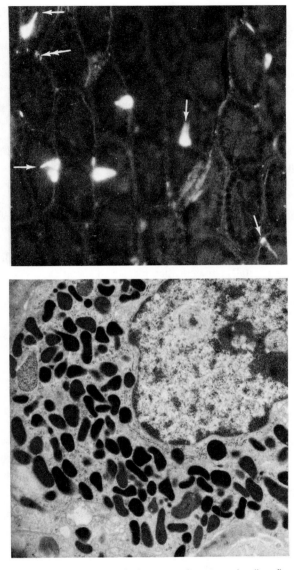

FIG. 1b. Top: Fluorescence micrograph demonstrating several yellow fluorescent triangular enterochromaffin cells in transversely cut feline jejunal crypts *(single arrows)* and surrounding green fluorescent adrenergic nerve terminals *(double arrows)*. Each enterochromaffin cell is about 20 to 25 μm in length. **Bottom:** Electronmicrograph demonstrating details of osmiophilic secretory granules of feline enterochromaffin cells. (Diameter of granules 100−600 nm).

microscope (either trans- or epi-illumination type), equipped with filter combinations for the demonstration of the yellow 5-hydroxytryptamine fluorophore (2,20,54). The enterochromaffin cells of the gut mucosa were identified by fluorescence microscopy by the presence of strongly fluorescent yellow granules in the cytoplasm. Adrenergic nerves can also be studied with the same method because they contain the strongly fluorescent green product of norepinephrine and paraformaldehyde (Fig. 1). Since the intensity of the formaldehyde-induced 5-hydroxytryptamine fluorescence is relative to the intracellular concentration of the amine under certain conditions (see refs. 2,34,54), cytofluorimetric measurements of individual enterochromaffin cells were performed. A schematic illustration of this procedure is shown in Fig. 2. After identification of enterochromaffin cells in crypts of the intestinal mucosa, individual cells were positioned within a measuring diaphragm, with a diameter to encompass the entire cell. The intensity of 5-hydroxytryptamine fluorescence was recorded with a photometer tube and registered on a digital voltmeter and finally fed into a computer (Hewlett-Packard). Background fluorescence was also measured and subtracted from the actual reading of individual cells. In each specimen 20 to 30 cells, randomly chosen, were measured. The fluorescence intensities of experimentally treated specimens (all samples coded), expressed in arbitrary units, were then compared with controls and normalized. The effect of various treatments on the relative content of 5-hydroxytryptamine (increase or decrease over control) could thus be evaluated.

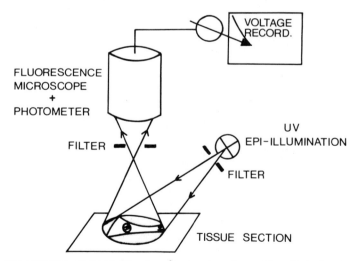

FIG. 2. The principles of cytofluorimetry, where enterochromaffin cells in tissue section, are activated with ultraviolet incident light. The fluorescence intensity emitted from each cell is recorded by means of a photometer and voltmeter. (With permission of *Acta Physiologica Scandinavica*.)

IN VIVO STUDIES ON THE ADRENERGIC INNERVATION OF THE INTESTINAL MUCOSA

Vagal Adrenergic Input

In the guinea pig, when the vagal nerves are stimulated at the cervical level, the 5-hydroxytryptamine level in gut homogenates decreases, and the number of argentaffin granules in the enterochromaffin cells is reduced (31,60). In cats, with bilaterally ligated adrenals to reduce circulating catecholamines (which may influence the tryptamine concentration in enterochromaffin cells), similar stimulations cause a clear decrease in the content of enterochromaffin cells at three different levels of the small intestine (3), indicating the release of 5-hydroxytryptamine. This vagally-induced decrease was not blocked by atropine, but could be inhibited with pro-pranolol, a beta-adrenoceptor blocking agent. Alpha-adrenergic blocking drugs, e.g., phenoxybenzamine and phentolamine, did not inhibit the decrease; on the contrary, in their presence the 5-hydroxytryptamine content was often significantly increased (4). Removal of the superior cervical ganglion prior to stimulation also blocked the decrease in 5-hydroxytryptamine content of the enterochromaffin cells, suggesting that an *adrenergic* mechanism was activated upon vagal stimulation.

In order to study if the vagal nerves contain adrenergic fibers, the vagi were crush-operated at the cervical level in cats. Crushing of a nerve causes an immediate arrest in the rapid intraaxonal transport of material synthesized in the nerve soma and transported distally toward the nerve endings (21,27). Due to this blockade, substances moving toward the nerve terminals accumulate proximal to the crush, where they can be measured biochemically or studied histochemically. In the feline crushed vagal nerve, numerous adrenergic axons with prominent accumulations of norepinephrine (green fluorescence after formaldehyde treatment; see the following section) were demonstrated. After removal of the superior cervical ganglion these adrenergic fibers were absent at the cervical level. At the subdiaphragmatic level branches of the vagal nerve (e.g., the nerve of Latarjet) also contained adrenergic fibers (4). Studies on human nerve specimens, removed during surgery, demon-strated that the vagal nerve carries many adrenergic postganglionic fibers in man also (44).

The presence of adrenergic fibers in the vagal nerve, demonstrated also previously for dog and cat (43,48), appeared remarkable at that time, since the vagus was generally considered to be a pure parasympathetic nerve. Stimulation experiments indicated that some of these adrenergic fibers probably innervated not only the gut mucosa, but also smooth muscle cells (47). In order to establish the existence of a nervous pathway between the sympathetic ganglia of the neck and the small intestine, experiments using the retrograde horseradish peroxidase technique were performed. Horseradish peroxidase is a protein taken up by nerve terminals by pinocytotic mechanisms and transported by retrograde axonal transport to the cell body where horseradish peroxidase-activity can be demonstrated with cytochemical techniques (39). Cats and guinea pigs were used for the study. Under anesthesia, a horseradish peroxidase solution was injected at multiple sites into the gut wall along the duodenum and jejunum. At various times after this procedure the animals were killed by perfusion fixation and the superior cervical, stellate, nodose, and celiac ganglia (Fig. 3) were dissected and examined for the presence of horseradish peroxidase positive cells (45). All guinea pig ganglia contained horseradish peroxidase positive cells 24 hr after the injection; the celiac and the nodose ganglia contained a large, but the stellate and superior cervical ganglion a rather small number of positive cells. In the cat, only the celiac ganglion contained horseradish peroxidase-labeled cells at 24 hr but at 60 hr the stellate, and at 72 hr the nodose and superior cervical ganglion also contained labeled cells, reflecting the longer transport distance in the cat than in the guinea pig. If the cervical vagal nerve was crush-operated at the time of the injection, this prevented the occurrence of horseradish peroxidase in the ipsilateral superior cervical and nodose ganglion after sufficient transport time (Fig. 3). Crushing the preganglionic sympathetic trunk alone did not prevent the appearance of horseradish peroxidase in the superior cervical ganglion. This demonstrates that: (a) The horseradish peroxidase in the superior cervical ganglion was not taken up from the blood; (b) the horseradish peroxidase reached this ganglion via a nervous pathway; and (c) axons in the vagus, not in the preganglionic sympathetic trunk, carried the horseradish peroxidase up to the superior cervical ganglion. Horseradish peroxidase could also be demonstrated in the vagal nerve distal to the crush-operation (45). The pathway between cervical sympathetic ganglia via the vagal nerve to the wall of the small intestine was thus established both by anterograde and retrograde techniques. The results were corroborated in another series of anterograde studies by fluorescence histochemistry, where ipsilateral removal of the superior cervical and stellate ganglion, respectively, caused a marked reduction in the number of vagal adrenergic fibers at the subdiaphragmatic level (6).

However, in order to postulate a stimulatory effect on the enterochromaffin cells in the gut mucosa, one must demonstrate the presence of nervous elements near these enterochromaffin cells. With the fluorescence microscopy, adrenergic nerve terminals were frequently observed very close to the base of enterochromaffin cells (Fig. 1).

In order to study this relationship at the ultrastructural level, guinea pigs were treated with 5-OH-dopamine, i.v., 1 or 24 hr before sacrifice, using the perfusion fixation technique. The 5-OH-dopamine is taken up into adrenergic nerve terminals and incorporated into the amine granules, inducing a very marked electron density upon osmification (62). Examination of serial sections revealed that every enterochromaffin cell, and often also neighboring "intestinocytes" (absorptive cells), were accompanied by bundles of nerve fibers incompletely ensheathed in Schwann cells. The nerve processes consisted of at least four different kinds: (a) filled with mainly small clear vesicles and a few large dense core vesicles; (b) processes with many small electron dense vesicles, probably adrenergic terminals having taken up the 5-OH-dopamine; (c) boutons with many large opaque to dense vesicles, probably "p-type" boutons; and (d) nerve processes with a clear cytoplasm with a few irregular

CRUSH OP.	CELIAC GGL. BILATERAL	STELLATE GGL. IPSI	CONTRA	SCG IPSI	CONTRA
(N=2)	+	+	+	+	+
CERV. VAGUS UNILAT. (N=2)	+	+	+	-	+
CERV. VAGUS BILAT. (N=2)	+	+	+	-	-
CERV. VAGUS SYMP. CHAIN UNILAT. (N=2)	+	+	+	-	+
CERV. SYMP. CHAIN BILAT	+	+	+	+	+

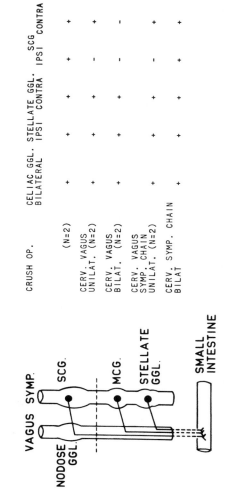

FIG. 3. Table summarizing the presence (+) or absence (−) of the horseradish peroxidase reaction product in various sympathetic ganglia (ggl) (superior cervical ggl = SCG; mediate cervical ggl = MCG; stellate ggl) 24 hr after local injection of horseradish peroxidase into the guinea pig duodenal wall, when various types of nerve crushes uni- or bilaterally were performed at a level just below the vagal nodose ganglion (*dashed line*).

vesicles, mitochondria and, occasionally, ribosomes, probably representing dendrites (46). These bundles of nerve fibers were present near the base of the enterochromaffin cells, but well within the distance of the so called "autonomic gap" of 500 nm, considered to be of functional importance in the autonomic nervous system (16). Synapse-like contacts between efferent nerve terminals and enteroendocrine cells were observed later (49) (Fig. 4). Thus, the morphological evidence for a nerve-mediated influence on enterochromaffin cells is established.

Splanchnic Adrenergic Input

The major part of the extrinsic adrenergic supply to the gastrointestinal tract runs with the splanchnic nerves. This was confirmed in the horseradish peroxidase experiments, where a large number of ganglion cells in the celiac ganglion were retrogradely labeled with horseradish peroxidase following injection of the enzyme into the gut wall. In the cat with both adrenals ligated, stimulation of the splanchnic nerve at the preganglionic level also caused a significant reduction of the 5-hydroxytryptamine content in enterochromaffin cells at different levels of the small intestine (42). This decrease could not be blocked by atropine; however, propranolol, and to a certain extent, alpha-adrenoceptor blocking drugs, could inhibit this effect (42). Thus, the adrenergic input from the splanchnic nerves also seems to participate in the extrinsic neural control of the release of 5-hydroxytryptamine of enterochromaffin cells in the gut.

IN VITRO STUDIES

Incubations of gut specimens from the rat were performed in 10 ml vials containing oxygenated Krebs' solution with various drugs added (53). Control specimens were incubated in Krebs' solution alone for the same period of time as the experimental specimens. Various receptor agonists were added to the bath in concentrations ranging between 10^{-9} to 10^{-5} M, and the incubation time was 30 min at 37 to 39°C. The beta-adrenoceptor agonists epinephrine and isoprenaline caused a significant dose-dependent decrease in 5-hydroxytryptamine of enterochromaffin cells at all concentrations studied, even at 10^{-9} M, epinephrine being the most potent in lowering the 5-hydroxytryptamine fluorescence intensity (to 35–45% of control). Norepinephrine, a potent alpha-adrenoceptor agonist, was effective at a concentration as low as 10^{-7} M. Dopamine did not lower 5-hydroxytryptamine in the enterochromaffin cells, while acetylcholine incubation induced a small but significant decrease in the 5-hydroxytryptamine level (by about 14–16%) (53).

In order to study the type of receptor activated by epinephrine in these *in vitro* studies, preincubation with various adrenoceptor-blocking agents was performed. The epinephrine (10^{-7} M)-induced decrease in 5-hydroxytryptamine was blocked by d,l-propranolol (10^{-6} M) if present in the incubation medium for 15 min before the agonist was added; d-propranolol did not block the epinephrine effect, showing that the d,l-propranolol blockade was not due to membrane stabilizing properties of the compound. The selective beta$_1$-antagonist metoprolol (10^{-6} M) did not prevent

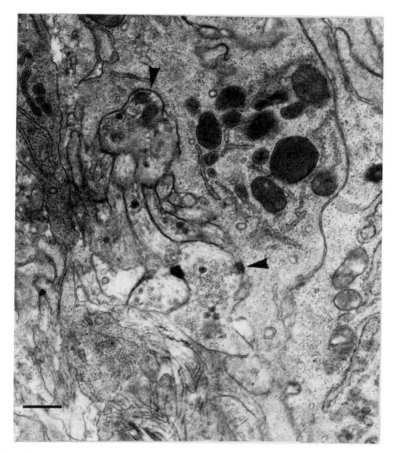

FIG. 4. Between two crypts of the rat ileal mucosa close to an enterochromaffin cell (with large granules to the *right*) two nerve terminal varicosities *(arrow heads)* can be seen. The lower one has a true synaptic specialization on the enterochromaffin cell membrane. Both large dense core vesicles and small round clear vesicles are present in the varicosity. *Bar* represents 400 nm. (With permission of *Acta Physiologica Scandinavica.*)

the epinephrine effect, nor did the alpha-adrenoceptor antagonists phentolamine and phenoxybenzamine. Thus, the effect of epinephrine incubation on the 5-hydroxytryptamine levels in the enterochromaffin cells must be mediated by beta$_2$-adrenoceptors (53).

If a nervous adrenergic mechanism participated in the regulation of 5-hydroxytryptamine in these cells, field stimulation of gut strips *in vitro* should cause a similar decrease of 5-hydroxytryptamine in the enterochromaffin cells. This was tested in an experimental model (Fig. 5), where a gut strip was mounted between two parallel platinum meshwork electrodes, 7 mm apart, in an open plexiglass chamber submerged in oxygenated Krebs' solution. The upper free end of the specimen strip was connected to a force displacement transducer in order to obtain

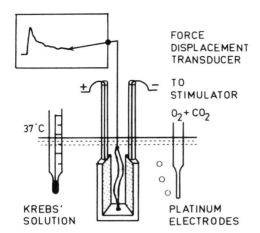

FIG. 5. Experimental model for transmural field stimulation. The gut strip was mounted between two meshwork electrodes in an open plexiglass chamber submerged in oxygenated Krebs' solution with the drug to be tested. Upper end of gut specimen connected to a force displacement transducer to record contractility during stimulation. (With permission of *Acta Physiologica Scandinavica.*)

recordings of smooth muscle contraction (55). Stimulation of control specimens (18V, 2 msec, 10 Hz for 15 min, inducing a current of 5 to 6 mA/mm²/2 msec) caused a marked contractile response of the gut strips and a significant decrease in the 5-hydroxytryptamine level of the enterochromaffin cells (by 18–53%). The addition of tetrodotoxin (10^{-6} M) to the incubation system abolished both the field stimulation-induced contractions of the specimens and the 5-hydroxytryptamine decrease in the enterochromaffin cells. This indicates that the field stimulation procedure influenced both smooth muscle cells and mucosa of the gut strip via a nervous mechanism, since tetrodotoxin inhibits action potentials of nerves by blocking the Na^+-channels of the axolemma (35); *d,l*-propranolol blocked the 5-hydroxytryptamine decrease in the enterochromaffin cells, but had no influence on the smooth muscle contraction. When the adrenergic nerves of the gut were selectively destroyed by pretreatment of the rats with 6-OH dopamine 1 week prior to the experiments, the field stimulation-induced 5-hydroxytryptamine reduction was prevented in 5 of 6 rats (Fig. 6). These field stimulation experiments thus demonstrate that the decreased 5-hydroxytryptamine levels in enterochromaffin cells are caused by a neurogenic mechanism mediated by beta-adrenoceptors (54,55).

RELEASE OF 5-HYDROXYTRYPTAMINE FROM ENTEROCHROMAFFIN CELLS INTO THE PORTAL CIRCULATION

The marked reduction in the 5-hydroxytryptamine levels of enterochromaffin cells upon vagal or splanchnic nerve stimulation suggests that the cells release the amine when extrinsically stimulated. A marked intracellular deamination and/or a reduced synthesis may, of course, also contribute to the stimulation induced decrease in 5-hydroxytryptamine content of the enterochromaffin cells, but the potent biological effects of 5-hydroxytryptamine in the gastrointestinal tract (10,14,15,33,54) make it more likely that this amine is released extracellularly together with the peptide(s) which are also stored in the large osmophilic granules (7).

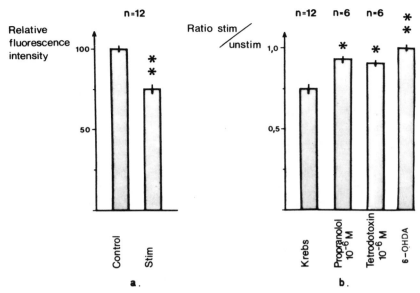

FIG. 6. **(a):** The effect of field stimulation (see text) on 5-hydroxytryptamine fluorescence in duodenal enterochromaffin cells from normal rats. Mean values and SEM. Difference from unstimulated controls indicated by *two asterisks* ($p < 0.01$). **(b):** The influence of propranolol, tetrodotoxin, and 6-OH-dopamine on 5-hydroxytryptamine fluorescence in enterochromaffin cells. Mean values and SEM of the ratios stimulated/unstimulated are given for each group. *Single asterisk:* differences from gut specimens stimulated in Krebs' solution ($p < 0.05$). *Two asterisks* are significant $p < 0.01$.

Since the storage granules are usually localized near the base of the cells, a release across the basolateral membrane is likely. The amine may then either escape into the portal circulation, or be metabolized locally after uptake into neighboring cells. However, there is no evidence from fluorescence histochemical studies for the marked uptake of 5-hydroxytryptamine into "intestinocytes," fibroblasts, or other connective tissue cells which would be needed to handle the large amounts released from the enterochromaffin cells. Therefore, measurements of the 5-hydroxytryptamine levels in the portal plasma before, during, and after vagal nerve stimulation were performed. Cats, fasted for 24 hr with free access to water, were studied under chloralose anesthesia. Blood samples (2–2.5 ml each) were drawn through a heparinized catheter inserted in the portal vein with the tip in the hilus region. Saline was given, i.v., before and during the experiment to maintain blood volume. The blood samples were collected on ice and centrifuged at the end of the experiment to remove all blood corpuscles, and the plasma was then frozen until the 5-hydroxytryptamine concentration in the plasma was assayed fluorimetrically using modified Cox and Perhach method (41,56).

Vagal nerve stimulation induced a rapid rise in plasma 5-hydroxytryptamine, from a basal level of about 200 ng/ml up to 487 ± 56 ng/ml after 15 min of nerve stimulation. After stimulation the levels normalized within 10 to 15 min (56).

Propranolol, which should be effective in blocking 5-hydroxytryptamine release from the enterochromaffin cells if a beta-adrenoceptor mechanism is involved, significantly reduced, but did not abolish, the 5-hydroxytryptamine increase in portal plasma at low doses (0.1 and 1 mg/kg); higher doses (2 mg/kg) seemed to be less effective (Fig. 7). This lack of dose-response relationship, together with the incomplete blockade with "optimal" doses of propranolol, may be due to, e.g., facilitation of other release mechanisms with higher doses of the beta-adrenergic blocking drug, or, more likely, to the membrane-stabilizing effect of propranolol which causes inhibition of the uptake of 5-hydroxytryptamine into blood platelets (28).

Splanchnic nerve stimulation caused a significant rise in the 5-hydroxytryptamine concentrations of portal plasma during stimulation (from a basal level of about 300 ng/ml to about 500 ng/ml after 15 min). The values normalized within 15 min after cessation of the stimulation (41). In this study the levels of substance P were also measured, since some enterochromaffin cells may store this peptide (e.g., ref. 57). No change in the levels of substance P were observed with splanchnic nerve stimulation, which may be explained by the immunohistochemical observation that feline enterochromaffin cells do not appear to contain measurable levels of this peptide (J. M. Lundberg et al., *unpublished*).

RELEASE OF 5-HYDROXYTRYPTAMINE INTO THE GUT LUMEN

Occasionally, and especially after vagal nerve stimulation, one may observe both in fluorescence microscopic sections (32) and in electron micrographs (5) that the 5-hydroxytryptamine storing granules are located in the apical portion, rather than at the base of the cells. This indicates that the granules have migrated towards apical parts of the cell. Therefore, the possibility of an apical release 5-hydroxytryptamine from the enterochromaffin cells into the gut lumen was investigated. Early *in vitro* experiments by Bülbring and colleagues (14,15) had already suggested that a 5-hydroxytryptamine-like material is released into the lumen of the guinea pig ileum and the rabbit jejunum during chemical or mechanical stimulation. With combined electron microscopy and autoradiography after injection of ^{3}H-5-hydroxytryptophan, a release of the radioactive tracer into the gut lumen was demonstrated in response to electrical vagal nerve stimulation (8) (Fig. 8).

During *in vivo* perfusion of proximal jejunal segments of fasted cats there was a constant basal rate of intraluminal secretion of the amine (64 ± 12 ng/5 min at a perfusion rate of 1 ml saline/min) as measured by a sensitive radioimmunoassay (36).

During efferent electrical stimulation of the cut cervical vagal nerves, 5-hydroxytryptamine significantly increased (by 120%) in the perfusate. This stimulatory effect was not altered following bilateral adrenalectomy in the same animals (9). Vagal nerve stimulation at the thoracic level was compared with cervical stimulation in the same animals because the cervical stimulation causes a decreased mucosal blood flow in the small intestine. Vagal nerve stimulation at the thoracic level

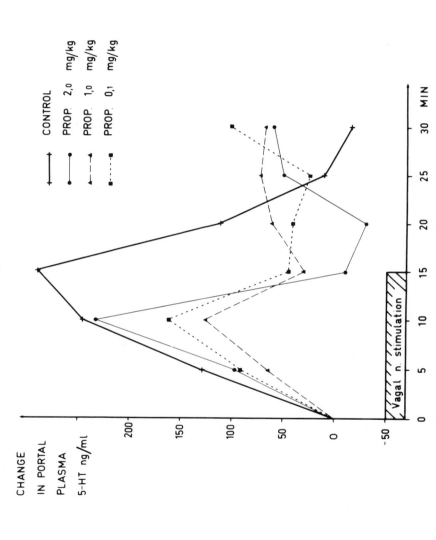

FIG. 7. Diagram demonstrating the increase in portal plasma. 5-hydroxytryptamine concentration upon vagal nerve stimulation in untreated controls ($n = 7$) and cats treated with propranolol ($n = 3$ at each dose tested). Note maximal inhibition at the two lowest doses. (With permission of *Acta Physiologica Scandinavica*.)

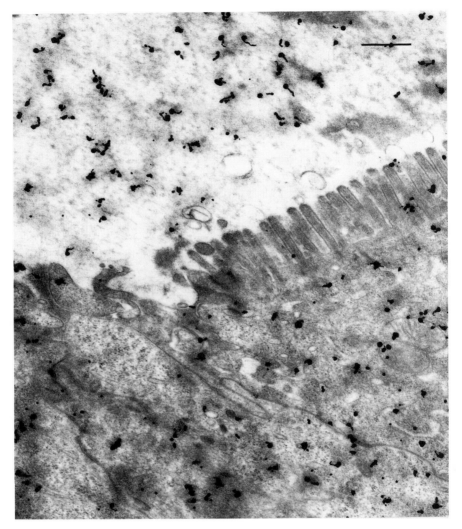

FIG. 8. Electronmicroscopic autoradiograph from rat duodenal mucosa 3 hr after injection of tritiated 5-hydroxytryptophan (1 m Ci, i.v.) and a 10 min period of vagal nerve stimulation. Numerous silver grains are present in the apical portion of the intestinal epithelium both in enteroendocrine cells and "intestinocytes" (absorptive cells) but also in the gut lumen. *Bar* represents 800 nm. (With permission of *Acta Physiologica Scandinavica*.)

caused a similar increase of luminal 5-hydroxytryptamine, which supports the hypothesis of a true neurogenic release mechanism (63).

THE EFFECT OF CHOLERA TOXIN ON THE
5-HYDROXYTRYPTAMINE OF ENTEROCHROMAFFIN CELLS

Cholera toxin may induce diarrhea secretion in the small intestine by directly acting on the "intestinocytes," inducing increased concentrations of cyclic adenosine monophosphate (22). However, other nervous mechanisms may also play an important role (17,18). The absorption/secretion of fluid was measured in isolated, weighed segments of the feline small intestine after instillation of crude cholera toxin into the lumen of the segment for 30 min. The toxin was then washed out. The pronounced secretion caused by cholera toxin could be blocked and turned into a normal absorptive pattern by administration of tetrodotoxin, or by local anesthetic agents applied to the mucosal surface (17). Furthermore, rendering the gut tachyphylactic to 5-hydroxytryptamine by repeated high doses of the amine also markedly reduced the cholera toxin-induced secretion (18). This indicates that 5-hydroxytryptamine may play a role in the cholera-associated diarrhea. Therefore, the effect of cholera toxin on 5-hydroxytryptamine levels in enterochromaffin cells of the feline jejunum was determined with simultaneous recording of the absorption/secretion. Either cholera toxin or heat-inactivated toxin were instilled in gut segments. Small biopsies were taken 1 to 5 hr after the onset of the cholera toxin administration. They were frozen and treated for fluorescence histochemistry as described in the first section. Cytofluorimetric estimations of 5-hydroxytryptamine in enterochromaffin cells, located in crypts and in villi, revealed that almost every animal showed a marked decrease (in some cats by as much as 70% of control) in intracellular 5-hydroxytryptamine. This decrease occurred in some cats after 1 hr, in other cats the maximal decrease was observed 4 to 5 hr after the toxin instillation. The results from the physiological part of the experiments demonstrated a remarkable parallelism in the secretory response of the gut (Fig. 9). In cats where the cellular content of 5-hydroxytryptamine was the lowest at 1 hr, the secretory response was maximal at this time, then slowly returned toward zero secretion. Accordingly, in animals where the cellular content of 5-hydroxytryptamine was lowest at 5 hr, the secretion was most pronounced at this time. In one cat where cholera toxin instillation had no significant effect on the 5-hydroxytryptamine content in the enterochromaffin cells, no secretory response was recorded. Heat-inactivated cholera toxin had no effect on the 5-hydroxytryptamine levels, nor on the absorption of fluid (50).

The results demonstrate that cholera toxin is the most powerful 5-hydroxytryptamine-releasing agent so far tested on enterochromaffin cells, and that the timing of the effect on 5-hydroxytryptamine in enterochromaffin cells is strikingly congruent with the effect on intestinal secretion. Further experiments will give information if these two responses are causally related.

THE BIOLOGICAL SIGNIFICANCE OF 5-HYDROXYTRYPTAMINE RELEASED FROM THE GUT

The physiological significance of 5-hydroxytryptamine in the gut is still not understood. The rapid elimination of 5-hydroxytryptamine from plasma by uptake into platelets (12) and a postulated rapid degradation in liver and lung (61) seem to favor a local or paracrine role of the amine. It has been known for long that acidification of the duodenum results in a marked inhibition of the gastric acid secretion (58). 5-Hydroxytryptamine is released into the portal circulation following

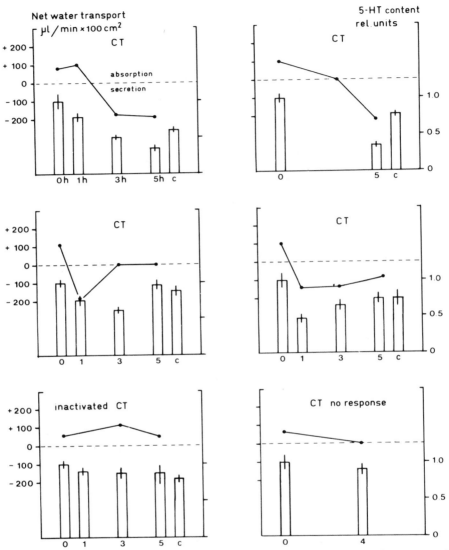

FIG. 9. The relation between intestinal secretion and 5-hydroxytryptamine fluorescence in samples of enterochromaffin cells (*n* = 20) in small intestinal segments from 6 cats at various times after exposure to cholera toxin. Note parallel changes in these parameters; e.g., in one cat treated with inactivated cholera toxin and in one cat nonresponsive to cholera toxin, no significant changes in intracellular 5-hydroxytryptamine occurred.

duodenal acidification (38). Several authors have demonstrated that the amine is a potent inhibitor of gastric acid secretion (11,29). Despite these properties, 5-hydroxytryptamine was never a serious candidate for the humoral mediation of this response due to the rapid hepatic inactivation, until Jaffe et al. (33) studied various fractions (whole blood, platelet-rich and platelet-poor plasma) of portal blood. These authors found that platelet-bound 5-hydroxytryptamine escaped hepatic inactivation in considerable amounts, and that endogenously liberated 5-hydroxytryptamine had acid inhibitory effects similar to those of exogenously administered 5-hydroxytryptamine, in support of the hypothesis that 5-hydroxytryptamine is involved in the physiological control of gastric acid secretion.

The peripheral 5-hydroxytryptamine levels are elevated following a meal (36). Biber et al. (10) have suggested that 5-hydroxytryptamine participates in the postprandial hyperemia of the gut and that an intrinsic vasodilator reflex involving a 5-hydroxytryptamine-mediated step is activated by mechanical stimulation of the mucosa. An intact vascular response to 5-hydroxytryptamine is necessary for the vasodilator effects of gastrointestinal hormones such as cholecystokinin and secretin. Early observations by Bülbring and Lin (14) had suggested that 5-hydroxytryptamine could modulate the peristaltic reflex; however, an almost complete depletion of mucosal 5-hydroxytryptamine did not abolish it (13). Cholera toxin could trigger 5-hydroxytryptamine release from enterochromaffin cells which, in turn, could activate submucosal nerve endings which presumably constitute the afferent link of an intrinsic reflex, the activation of which may result in increased secretion from the intestinal epithelium (see Fig. 10).

This "neurogenic" hypothesis is corroborated by the fact that the effect of cholera toxin is blocked by local anesthesia of the mucosa, tetrodotoxin, propranolol, and ganglionic blocking agents (17,18,22). The cholera toxin effect is also blocked by tachyphylaxis against 5-hydroxytryptamine and the use of 5-hydroxytryptamine-blocking agents such as methysergide and chlorpromazine (18).

The significance of intraluminal 5-hydroxytryptamine is not well known. Bülbring and Lin (14) reported that when 5-hydroxytryptamine was added to the fluid passing through the lumen of the gut, peristalsis was stimulated. Among other roles the amine may exert trophic effects on the gastrointestinal mucosa, as demonstrated earlier for intraluminal gastrin. A luminal 5-hydroxytryptamine receptor may also be involved in the potent actions of the amine on motility and secretion in the postprandial response of the small intestine, especially since rapid degradation by intracellular monoamine oxidase may be avoided in the case of luminal secretion (9).

In preliminary investigations of rat lungs *in vivo*, we found that, after endothelial passage, exogenous 5-hydroxytryptamine was taken up and stored in pulmonary mast cells. However, *in vitro* experiments demonstrated a significant uptake-retention of 5-hydroxytryptamine from the incubation medium into cultured endothelial cells from the rat pulmonary artery. The 5-hydroxytryptamine content of the cells was increased after monoamine oxidase inhibition, indicating an intracellular metabolization of the amine. It is, therefore, possible that *in vivo* also, the endothelial cells can metabolize 5-hydroxytryptamine by oxidation, but that 5-hydroxytryptamine can be transported across the endothelium into the pulmonary parenchyma (mast cells) when the concentration of circulating 5-hydroxytryptamine is high enough (37).

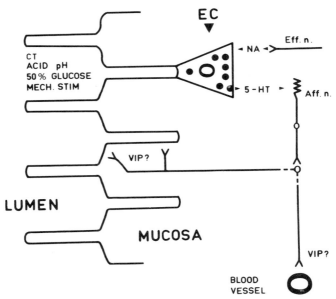

FIG. 10. Hypothetical relationship between nerves and enterochromaffin cells, and participation of 5-hydroxytryptamine from enterochromaffin in intrinsic reflexes of the intestine, where a final vasoactive intestinal polypeptide (VIP) containing neuron has been suggested (refs. 10,17, 18; C. Lundgren and M. Jodal, *personal communication*).

The clinical role of 5-hydroxytryptamine released from the gut has been recognized in patients with carcinoid tumors and the postgastrectomy dumping syndrome. In patients with inflammatory bowel disease there is an inverse relation between the density of the adrenergic innervation and the number of enterochromaffin cells found (40). Catecholamines are potent flush-inducing agents in patients with the carcinoid syndrome (51).

ACKNOWLEDGMENTS

This work was supported by grants from the Swedish Medical Research Council (17X5220, 14X2207, 04P-4173). The Medical Faculty, University of Göteborg, Göteborg Medical Society, M. Bergwalls Foundation, and H. and G. Jeanssons Foundation.

REFERENCES

1. Ahlman, H., and Enerbäck, L. (1974): A cytofluorometric study of the myenteric plexus in the guinea pig. *Cell Tissue Res.*, 153:419–434.
2. Ahlman, H. (1976): Fluorescence histochemical studies on serotonin in the small intestine and the influence of vagal nerve stimulation. *Acta Physiol. Scand. (Suppl.)*, 437.
3. Ahlman, H., Dahlström, A., Kewenter, J., and Lundberg, J. (1976): Vagal influence on serotonin concentration in enterochromaffin cells in the cat. *Acta Physiol. Scand.*, 97:362–368.
4. Ahlman, H., Lundberg, J., Dahlström, A., and Kewenter, J. (1976): A possible vagal adrenergic release of serotonin from enterochromaffin cells in the cat. *Acta Physiol. Scand.*, 98:366–375.

5. Ahlman, H., Bhargava, H. N., Donahue, P. E., Newson, B., Das Gupta, T. K., and Nyhus, L. M. (1978): The vagal release of 5-HT from enterochromaffin cells in the cat. *Acta Physiol. Scand.*, 104:262–270.
6. Ahlman, H., Larson, G. M., Bombeck, C. T., and Nyhus, L. M. (1979): Origin of the adrenergic nerve fibers in the subdiaphragmatic vagus in the dog. *Am. J. Surg.*, 137:116–122.
7. Ahlman, H., Newson, B., Das Gupta, T. K., and Nyhus, L. M. (1979): Secretory granules of the duodenal enterochromaffin cells of the cat. *J. Surg. Res.*, 27:145–147.
8. Ahlman, H., Bhargava, H. N., Dahlström, A., Larsson, I., Newson, B., and Pettersson, G. (1981): On the presence of serotonin in the gut lumen and possible release mechanisms. *Acta Physiol. Scand.*, 112:263–269.
9. Ahlman, H., De Magistris, L., Zinner, M., and Jaffe, B. M. (1981): Release of immunoreactive serotonin into the gut lumen of the feline gut in response to vagal nerve stimulation. *Science*, 213:1254–1255.
10. Biber, B., Fara, J., and Lundgren, O. (1974): A pharmacological study of intestinal vasodilator mechanisms in the cat. *Acta Physiol. Scand.*, 90:673–683.
11. Black, J. W., Fisher, E. W., and Smith, A. N. (1958): The effect of 5-HT on gastric secretion in anesthetized dogs. *J. Physiol. (Lond.)*, 141:27–34.
12. Born, G. V. R., and Gillson, R. E. (1959): Studies on the uptake of 5-HT by blood platelets. *J. Physiol. (Lond.)*, 146:472–491.
13. Boullin, D. J. (1964): Observations on the significance of 5-HT in relation to the peristaltic reflex of the rat. *Br. J. Pharmacol.*, 23:14–33.
14. Bülbring, E., and Lin, R. C. Y. (1958): The effect of intraluminal application of 5-HT and 5-HTP on peristalsis; the local production of 5-HT and its release in relation to intraluminal pressure and propulsive activity. *J. Physiol. (Lond.)*, 140:381–407.
15. Bülbring, E., and Crema, A. (1959): The release of 5-HT in relation to pressure exerted on the mucosa. *J. Physiol. (Lond.)*, 146:18–28.
16. Burnstock, G., and Costa, M. (1975): *Adrenergic Neurons, Their Organization, Function and Development in the Peripheral Nervous System*. Chapman & Hall, London.
17. Cassuto, J., Jodal, M., Tuttle, R., and Lundgren, O. (1979): The effect of lidocaine on the secretion induced by cholera toxin in the cat small intestine. *Experientia*, 35:1467–1468.
18. Cassuto, J., Fahrenkrug, J., Jodal, M., Tuttle, R., and Lundgren, O. (1980): The role of 5-HT and vasoactive intestinal polypeptide in the pathogenesis of choleraic secretion. *Proc. Scand. Soc. Physiol.*, D 40.
19. Ciaccio, C. (1906): Sur une nouvelle espèce cellulaire dans les glandes de Lieberkühn. *C. R. Soc. Biol. (Paris)*, 60:76–77.
20. Dahlström, A., and Fuxe, K. (1964): A method for the demonstration of adrenergic nerve fibers in peripheral nerves. *Z. Zellforsch.*, 62:602–607.
21. Dahlström, A. (1971): Axoplasmic transport (with particular respect to adrenergic neurons). In: *Subcellular and Macromolecular Aspects on Synaptic Transmission*, edited by H. Blaschko and A. D. Smith, pp. 325–358. Philos. Trans. R. Soc. (Lond.).
22. Donowitz, M., Charney, A. N., and Hynes, R. (1979): Propranolol prevention of choleraenterotoxin-induced intestinal secretion in the rat. *Gastroenterology*, 76:482–491.
23. Erspamer, V. (1954): Quantitative estimation of 5-HT in gastrointestinal tract, spleen and blood of vertebrates. In: *CIBA Symposium on Hypertension*, edited by G. Wolstenholme and M. P. Cameron, pp. 78–84. Churchill, London.
24. Feyrter, F. (1938): Über diffuse endokrine epitheliale Organe. Barth, Leipzig.
25. Gershon, M. D., Drakontides, A. B., and Ross, L. L. (1965): Serotonin: Synthesis and release from the myenteric plexus of the mouse intestine. *Science*, 149:197–199.
26. Gershon, M. D. (1981): Enteric serotoninergic neurons. *Annu. Rev. New Sci.*, 4:227–272.
27. Grafstein, B., and Forman, D. S. (1980): Intracellular transport in neurons. *Physiol. Rev.*, 60(4):1167–1283.
28. Grobecker, H., Lenner, B., Hellenbrecht, D., and Wiethold, G. (1973): Inhibition by anti-arrhythmic and betasympatholytic drugs of serotonin uptake by human platelets: Experiments *in vitro* and *in vivo*. *Eur. J. Clin. Pharmacol.*, 5:145–150.
29. Haverback, B. J., Bogdanski, D., and Hogben, C. A. M. (1958): Inhibition of gastric acid secretion in the dog by the precursor of 5-HT, 5-HTP. *Gastroenterology*, 37:188–192.
30. Heidenhain, R. (1870): Untersuchungen über den Bau den Labdrüsen. *Arch. Mikr. Anat.*, 6:368–406.

31. Hohenleitner, F., Tansy, M., and Golder, R. (1971): Effect of vagal stimulation on duodenal serotonin in the guinea-pig. *J. Pharmacol. Sci.*, 60:471–472.
32. Izumikawa, F. (1980): Release mechanisms of 5-HT from the gastrointestinal tract in rats. *Arch. Jap. Clin.*, 49(5):572–594.
33. Jaffe, B. M., Kopen, D. F., and Lazan, D. W. (1977): Endogenous serotonin in the control of gastric acid secretion. *Surgery*, 82:156–163.
34. Jonsson, G. (1971): *Quantitation of Fluorescence of Biogenic Monoamines Demonstrated by the Formaldehyde Fluorescence Method.* G. Fischer Verlag, Stuttgart.
35. Kao, C. Y. (1966): Tetrodotoxin, sacitoxin and their significance in the study of excitation phenomena. *Pharmacol. Rev.*, 18:997–1049.
36. Kellum, J. M., and Jaffe, B. M. (1976): Validation and application of a radioimmunoassay for serotonin. *Gastroenterology*, 70:516–522.
37. Kjellström, T., Ahlman, H., Dahlström, A., and Risberg, B. (1982): The cellular uptake of 5-HT in the rat lung in vivo—a histochemical study. *Acta Physiol. Scand. (in press)*.
38. Koren, E., Wapnick, S., and Solowiejczyk, M. (1976): 5-HT in the portal vein after acidification. *Intern. Surg.*, 61:370–372.
39. Kristensson, K., and Olsson, Y. (1973): Diffusion pathways and retrograde axonal transport of protein tracers in peripheral nerves. *Prog. Neurobiol.*, 1:85–109.
40. Kyösola, K., Penttilä, O., and Salaspuro, M. (1977): Rectal mucosal innervation and enterochromaffin cells in ulcerative colitis and irritable colon. *Scand. J. Gastroenterol.*, 12:363–367.
41. Larsson, I., Ahlman, H., Bhargava, H. N., Dahlström, A., Pettersson, G., and Kewenter, J. (1979): The effects of splanchnic nerve stimulation on the plasma levels of 5-HT and substance P in the portal vein of the cat. *J. Neural Transm.*, 46:105–112.
42. Larsson, I., Dahlström, A., Pettersson, G., Larsson, P. A., Kewenter, J., and Ahlman, H. (1980): The effects of adrenergic antagonists on the 5-HT levels of the feline enterochromaffin cells after splanchnic nerve stimulation. *J. Neural Transm.*, 47:89–98.
43. Liedberg, G. I., Nielsen, K. C., Owman, C. H., and Sjöberg, N-O. (1973): Adrenergic contribution to the abdominal vagus nerves in the cat. *Scand. J. Gastroenterol.*, 8:177–180.
44. Lundberg, J., Ahlman, H., Dahlström, A., and Kewenter, J. (1976): Catecholamine-containing nerve fibres in the human abdominal vagus. *Gastroenterology*, 70:472–474.
45. Lundberg, J. M., Dahlström, A., Larsson, I., Pettersson, G., Ahlman, H., and Kewenter, J. (1978): Efferent innervation of the small intestine by adrenergic neurons from the cervical sympathetic and stellate ganglia studied by retrograde transport of peroxidase. *Acta Physiol. Scand.*, 104:33–42.
46. Lundberg, J. M., Dahlström, A., Bylock, A., Ahlman, H., Pettersson, G., Larsson, I., Hansson, H-A., and Kewenter, J. (1978): Ultrastructural evidence for an innervation of epithelial enterochromaffin cells in the guinea-pig duodenum. *Acta Physiol. Scand.*, 104:3–12.
47. Martin, J., Innes, D., and Tansy, M. (1974): A demonstration of vagal adrenergic vascular and motor influences in the small intestine of the dog. *Surg. Gynecol. Obstet.*, 138:6–12
48. Muryobayashi, T., Mori, J., Fujiwara, M., and Shimamoto, K. (1968): Fluorescence histochemical demonstration of adrenergic nerve fibres in the vagus nerve of cats and dogs. *Jpn. J. Pharmacol.*, 18:285–293.
49. Newson, B., Ahlman, H., Dahlström, A., Das Gupta, T. K., and Nyhus, L. M. (1979): On the innervation of the ileal mucosa in the rat-a synapse. *Acta Physiol. Scand.*, 105:387–389.
50. Nilsson, O., Lidberg, P., Ahlman, H., Cassuto, J., Dahlström, A., Jodal, M., Larsson, P. A., Lundgren, O., and Pettersson, G. (1980): Effect of choleratoxin in 5-HT content EC in the cat small intestine. *Proc. Scand. Soc. Physiol.*, C 16.
51. Peart, W. S., Robertson, J. I. S., and Andrews, T. M. (1959): Facial flushing produced in patients with the carcinoid syndrome by intravenous adrenaline and noradrenaline. *Lancet*, 2:715–716.
52. Penttilä, A. (1966): Histochemical reactions of the enterochromaffin cells and the 5-HT content of the mammalian duodenum. *Acta Physiol. Scand. (Suppl.)*, 281.
53. Pettersson, G., Dahlström, A., Larsson, I., Lundberg, J. M., Ahlman, H., and Kewenter, J. (1978): The release of serotonin from rat duodenal enterochromaffin cells by adrenoceptor agonists studied in vitro. *Acta Physiol. Scand.*, 103:219–224.
54. Pettersson, G. (1979): The neural control of the 5-HT content in mammalian enterochromaffin cells. *Acta Physiol. Scand. (Suppl.)*, 470.
55. Pettersson, G., Ahlman, H., Dahlström, A., Kewenter, J., Larsson, I., and Larsson, P. A. (1979): The effect of transmural field stimulation on the serotonin content in rat duodenal enterochromaffin cells in vitro. *Acta Physiol. Scand.*, 107:83–87.

56. Pettersson, G., Ahlman, H., Bhargava, H. N., Dahlström, A., Kewenter, J., Larsson, I., and Siepler, J. K. (1979): The effect of propranolol on the vagal release of 5-HT into the portal blood in the cat. *Acta Physiol. Scand.*, 107:327–331.
57. Polak, J. M., Heitz, P., and Pearse, A. G. E. (1976): Differential localization of substance P and motilin. *Scand. J. Gastroenterol.*, 11:39–42.
58. Shemaikin, A. I. (1904): Thesis, St. Petersburg. Cited in: *Secretory Mechanisms of the Digestive Glands*, B. P. Babkin, 1950. Paul B. Hoeber, New York.
59. Tafuri, W. L., and Raick, A. (1964): Presence of 5-HT in the intramural nervous system of guinea-pigs intestine. *Z. Naturforsch.*, 19:1126–1128.
60. Tansy, M. F., Rothman, G., Bartlett, J., Farber, P., and Hohenleitner (1971): Vagal adrenergic degranulation of enterochromaffin cell system in guinea pig duodenum. *J. Pharm. Sci.*, 60:81–84.
61. Thompson, J. H. (1971): Serotonin and the alimentary tract. *Res. Commun. Chem. Pathol. Pharmacol.*, 2:687–781.
62. Tranzer, J. P., and Thoenen, R. L. (1967): Electromicroscopic localization of 5-OHDA, a new "false" sympathetic transmitter. *Experientia*, 23:743–745.
63. Zinner, M. J., Jaffe, B. M., DeMagistris, L., Dahlström, A., and Ahlman, H. (1982): The effect of cervical and thoracic vagal stimulation of luminal serotonin release and regional blood flow in cats. *Gastroenterol. (in press)*.

5-Hydroxytryptamine in Peripheral Reactions,
edited by Fred De Clerck and Paul M.
Vanhoutte. Raven Press, New York © 1982.

5-Hydroxytryptamine in Mucosal Endocrine Cells of the Gut and Lung

*J. M. Polak, **J. De Mey, and *S. R. Bloom

*Histochemistry Unit (Department of Histopathology) and Department of Medicine,
Royal Postgraduate Medical School, Hammersmith Hospital, London W12 OHS,
United Kingdom, and **Janssen Pharmaceutica Research Laboratories,
B-2340 Beerse, Belgium

The argentaffin and chromaffin agent contained in the enterochromaffin cells, responsible for their reaction with diazonium compounds, previously thought to be an enteramine, was identified as 5-hydroxytryptamine by Erspamer and Asero (3) in 1952. 5-Hydroxytryptamine-containing enterochromaffin cells are widely distributed throughout the body. Tissues rich in enterochromaffin cells include the gastrointestinal tract, the pancreas of certain mammals, the lung and, in some species, the thyroid, thymus, and urogenital tract. 5-Hydroxytryptamine is also found in central and peripheral neurons. The latter have been investigated particularly in the gastrointestinal tract by means of uptake mechanisms and the determination of 5-hydroxytryptamine binding proteins (6).

The enterochromaffin cells have, so far, been investigated by means of their staining properties, i.e., argentaffin and/or diazonium reaction (16), or formaldehyde-induced fluorescence (5). Recent studies using specific antibodies to 5-hydroxytryptamine indicate this to be the method of choice for the accurate and reliable identification of enterochromaffin cells. Few studies have so far been carried out using specific antibodies to 5-hydroxytryptamine; we, therefore, wish to describe the distribution of 5-hydroxytryptamine-containing endocrine cells in the gastrointestinal tract, in view of the reported large concentrations of the monoamine in mucosal extracts, and in the lung, where the presence of numerous mucosal argentaffin cells has been well documented (8).

ANTISERA

Antibodies to 5-hydroxytryptamine were raised in rabbits by coupling 5-hydroxytryptamine creatinine sulphate to bovine serum albumin using formaldehyde, following the procedure described by Steinbush et al. (19). The characteristics of the 5-hydroxytryptamine antibodies are shown in Table 1.

In order to investigate the anatomical relationships between enterochromaffin cells containing 5-hydroxytryptamine and endocrine cells containing regulatory

TABLE 1. *Characterization of antiserum to 5-hydroxytryptamine*

Antigen/analog tested	Concentration of antigen/analog (μmole/ml of diluted antiserum)		
	0.1	1.0	10.0
5-Hydroxytryptamine HCl	+	−	−
Tryptamine	+	−	−
6-Hydroxytryptamine HCl	−	−	−
5-Methoxytryptamine	+	+	−
Tryptophan	+	+	+
5-Hydroxytryptophan	+	+	+

Final dilution of antiserum—1:150,000.
+ = positive immunostain.
− = negative immunostain.

TABLE 2. *Antiserum characteristics*

Antiserum to:	Dilution		Region specificity	Absorption value (μM)
	IMF	PAP		
Motilin	1:200	1:1,000	C-terminus	5.0
Motilin	1:200	1:1,000	N-terminus	10.0
Substance P	1:2,000	1:16,000	C-terminus	10.0
VIP	1:2,000	1:20,000	Whole molecule	5.0
Bombesin	1:400	1:10,000	C-terminus	10.0
Somatostatin	1:400	1:4,000	Whole molecule	0.1
Gastrin	1:400	1:4,000	C-terminus	10.0
NSE	1:800	1:4,000	Whole molecule	1.0

Absorption value = Concentration of antigen required to prevent immunostaining.
PAP = Indirect immunoperoxidase.
IMF = Indirect immunofluorescence.

peptides, known also to be present in autonomic nerves of the gut and lung, specific antibodies to Vasoactive Intestinal Polypeptide (VIP) (1), motilin (10), bombesin (25), gastrin (2), somatostatin (14), and substance P (23) were also employed. In addition, the further characterization of 5-hydroxytryptamine-containing cells was carried out using antibodies to a neuronal enzyme, neuron-specific enolase, recently found to be a good and reliable marker for all components of the diffuse neuroendocrine system (21), to which 5-hydroxytryptamine-containing endocrine cells belong. The details of the specificity of antibodies to peptides and enzyme are presented in Table 2.

IMMUNOCYTOCHEMISTRY

Immunocytochemistry was carried out by the use of the peroxidase-antiperoxidase (PAP) technique (20) or the immunogold staining method (IGS) (7). The specificity of the immunoreaction was tested by numerous control experiments, including the quenching of the immunostain by preabsorption of the antibodies with the corresponding antigen (see Tables 1 and 2). For comparative studies of the possible co-storage of regulatory peptides/enzyme and 5-hydroxytryptamine in cells and the putative interrelationships between peptide-containing autonomic nerves or endocrine cells with 5-hydroxytryptamine cells, a combination of double immunostaining procedures was carried out. These included the use of serial semithin (3 μm) paraffin wax sections, the elution procedure of Tramu et al. (22) on a single tissue section and a newly developed double immunostaining technique, incorporating both the PAP method, using 4-chloro-1-naphtol (blue product) as coupler, and the IGS (red product) technique (7).

TISSUES

The material obtained from fetuses, neonates, and adults consisted of pieces of gastrointestinal tract (fundus, antrum, duodenum, jejunum, ileum, and colon) and lung (trachea, main bronchi, as well as inner, middle, and outer lung) from a variety of mammals (rats, $n = 6$; guinea-pigs, $n = 6$; cats, $n = 6$), as well as man ($n = 5$). Pathological material consisted of carcinoid tumors ($n = 25$) of both the gut ($n = 22$) and the lung ($n = 3$). The tissues were fixed in a variety of different fixatives, in both liquid and vapor phases, including Bouin's solution, formaldehyde, and benzoquinone (13).

DISTRIBUTION

Gastrointestinal Tract

5-Hydroxytryptamine-containing mucosal cells were found in all areas of the bowel with interspecies variations closely matching those reported by other workers using other histological stains (17).

5-Hydroxytryptamine-containing cells often display a triangular shape with the narrow end terminating at the bowel lumen (Fig. 1). Frequently, 5-hydroxytryptamine-containing cells show a basal elongation analogous to the basal cytoplasmic extension described in other endocrine cells (12). They were localized mainly in the crypt compartment, although scattered cells were also seen in the villous area. 5-Hydroxytryptamine-containing cells were almost invariably found as a separate population of cells, intermingled with other mucosal endocrine cells producing regulatory peptides (Fig. 2).

5-Hydroxytryptamine and Peptide Co-storage and Relationships

Although possible co-storage of a regulatory peptide (motilin or substance P) with 5-hydroxytryptamine in cells has been postulated, this is only evident in a few species (e.g., substance P in mouse colon) or, in the case of motilin, by the use of N-terminally reactive antisera (10). In addition, despite the increasing demonstration of the production of regulatory peptides by amine-containing cells or nerves

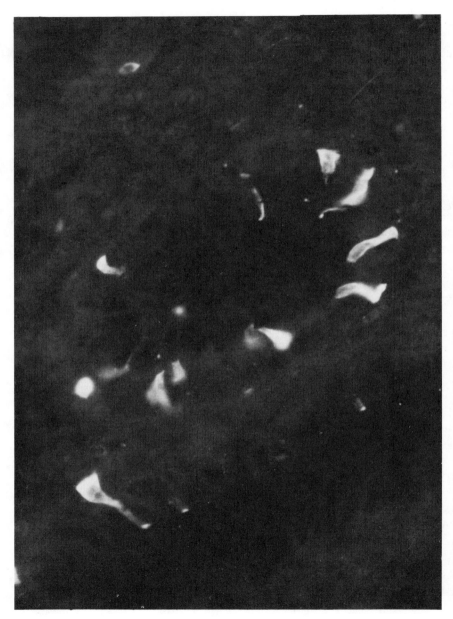

FIG. 1. 5-Hydroxytryptamine-containing cells in the mucosal epithelium of the human colon (×400).

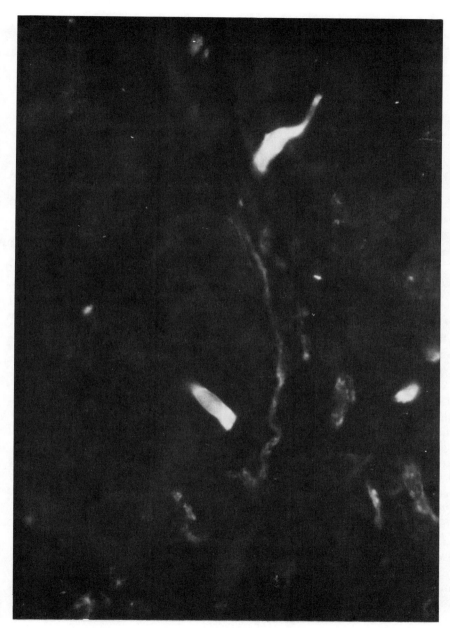

FIG. 2. VIP nerve fibers running around the mucosal crypts of human colon, in close proximity to 5-hydroxytryptamine cells in the epithelium (×420).

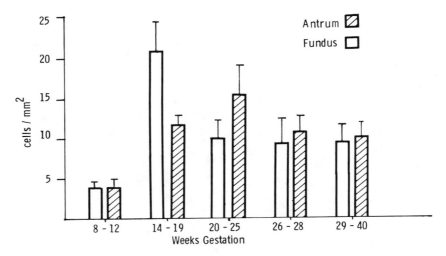

FIG. 3. Cell quantification showed an initial rise up to 20 weeks (especially in the fundus) which reached a plateau after 25 weeks, continuing at this level to birth.

(5-hydroxytryptamine and substance P in central neurons of the medulla oblongata (9), enkephalins in amine-producing cells of the carotid body (24) and adrenal medulla) there is, as yet, no firm evidence for co-storage of peptide and 5-hydroxytryptamine in mucosal endocrine cells.

The presence of the neuronal enzyme, neuron-specific enolase, is, however, undisputed. This enzyme is found in all peptide/amine-producing cells and nerves of the diffuse neuroendocrine system (21). The possible anatomical associations between 5-hydroxytryptamine-containing cells and peptide-containing endocrine cells and autonomic nerves have also been investigated by means of a variety of immunocytochemical procedures, especially by combining the PAP and the immunogold staining method (7). Using this procedure it was possible to see 5-hydroxytryptamine-containing cells in close association with other endocrine cells and autonomic nerves, in particular with somatostatin cells and VIPergic nerves, the latter frequently lying underneath the epithelium. This anatomical relationship between 5-hydroxytryptamine cells and VIPergic nerves is of interest in view of the recent postulate that release of 5-hydroxytryptamine from enterochromaffin cells activates VIP fibers in the gut (4).

The recent demonstration of 5-hydroxytryptamine in autonomic nerves of the bowel wall, albeit in much lesser concentrations than those found in the mucosal layer, fits well with the reports of the neurally mediated effects of 5-hydroxytryptamine in gut motility (6–15).

Development

Examination of human fetal and neonatal gut tissues revealed that 5-hydroxytryptamine-producing cells can first be detected by immunocytochemistry at the

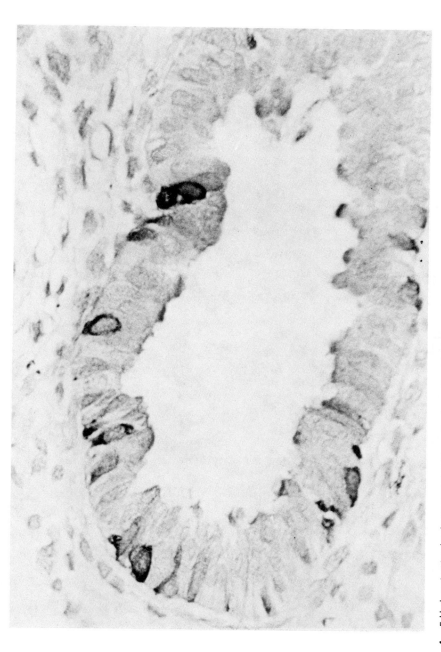

FIG. 4. 5-Hydroxytryptamine immunostained in endocrine cells of the bronchial epithelium of human fetal lung. Immunoreactive cells are seen singly or in small groups (×420).

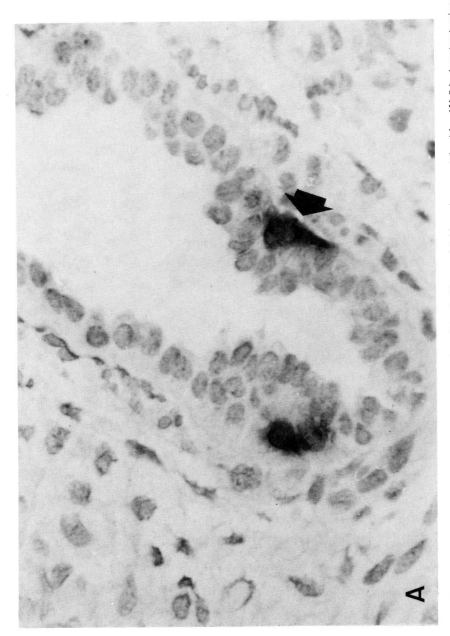

FIG. 5. Endocrine cells of the bronchial epithelium, in serial sections (3 μm) of human fetal lung, immunostained for: **(A)** 5-hydroxytryptamine; **(B)** bombesin.

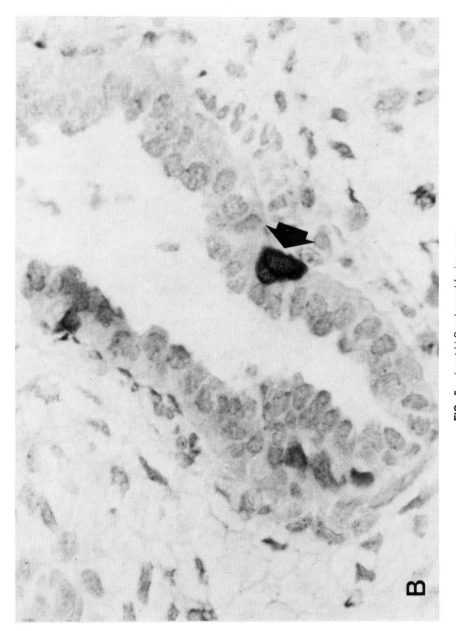

FIG. 5. *(contd.)* See legend facing page.

eleventh week of gestation. The number of cells increase progressively with age to reach adult level by the twentieth week (18) (Fig. 3). Comparative immunocytochemical investigations reveal that, as in adult life, 5-hydroxytryptamine cells correspond to a population of cells separate from those producing regulatory peptides. This is in contradistinction to earlier publications suggesting a co-storage of 5-hydroxytryptamine and peptide during embryonic life (11).

Respiratory Tract

The presence in bronchial epithelium of typical mucosal endocrine cells capable of reducing silver salts (argentaffin) and displaying ultrastructurally distinguishable, irregular secretory granules, similar to the 5-hydroxytryptamine-containing secretory granules of the gut enterochromaffin cells, has been recognized for some time (8). However, their content of 5-hydroxytryptamine was not fully confirmed until the advent of specific immunostaining for the monoamine.

5-Hydroxytryptamine-containing cells of the bronchial epithelium are scattered and intermingled with other endocrine and nonendocrine mucosal cells. As with other bronchial endocrine cells they are most abundant in the fetal and neonatal periods (Fig. 4) and are first seen in man at twelve weeks of gestation (25). Unlike 5-hydroxytryptamine-containing cells of the gut mucosa, some (approximately one-third) of the bronchial 5-hydroxytryptamine-containing cells co-store bombesin, a newly discovered regulatory peptide with potent bronchoconstrictor properties (Fig. 5) (25).

Carcinoids

Carcinoid tumors of several tissues (stomach, small or large bowel, respiratory tract) known to produce and release 5-hydroxytryptamine, are frequently highly reactive to specific 5-hydroxytryptamine antibodies (Fig. 6). The use of these antibodies has proved to be the most specific and sensitive histological method for the accurate characterization of carcinoid tumors, when compared with the more classical techniques, including silver impregnation and formaldehyde-induced fluorescence (5).

CONCLUSIONS

In spite of its discovery almost 35 years ago and of its reported potent actions in most organ systems, little is known of the precise distribution of 5-hydroxytryptamine in the body. This was, until recently, largely due to the lack of specific antibodies to the monoamine. The increasing use of such antibodies will, undoubtedly, lead to further knowledge of 5-hydroxytryptamine storage sites, many of which are as yet unknown. Anatomical evidence is badly needed to support the massive amount of data on the actions of 5-hydroxytryptamine. The use of specific antibodies will also allow the further determination of possible co-storage, with regulatory peptides or anatomical associations of 5-hydroxytryptamine cells with

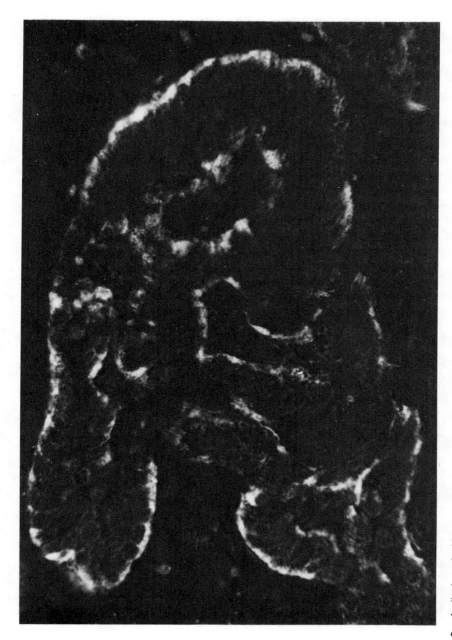

FIG. 6. An ileal carcinoid tumor, showing typical histological features, immunostained for 5-hydroxytryptamine. Note the characteristic distribution of 5-hydroxytryptamine immunoreactivity.

peptide-containing endocrine cells or nerves, where close functional interrelationships are beginning to be described. Clear understanding of the precise tissue distribution of this fascinating amine will undoubtedly lead to a better understanding of disease states in which 5-hydroxytryptamine plays a key role, leading to improved therapeutic prospects.

REFERENCES

1. Bishop, A. E., Polak, J. M., Green, I. C., Bryant, M. G., and Bloom, S. R. (1980): The location of VIP in the pancreas of man and rat. *Diabetologia*, 18:73–78.
2. Buchan, A. M. J., Polak, J. M., Solcia, E., and Pearse, A. G. E. (1979): Localisation of intestinal gastrin in a distinct endocrine cell type. *Nature*, 277:138–140.
3. Erspamer, V., and Asero, B. (1952): Identification of enteramine, the specific hormone of the enterochromaffin cell system, as 5-hydroxytryptamine. *Nature*, 169:800–801.
4. Fahrenkrug, J. (1981): Physiological role of VIP in digestion. In: *Gut Hormones*, 2nd ed., edited by S. R. Bloom and J. M. Polak, pp. 385–391. Churchill Livingstone, Edinburgh.
5. Falck, B. (1962): Observations on the possibilities of the cellular localisation of monoamines by a fluorescence method. *Acta Physiol. Scand.*, 56:1–25.
6. Gershon, M. D. (1981): Storage and release of serotonin and serotinin-binding protein by serotonergic neurons. In: *Cellular Basis of Chemical Messengers in the Digestive System*, edited by Morton I. Grossman, Mary A. B. Brazier, and Juan Lechago, pp. 285–298. Academic Press, New York.
7. Gu, J., De Mey, J., Moeremans, M., and Polak, J. M. (1981): Sequential use of the PAP and immunogold staining methods for the light microscopical double staining of tissue antigens. *Reg. Pep.*, 1:No.6, 365–374.
8. Hage, E. (1974): Histochemistry and fine structure of endocrine cells in foetal lungs of the rabbit, mouse and guinea pig. *Cell Tissue Res.*, 149:513–524.
9. Hokfelt, T., Ljungdahl, A., Steinbusch, H., Verhofstad, A., Nilsson, G., Brodin, E., Pernow, B., and Goldstein, M. (1978): Immunohistochemical evidence of substance P-like immunoreactivity in some 5-HT containing neurons in the rat central nervous system. *Neuroscience*, 3:517–538.
10. Kishimoto, S., Polak, J. M., Buchan, A. M. J., Verhofstad, A. A. J., Steinbusch, H. W. M., Yanaihara, N., Bloom, S. R., and Pearse, A. G. E. (1981): Motilin cells investigated by the use of region-specific antisera. *Virchows Arch. (B)*, 36:207–218.
11. Larsson, L.-I., and Jorgensen, L. M. (1978): Ultrastructural and cytochemical studies on the cytodifferentiation of duodenal endocrine cells. *Cell Tissue Res.*, 194:79–102.
12. Larsson, L-I. (1981): Somatostatin cells. In: *Gut Hormones*, 2nd ed., edited by Stephen R. Bloom and Julia M. Polak, pp. 350–353. Churchill Livingstone, Edinburgh.
13. Pearse, A. G. E., and Polak, J. M. (1975): Bifunctional reagents as vapour- and liquid-phase fixatives for immunohistochemistry. *Histochem. J.*, 7:179–186.
14. Polak, J. M., Pearse, A. G. E., Grimelius, L., Bloom, S. R., and Arimura, A. (1975): Growthhormone releasing-inhibiting hormone (GH-RIH) in gastrointestinal and pancreatic D cells. *Lancet*, I:1220–1222.
15. Robertson, P. A. (1953): Antagonism of 5-hydroxytryptamine by atropine. *J. Physiol. (Lond.)*, 121:54–55.
16. Solcia, E., Sampietro, R., and Vassallo, G. (1966): Indole reactions of enterochromaffin cells and mast cells. *J. Histochem. Cytochem.*, 14:691–692.
17. Solcia, E., Capella, C., Buffa, R., Usellini, L., Frigerio, B., and Fontana, P. (1979): Endocrine cells of the gastrointestinal tract and related tumors. In: *Pathobiology Annual*, edited by H. L. Ioachim, (9) pp. 163–202. Raven Press, New York.
18. Stein, B. A., Buchan, A. M. J., Morris, J. F., and Polak, J. M. (1982): Development of gastrin-, somatostatin-, glucagon- and serotonin-containing cells in the human foetal stomach. *J. Pathol. (in press)*.
19. Steinbusch, H. W., Verhofstad, A. A., and Joosten, H. W. (1978): Localisation of serotonin in the central nervous system by immunohistochemistry: Description of a specific and sensitive technique and some applications. *Neuroscience*, 3(9):811–819.

20. Sternberger, L. (1974): *The Unlabelled Antibody Enzyme Method*, pp. 142–161. Prentice Hall, Englewood Cliffs.
21. Tapia, F. J., Barbosa, A. J. A., Marangos, P. J., Polak, J. M., Bloom, S. R., Dermody, C., and Pearse, A. G. E. (1981): Neurone-specific enolase is produced by neuroendocrine tumours. *Lancet I*, 808–811.
22. Tramu, G., Pillez, A., and Leonardelli, J. (1978): An efficient method of antibody elution for the successive or simultaneous location of two antigens by immunocytochemistry. *J. Histochem. Cytochem.*, 26:322–324.
23. Wharton, J., Polak, J. M., Bloom, S. R., Will, J. A., Brown, M. R., and Pearse, A. G. E. (1979): Substance P-like immunoreactive nerves in mammalian lung. *Invest. Cell Pathol.*, 2:3–10.
24. Wharton, J., Polak, J. M., Pearse, A. G. E., McGregor, G. P., Bryant, M. G., Bloom, S. R., Emson, P. C., Bisgard, G. E., and Will, J. A. (1980): Enkephalin-, VIP- and substance P-like immunoreactivity in the carotid body. *Nature*, 184:269–271.
25. Wharton, J., Polak, J. M., Cole, G. A., Marangos, P. J., and Pearse, A. G. E. (1981): Neuron specific enolase as an immunocytochemical marker for the diffuse neuroendocrine system in human foetal lung. *J. Histochem. Cytochem.*, 29:1359–1364.

5-Hydroxytryptamine in Peripheral Reactions,
edited by Fred De Clerck and Paul M.
Vanhoutte. Raven Press, New York © 1982.

Captation of 5-Hydroxytryptamine and Effects on Endothelial Cell Metabolism

*Patricia D'Amore and **David Shepro

*Department of Ophthalmology, Johns Hopkins University School of Medicine,
Baltimore, Maryland 21205; and **Departments of Biology and Surgery, Boston
University, Boston, Massachusetts 02115*

Endothelial cells line the heart and large blood vessels and are the principal cellular components of the microvascular system. In this central location they are the first cells to come into contact, and therefore interact with, any circulating substances. The list of substances that circulate in the plasma is long and varied. It is known from many recent studies on the biochemistry and physiology of endothelial cells (see ref. 12 for review) that these cells have specialized functions through which they deal with their environment. These functions operate via receptors, surface enzymes, and secreted molecules.

5-Hydroxytryptamine, a ubiquitous monoamine, is found in the blood. Platelet-free plasma levels of 5-hydroxytryptamine that have been reported range from 58 to 221 pmoles/g (6). Because of the relatively slow blood flow rate at the microvascular level and the small area of the capillary lumen, it is feasible that the effective concentrations of 5-hydroxytryptamine in the microcirculation are even higher than those measured in plasma. Furthermore, at the site of large vessel injury, platelets adhere to the exposed subendothelium where they aggregate and undergo the release reaction. During the release reaction platelets liberate from their dense granules large amounts of 5-hydroxytryptamine (0.21–5.95 nmoles/10^9 platelets) (6). This localized release causes a transient increase in 5-hydroxytryptamine concentration in the area of the wound.

In order to examine the effects that 5-hydroxytryptamine may have on vascular endothelial cells, the response of a number of physiological parameters of vascular endothelial cells *in vitro* to added 5-hydroxytryptamine have been studied. The cells used in these studies were endothelial cells isolated from neonatal bovine aortas. The parameters that were studied included: (a) proliferation, (b) calcium influx, and (c) ornithine decarboxylase activity.

---

*Current address: Department of Surgery, Children's Hospital Medical Center, Harvard Medical School, Boston, Massachusetts 02115

The rationale for choosing these three phenomena stems from the following lines of reasoning. First, since there is (as was discussed previously) a transient increase in 5-hydroxytryptamine concentration at the site of an injury, it would be interesting to see if the presence of 5-hydroxytryptamine could stimulate proliferation of sub-confluent endothelium. Second, calcium is known to function as a second messenger (1), thereby mediating a number of cellular processes (7,9). The effect of 5-hydroxytryptamine on calcium influx would shed some light on possible 5-hydroxytryptamine effects. Third, ornithine decarboxylase is the rate-limiting enzyme in the production of the polyamines. The polyamines are a group of polycationic molecules that are known to function in a wide variety of basic cellular processes including stabilization of polyribosomes and nucleic acids, facilitation of nucleic acid and protein synthesis, and stabilization of membranes (14). Thus, the ornithine decarboxylase activity in a cell should be a valid reflection of the cell's metabolic state.

MATERIALS AND METHODS

Endothelial Cell Culture

Endothelial cell cultures were established and maintained as previously described (3). Briefly, the aortas from neonatal calves were collected into sterile balanced salt solution (Grand Island Biological Company, GIBCO) and transported from the abbatoir on ice. The aorta was cleared of adventita and rinsed with several washes of balanced salt solution. The intercostal vessels and one end of the aorta were clamped and the vessel was filled with 0.2% collagenase (Sigma, Type IV) in balanced salt solution for 15 min at 37°C. The solution was removed and the cells centrifuged out at $2,000 \times g$ for 5 min. The cells were grown in RPMI 1640 with 17% fetal calf serum (FCS) (RPMI/17, both from GIBCO) supplemented with 100 units/ml penicillin/streptomycin, 200 units/ml neomycin and glutamine to a final concentration of 2 mM before use.

Growth Studies

Endothelial cells (1.2×10^4) in RPMI/17 were plated into 35-mm petri dishes and allowed to attach overnight. On day 1 of the test the media was changed and fresh RPMI/17 with 5-hydroxytryptamine (5-hydroxytryptamine hydrochloride, Calbiochem) was added. At 3-day intervals the cells were removed, dissociated with 0.2% trypsin (Difco Laboratories) and 0.02% EDTA, and counted using a hemocytometer. The media and 5-hydroxytryptamine were changed every 3 days. Cell counts are expressed as a percent of controls.

Calcium Influx Studies

Flasks (25 cm²) at 1 to 3 days postconfluence, containing an average of 2.5–3.0 $\times$ 10⁶ cells/flask, were used in these experiments. The ⁴⁵CaCl₂ (13–15 Ci/mg,

New England Nuclear) and the 5-hydroxytryptamine were added simultaneously and allowed to incubate at 37°C for given time intervals. The media was then decanted and the cells washed ten times with 2 ml aliquots of ice-cold 0.1 M Tris-HCl (pH 7.2). The tenth wash was sampled to determine remaining counts and this value was subtracted from the final value. Each time point was assayed in triplicate. The cells were counted, dissolved with 1 N NaOH, neutralized, and counted for $^{45}Ca^{2+}$.

Ornithine Decarboxylase Assay

For each time point in a given experiment duplicate flasks were sampled. The medium was decanted and the flasks were frozen with 2 ml of incubation medium (50 mM Tris-HCl, 0.1 mM EDTA, 0.05 mM pyridoxal phosphate, and 10 mM dithiothreitol, pH 7.4). At the termination of the experiment the cells were thawed, scraped from the flask, and pipetted into a 10-ml plastic centrifuge tube. The suspension was frozen by immersion into liquid nitrogen for 15 sec, thawed at room temperature, and centrifuged at $10,000 \times g$ for 10 min. The supernatant, the enzyme sample, was assayed for ornithine decarboxylase activity by monitoring the release of $^{14}CO_2$ from the ^{14}C-ornithine substrate (11). The reaction mixture (1.0 ml enzyme sample, 50 nmoles of ornithine including 0.2 μCi ornithine mono-hydrochloride, DL-1-^{14}C, final concentration: $5 \times 10^{-5}M$) was incubated for 60 min in a test tube capped tightly with a rubber stopper holding a plastic center well (Kontes) containing 0.3 ml of 1 M hyamine hydroxide. After the 1 hr incubation time, 1 ml of 10% trichloroacetic acid was added by syringe through the stopper to terminate the reaction and to drive any remaining $^{14}CO_2$ from the solution. The mixture was then left for an additional 60 min to insure complete absorption of the $^{14}CO_2$ by the hyamine hydroxide. The center well was then placed into a vial containing 10 ml of scintiverse and counted for ^{14}C.

Postconfluent endothelial cell cultures were incubated overnight with RPMI 1640/2. At time zero, 5-hydroxytryptamine was added to duplicate flasks at the appropriate concentrations (the medium is not changed). At 1 hr time intervals over an 8 hr time course, duplicate flasks were processed for the ornithine decarboxylase assay. For studies employing imipramine or fluoxetine, the substances were added to the flasks 30 min before the addition of the 5-hydroxytryptamine.

Calcium/Ornithine Decarboxylase Studies

The experiment testing the relationship of calcium influx to the stimulation of ornithine decarboxylase activity contained three groups of flasks. The cells in all the flasks were rinsed five times with 50 mM Tris-HCl (pH 7.2) to remove the residual medium whose phosphate would precipitate with the lanthanum ions. At zero time, the appropriate medium was added to each flask. One set of flasks was prepared immediately to determine baseline values. The other two groups were incubated for 30 min with 2 mM $LaCl_3$. Following the $LaCl_3$ treatment one group received RPMI 1640 with 35% fetal calf serum while the second group was washed five times with 2.5 mM EDTA in Tris-HCl to remove the lanthanum ions before the addition of the medium. The experiment was carried out over a 4 hr time course with duplicate flasks assayed at 1 hr intervals. There was a fourth group of flasks in this experiment. The cells of this group were not preincubated with LaCl$_3$. Instead, at time zero, the medium was changed and replaced with RPMI 1640/35 containing 3 mM EGTA, to chelate the available calcium.

Endothelial Integrity

In order to demonstrate that neither colchicine nor LaCl$_3$ treatment adversely affected the cell physiology over the time course of the experiment the effect of these two compounds on 5-hydroxytryptamine and adenine uptake by the cultured cells was determined. Postconfluent flasks that had been incubated overnight with RPMI 1640/2 were preincubated with colchicine (10^{-6} M) or 3 mM LaCl$_3$. At time zero, [^{3}H]5-hydroxytryptamine or [^{3}H]adenine were added to the flasks. At given time intervals triplicate flasks were rinsed seven times with ice-cold phosphate-buffered saline, the cells dissolved with NaOH and counted for ^{3}H. Experimental values were corrected for counts remaining in the final wash as was done for the calcium studies.

RESULTS

Growth Studies

The addition of 5-hydroxytryptamine at a final concentration of 10^{-6} M to growing endothelial cell cultures caused an increase in the number of cells at days 3, 6, and 9 of the experiment (Fig. 1). By day 9, the cells receiving the 5-hydroxytryptamine

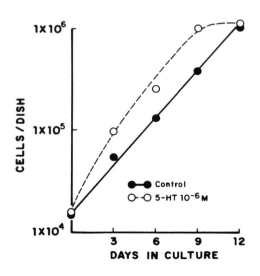

FIG. 1. Effect of 5-hydroxytryptamine (5-HT; 10^{-6}M) on the growth of endothelial cells *in vitro*. Endothelial cells (1.2×10^4) in RPMI/17 were plated into triplicate 35-mm petri dishes and allowed to attach overnight. On day 1 5-hydroxytryptamine in RPMI/17 was added to test dishes. At 3-day intervals the cells were dissociated with trypsin-EDTA and counted using a hemocytometer. Values are expressed as a percent of controls which received equivalent volumes of buffer,

were confluent and ceased dividing, whereas the control culture which had received equivalent volumes of the buffer required an additional 3 days to reach confluence.

Calcium Studies

Because calcium is known to function in a number of cellular processes including division and secretion (1), the effect of 5-hydroxytryptamine on calcium influx into the cells was examined. As is evident from Fig. 2 the influx of radiolabeled calcium into the endothelial cells was immediate, peaking at 4.5-fold control levels within 15 sec of the 5-HT/[45] calcium addition. During the 10 min following the peak of influx the calcium levels fell to control levels. To test the specificity of this influx the same experiment was conducted following a 30 min preincubation with $LaCl_3$. This treatment blocked both stimulated and baseline calcium influx (data not shown).

Ornithine Decarboxylase Studies

The addition of various concentrations of 5-hydroxytryptamine stimulated ornithine decarboxylase activity in endothelial cells (Fig. 3). The minimal concentrations at which stimulation was measured was $10^{-7}M$ 5-hydroxytryptamine. Maximal stimulation of ornithine decarboxylase occurred at 10^{-5} M 5-hydroxytryptamine and increases in 5-hydroxytryptamine concentrations above this level did not alter ornithine decarboxylase activity significantly. Preincubation of the cells for 30 min in the presence of fluoxetine ($10^{-6}M$) or imipramine (10^{-5} M) depressed the 5-hydroxytryptamine-inducible ornithine decarboxylase activity (Fig. 4).

LaCl₃/Ornithine Decarboxylase Studies

In order to determine if there was any relationship between the influx of calcium that was measured in response to addition of 5-hydroxytryptamine and the induction

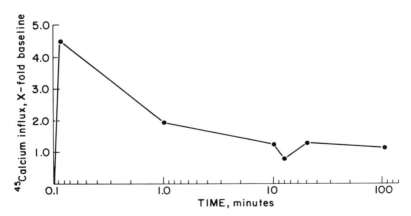

FIG. 2. Time course of [45]calcium influx in 5-hydroxytryptamine-stimulated endothelial cells. Postconfluent flasks of endothelial cells were incubated overnight in RPMI/2. At time zero, 5-HT (10^{-5} M) and $^{45}Ca^{2+}$ were added simultaneously and incubated for given time intervals, the medium was decanted, and the cells were dissolved and counted for $^{45}Ca^{2+}$. Final counts were corrected for nonspecific binding and counts remaining in the final wash.

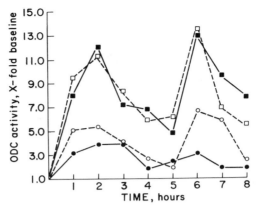

FIG. 3. Stimulation of ornithine decarboxylase (ODC) activity in endothelial cells by 5-hydroxy-tryptamine. Postconfluent flasks of endothelial cells were incubated overnight in RPMI/2. At time zero, 5-hydroxytryptamine was added at the appropriate concentrations. Duplicate flasks from each group were assayed for ornithine activity at 1-hr intervals over an 8-hr time course. *Closed circles:* 10^{-7} M, *open circles:* 10^{-6} M, *closed squares:* 10^{-4} M, *open squares:* 10^{-5} M.

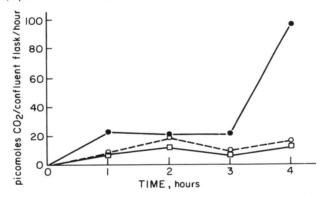

FIG. 4. Effect of fluoxetine and imipramine on stimulation of ornithine decarboxylase (ODC) in endothelial cells by 5-hydroxytryptamine. Experimental flasks were preincubated for 30 min at 37°C with fluoxetine (10^{-6} M) and imipramine (10^{-5} M). At time zero, 5-hydroxytryptamine (10^{-5} M) was added to both experimental and control flasks. Duplicate flasks from each group were assayed for ornithine decarboxylase at 1 hr intervals over a 4 hr time course. *Closed circles:* 5-HT control, *open circles:* fluoxetine, *open squares:* imipramine.

of ornithine decarboxylase activity by 5-hydroxytryptamine, LaCl$_3$ was used to block calcium influx. Lanthanum ions have a higher valence than calcium but a similar ionic radius and are capable of binding reversibly to external calcium binding sites. Thus, lanthanum can be used to examine mechanisms that are suspected to be calcium-dependent (15).

The addition of a number of agonists including serum, thrombin, and 5-hydroxy-tryptamine results in the stimulation of ornithine decarboxylase to levels from four to fifteen times baseline within 3 hr of their addition (4). Preincubation of the cells with 2 mM LaCl$_3$ for 30 min before the addition of the stimulus inhibited the stimulation (Fig. 5). In fact, the presence of the lanthanum ions apparently prevents even the basal levels of ornithine decarboxylase activity since at all four time points measured activity was below baseline levels. However, if the LaCl$_3$-preincubated cells were rinsed thoroughly with 2.5 mM EGTA prior to the addition of the stimulus the cells were once again capable of being stimulated (Fig. 5) to previous levels.

Furthermore, the inclusion of the calcium chelating agent, EGTA, in the medium at the time of stimulation resulted in sub-baseline levels of ornithine decarboxylase activity similar to that measured in the LaCl$_3$ preincubation experiment (Fig. 6). This is presumably due to the fact that the agent has bound up all of the available ionic calcium, preventing calcium influx.

Colchicine/Ornithine Decarboxylase

Finally, it has been postulated (5) that the microtubule-microfilament system is involved in the transduction of the stimulus from the receptor on the cell membrane

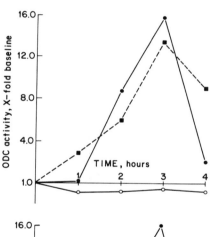

FIG. 5. Effect of lanthanum on ornithine decarboxylase (ODC) activity in endothelial cells. Postconfluent flasks were incubated overnight in RPMI/2. Two groups of flasks were preincubated with 2 mM LaCl$_3$ for 30 min at 37°C. The cells in one group of flasks were then rinsed five times with 2.5 mM EDTA and the cells in all flasks were washed with 0.1 M Tris-HCl before the addition of RPMI/35. Duplicate flasks from each group were assayed for ornithine decarboxylase activity at 1 hr intervals over a 4 hr time course. *Closed circles:* 35% RPMI control, *open circles:* LaCl$_3$ preincubated, *closed squares:* EGTA-washed.

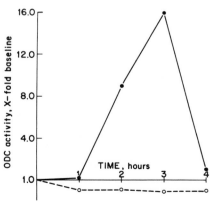

FIG. 6. Effect of calcium chelation on the stimulation of ornithine decarboxylase (ODC) activity in endothelial cells. Postconfluent flasks were incubated overnight in RPMI/2. At time zero, the experimental flasks received RPMI/35 to which EGTA had been added to a final concentration of 3 mM; controls received RPMI/35. Duplicate flasks from each group were assayed for ornithine decarboxylase activity at 1 hr intervals over a 4 hr time course. *Closed circles:* 35% RPMI control, *open circles:* 35% RPMI with 3 mM EGTA.

to sites within the cell. The microtubule disrupting agent, colchicine, was utilized to test the role of microtubules in the induction of ornithine decarboxylase activity by 5-hydroxytryptamine.

Cells maintained on RPMI/2 and stimulated with 35% fetal calf serum (v/v) displayed maximal ornithine decarboxylase activity within 2 to 3 hr of the addition of the fetal calf serum (v/v) (4). A dose curve of colchicine was tested to determine its effects on ornithine decarboxylase activity. Colchicine at a range of concentrations from 10^{-8} M to 5×10^{-3} M inhibited the ornithine decarboxylase activity to varying degrees with 50% inhibition at 5×10^{-8} M (data not shown). Maximal inhibitory activity occurred between 10^{-5} M and 10^{-4} M colchicine with 91% inhibition of the stimulated ornithine decarboxylase activity. Equivalent concentrations of lumicolchicine did not cause alterations of the stimulated ornithine decarboxylase activity.

Stimulation of colchicine-preincubated cells with 5-hydroxytryptamine did not result in the enhanced ornithine decarboxylase activity normally seen in the first 4 hr after 5-hydroxytryptamine addition (Fig. 7). In fact, whereas 5-hydroxytryptamine addition to the untreated culture caused ornithine decarboxylase levels to rise to five times baseline levels within 4 hr, colchicine preincubation prevented this rise and ornithine decarboxylase levels dropped as far as 30% below baseline activity. The cells that had been preincubated with lumicolchicine before the addition of 5-hydroxytryptamine responded in a manner similar to the controls.

DISCUSSION

The data illustrating increased proliferation in the presence of 5-hydroxytryptamine raise the question as to the "growth factor" capabilities of 5-hydroxytryptamine. According to an accepted definition of a growth factor put forth by Rudland

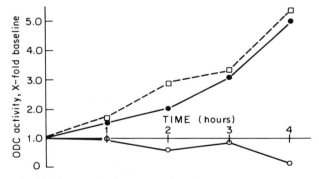

FIG. 7. Effect of colchicine on 5-hydroxytryptamine-stimulated ornithine decarboxylase (ODC) in endothelial cells. Postconfluent flasks of endothelial cells were incubated overnight in RPMI/2. One group of flasks was preincubated for 1 hr with colchicine (10^{-6} M); a second group with lumicolchicine (10^{-6} M). At time zero 5-hydroxytryptamine (10^{-5} M) was added to the flasks. Duplicate flasks from each group were assayed for ornithine decarboxylase activity at 1 hr intervals over a 4 hr time course. *Closed circles:* 5-HT control, *open circles:* colchicine, *open squares:* lumicolchicine.

and Jimenez de Asua (10), a true growth factor is capable of stimulating proliferation of a cell culture "in the absence of added serum components." In the light of these criteria, 5-HT does not constitute a valid growth factor. It, nevertheless, does appear to enhance proliferation of growing cultures. The mechanism of this enhancing effect is unknown and may occur via shortening of cell cycle or the recruitment of resting cells into cell cycle. In any case, a measurable effect of 5-hydroxytryptamine on endothelial cell growth does occur and may be significant in the case of wound repair when re-endothelialization of a denuded vessel surface is essential.

In addition to facilitating the proliferation of vascular endothelium in culture, 5-hydroxytryptamine causes an immediate influx of $^{45}Ca^{2+}$ into the cells. According to the stimulus-division coupling model of Berridge (1), stimulation of the plasma membrane causes a transient change in membrane permeability during which calcium influx may occur. Thus, the calcium influx measured in these experiments may be the beginning of a series of events which leads to division. Furthermore, we speculate that calcium may be functional in regulating, either directly or indirectly, a number of other endothelial cell functions including enzyme activities such as ornithine decarboxylase and the microtubule-microfilament systems.

These ideas led us to investigate the activity of ornithine decarboxylase in cultured endothelial cells. The addition of 5-hydroxytryptamine to postconfluent endothelial cells resulted in a biphasic increase in ornithine decarboxylase activity. This response is similar to the cycle of ornithine decarboxylase activity measured in synchronized culture of Chinese ovary fibroblasts (8). Although an increase in ornithine decarboxylase activity is a characteristic of proliferating tissue, stimuli that do not induce division, such as stress (2) or injury (16), can also increase ornithine decarboxylase activity. The inhibition of the 5-hydroxytryptamine-induced ornithine decarboxylase activity by fluoxetine and imipramine suggest that the stimulation is specific.

The data using the calcium blocking agent, lanthanum, indicate that the influx of calcium is functionally related to the induction of ornithine decarboxylase in cultured endothelial cells. Prevention of calcium influx by $LaCl_3$ preincubation or by removing the calcium from the medium via chelating agents not only prevented the stimulation of ornithine decarboxylase but decreased the activity to one-tenth of its baseline level. This observation indicates that calcium may be necessary as a signal in the stimulation of ornithine decarboxylase, but it may also be required to maintain baseline levels of ornithine decarboxylase activity.

According to the surface-modulating assembly model of Edelman (5), the submembranous cytoskeletal structures, microtubules and microfilaments, are functional in relaying messages from the extracellular environment to the interior of the cell. In an effort to determine the role of this "modulating assembly" in the induction of ornithine decarboxylase, we studied the effect of colchicine on 5-hydroxytryptamine-stimulated ornithine decarboxylase activity. Since colchicine, but not its inactive isomer lumicolchicine, was effective in preventing the stimulation, it appears that the microtubules are responsible for some phase of the enzyme activation.

Thus, 5-hydroxytryptamine may be functional both during injury and under normal physiological conditions. At the site of a wound 5-hydroxytryptamine that is released from platelets may act to stimulate proliferation of the endothelial cells at the wound edge. The first step in this sequence may be an influx in calcium, as was demonstrated in this series of studies.

Under physiological conditions circulating 5-hydroxytryptamine may contribute to the maintenance of the endothelial monolayer. The mechanism through which 5-hydroxytryptamine could contribute to the integrity of the vascular endothelial cells is not clear but it may involve the regulation of various enzyme activities (such as ornithine decarboxylase) or influencing the cytoskeletal system (13) using calcium as a second messenger.

ACKNOWLEDGMENTS

These investigations were supported by NIH grants HLB 16714 and GM 24891.

REFERENCES

1. Berridge, M. J. (1975): The interaction of cyclic nucleotides and calcium in the control of cellular activity. In: *Advances in Cyclic Nucleotide Research*, Vol. 6, edited by P. Greengard and G. A. Robison, pp. 1–98. Raven Press, New York.
2. Byus, C. V., and Russell, D. H. (1976): Possible regulation of ornithine decarboxylase in the adrenal medulla of the rat by a cAMP-dependent mechanism. *Biochem. Pharmacol.*, 25:1595–1600.
3. D'Amore, P., and Shepro, D. (1977): Stimulation of growth and calcium influx in cultured, bovine, aortic endothelial cells by platelets and vasoactive substances. *J. Cell. Physiol.*, 92:177–184.
4. D'Amore, P. A., Hechtman, H. B., and Shepro, D. (1978): Ornithine decarboxylase activity in cultured endothelial cells stimulated by serum, thrombin and serotonin. *Thromb. Haemost.*, 39:496–503.
5. Edelman, G. M. (1976): Surface modulation in cell recognition and cell growth. *Science*, 192:218–226.
6. Essman, W. B. (1978): Serotonin distribution in tissues and fluids. In: *Serotonin in Health and Disease*. Vol. 1. Availability, Localization and Disposition, edited by W. B. Essman, pp. 15–79. Spectrum, New York.
7. Goldberg, N. D., Haddox, M. K., Dunham, E., Lopez, E., and Hadden, J. W. (1974): The Ying Yang hypothesis of biological control: Opposing influences of cyclic GMP and cyclic AMP in the regulation of cell proliferation and other biological processes. In: *Control of Proliferation in Animal Cells*, edited by B. Clarkson and R. Baserga, pp. 609–625. Cold Spring Harbor Laboratory, New York.
8. Heby, O., Gray, J. W., Lindl, P. A., Marton, L. J., and Wilson, C. B. (1976): Changes in L-ornithine decarboxylase activity during cell cycle. *Biochem. Biophys. Res. Commun.*, 71:99–105.
9. Rasmussen, H., Goodman, D. B. P., and Tenenhouse, A. (1972): The role of cyclic AMP and calcium in cell activation. *CRC Crit. Rev. Biochem.*, 1:95–148.
10. Rudland, P. S., and Jimenez de Asua, L. (1979): Action of growth factors in the cell cycle. *Biochim. Biophys. Acta*, 56:91–133.
11. Russell, D., and Snyder, S. H. (1968): Amine synthesis in rapidly growing tissues: Ornithine decarboxylase activity in regenerating rat liver, chick embryo and various tumors. *Proc. Natl. Acad. Sci. USA*, 60:1420–1427.
12. Shepro, D., and D'Amore, P. (1982): Physiology and biochemistry of the vascular wall endothelium. In: *The American Physiological Society Handbook on the Microcirculation*, edited by E. M. Renkin, and C. C. Michel. American Physiological Society *(in press)*.
13. Sweetman, H. E., Shepro D., and Hechtman, H. B. (1981): Inhibition of thrombocytopenic petechiae by exogenous serotonin administration. *Haemostasis*, 10:65–78.

14. Tabor, C. W., and Tabor, H. (1976): 1,4-diaminobutane (putrescine), spermidine and spermine. *Annu. Rev. Biochem.*, 45:285–306.
15. Weiss, G. B. (1974): Cellular pharmacology of lanthanum. *Annu. Rev. Pharmacol.*, 14:343–354.
16. Wyatt, G. R., Rothaus, K., Lawler, D., and Herbst, E. J. (1973): Ornithine decarboxylase and polyamines in silkmoth pupal tissues: Effects of ecdysone and injury. *Biochem. Biophys. Acta*, 304:482–494.

5-Hydroxytryptamine in Peripheral Reactions,
edited by Fred De Clerck and Paul M.
Vanhoutte. Raven Press, New York © 1982.

5-Hydroxytryptamine and the Platelet: Specific Binding and Active Uptake

M. Schächter and D. G. Grahame-Smith

*MRC Unit and University Department of Clinical Pharmacology, Radcliffe Infirmary,
Oxford OX2 6HE, United Kingdom*

The platelet is extremely rich in 5-hydroxytryptamine. Almost all circulating 5-hydroxytryptamine is contained within platelets (29), mostly in specialized storage granules. It is thought that the main sources of the amine are the enterochromaffin cells of the gut (30). The platelet and 5-hydroxytryptamine can interact in several ways:

1. Storage of the amine, within organelles as well as in the cytoplasm (31);
2. Uptake, by passive diffusion and, more importantly, by a specific active uptake process effective against considerable concentration gradients (2,27);
3. Release, probably mainly by exocytosis *in vivo* (18); and
4. 5-Hydroxytryptamine-induced platelet shape change and aggregation, the latter usually accompanied by the release of 5-hydroxytryptamine, probably by exocytosis, and also of other cell constituents (e.g., ATP, β-thromboglobulin) and preceded by a change in cell shape from a flattened discoid form to a spherical one, with pseudopodia formation (1,13).

There are several similarities between these processes and the platelets as a model for such neurons has been extensively discussed [see reviews by Pletscher and Laubscher (24,25)].

Studies with drugs that are serotonergic antagonists in other systems have strongly suggested that 5-hydroxytryptamine induces platelet shape change and aggregation by interaction with a specific serotonergic receptor (13,25). A separate receptor is now believed to be involved in the active transport of 5-hydroxytryptamine across the cell membrane (8,29,34). This chapter deals mainly with the attempted characterization of these two receptors in human platelets using radioligand binding techniques, and with the quantitation of the active uptake process. Some clinical implications of these studies will also be discussed.

In 1975 Drummond and Gordon described the use of tritiated 5-hydroxytryptamine to label 5-hydroxytryptamine receptors on rat platelets (9). They defined three subgroups of receptors with, respectively, high, medium, and low affinities for the ligand. Boullin et al. (3), using a similar technique with human platelets, recognized high and low affinity receptors, probably corresponding to the high and medium affinity sites in the rat. This finding has been confirmed by Kim et al. (12) and by Peters and Grahame-Smith (23).

RADIOLIGAND BINDING AND HUMAN PLATELET SEROTONERGIC RECEPTORS

Platelet-rich plasma is prepared by low speed centrifugation from human blood anticoagulated with ethyldiaminetetraacetate (EDTA) (23). Aliquots of platelet-rich plasma are then incubated with varying concentrations of [^{3}H]5-hydroxytryptamine at 2°C for 2 min. To each incubate, either buffer or excess unlabeled 5-hydroxytryptamine is added. Specific binding is defined as the difference between the binding in the tubes containing only buffer (total binding) and that in tubes containing unlabeled 5-hydroxytryptamine (nonspecific binding). After a further 2 min equilibrium the reaction in all the incubates is stopped by high-speed centrifugation. The platelet pellet is lysed and radioactivity measured by liquid scintillation counting of samples of the lysate.

The existence of two binding sites was inferred from the following findings: (a) The addition of increasing concentrations of unlabeled 5-hydroxytryptamine, in the presence of the labeled amine, showed a biphasic displacement of [^{3}H]5-hydroxytryptamine from platelets (Fig. 1); and (b) Scatchard analysis of specific binding revealed a curvilinear plot (Fig. 2).

From these data the kinetic parameters of the two binding sites were estimated (see Table 1).

Peters and Grahame-Smith (23) attempted to relate site A binding to 5-hydroxytryptamine-induced platelet aggregation and site B binding to active 5-hydroxytryptamine uptake. They used known inhibitors of these physiological processors to inhibit [^{3}H]5-hydroxytryptamine binding. The results summarized in Tables 2 and 3 are consistent with the involvement of site A in aggregation and site B in uptake. It will be noted that IC_{50} values for the inhibition of aggregation are some 3 orders of magnitude greater than K_I figures for the inhibition of site A [^{3}H]5-hydroxytryptamine binding. This implies that a very high proportion of binding sites must be blocked by an inhibitor before aggregation is prevented.

CLINICAL STUDIES USING [^{3}H]5-HYDROXYTRYPTAMINE RECEPTORS BINDING

Not surprisingly, the clinical implications of this recently developed technique have been little explored. However, Peters and Grahame-Smith (23) have investigated platelet [^{3}H]5-hydroxytryptamine binding in three groups of subjects: (a) patients with the carcinoid syndrome *(unpublished)*; (b) migraine patients treated with the 5-hydroxytryptamine antagonist pizotifen *(unpublished)*; and (c) women taking the contraceptive pill (22). The findings were as follows:

1. Carcinoid patients have a high circulating level of 5-hydroxytryptamine, almost all of it within platelets. In these subjects there was a reduction in the receptor capacity at both site A and site B, without a change in affinity at either site. This

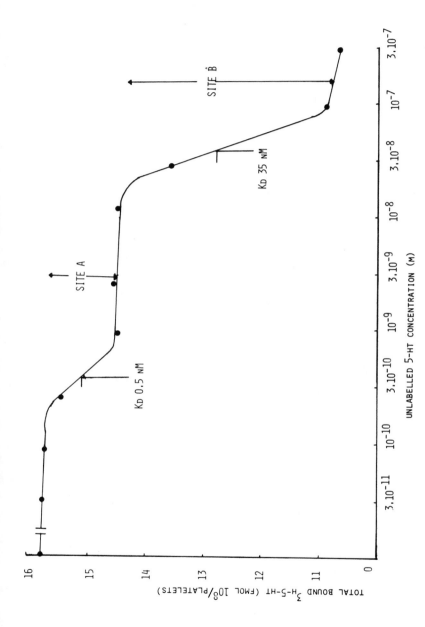

FIG. 1. Displacement of bound [³H]5-hydroxytryptamine from intact human platelets by addition of unlabeled 5-hydroxytryptamine. After reaching equilibrium at 2 min, specific bound [³H]5-hydroxytryptamine (final concentration 1 nM) was displaced by the addition of increasing concentrations of unlabeled 5-hydroxytryptamine. Values are means of four separate experiments performed in quadruplicate. (Reproduced from ref. 23.)

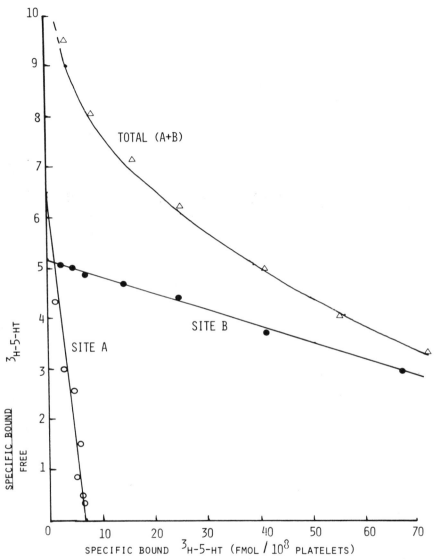

FIG. 2. Specific receptor binding of [³H]5-hydroxytryptamine to intact human platelets. Derivation of true asymptotes from curvilinear Scatchard analysis by differential displacement of specific bound [³H]5-hydroxytryptamine: 10^{-8} and 10^{-4} M unlabeled 5-hydroxytryptamine used for displacement at site A and sites A + B, respectively. For each free incubation concentration of [³H]5-hydroxytryptamine, the sum of [³H]5-hydroxytryptamine specifically bound to site A plus that to site B means of results from 8 normal subjects. (Reproduced from ref. 23.)

TABLE 1. *Kinetic parameters of human platelet 5-hydroxytryptamine receptors*

	B_{max} (sites/cell)	K_d (nM)
Site A	35–60	0.5–1
Site B	600–900	15–36

The values differ according to the method of calculation, i.e., whether displacement data, Scatchard analysis, or the adsorption isotherm is used. Data from ref. 23.

TABLE 2. *Inhibitory constants K_i for [³H]5-hydroxytryptamine (5-HT) receptor binding to site A and IC_{50} values for inhibition of 5-hydroxytryptamine (5-HT)-induced platelet aggregation*

Inhibitor	K_i [³H]5-HT site A binding (nM)	IC_{50} 5-HT aggregation (μM)
α-Flupenthixol	0.02	0.05
Methysergide	0.2	0.07
Mianserin	0.8	1.2
Pizotifen	1.1	2.3
β-Flupenthixol	2.0	11.0
5-Hydroxytryptamine	0.5	0.8

Reproduced from ref. 23.

TABLE 3. *Inhibitory constants for [³H]5-hydroxytryptamine (5-HT) receptor binding to site B and for active uptake of [³H]5-hydroxytryptamine (5-HT) under the same conditions*

Inhibitor	K_i site B [³H]5-HT binding (μM)	K_i uptake [³H]5-HT (μM)
Fluoxetine	0.004	0.003
5-Hydroxytryptamine	0.015	0.015
Chlorimipramine	0.13	0.08
Nortriptyline	0.50	0.25
Chlorpromazine	1.25	1.2
Mianserin	30.00	17.00
Pizotifen	85.00	70.00
Methysergide	250.00	75.00

Reproduced from ref. 23.

can be interpreted as a 'down regulation' in receptor number in response to a persistently raised blood level of 5-hydroxytryptamine. In addition, there was a decrease, or even abolition, of the aggregation response to 5-hydroxytryptamine.

2. Patients with migraine given the 5-hydroxytryptamine blocker, pizotifen, for prophylaxis show changes neither in capacity nor affinity at site B. However, affinity

at site A was reduced compared to that measured in the absence of drug. Site A capacity was unaffected. This indicates that pizotifen acts as a competitive antagonist at site A *in vivo*, confirming *in vitro* studies with the drug in other serotonergic systems.

3. The women studied were taking a combined estrogen-progestogen pill for 21 days in each menstrual cycle. During this 3-week period there was no significant variation in the binding parameters at either site. However, capacity at both sites was increased on day 21 as compared to day 28, i.e., after 7 days without treatment. Similarly, the aggregation response to 5-hydroxytryptamine, as well as active 5-hydroxytryptamine uptake, was greater on day 21 than on day 28. It is interesting to compare these findings with those reported by Elliott et al. (10). In rabbits treated with estrogens alone there was an increase in site A capacity, but there was a decrease following combined estrogen-progestogen treatment. These studies illustrate the possible relevance of this and similar binding techniques. Possible technical developments will be considered in the final section.

5-HYDROXYTRYPTAMINE UPTAKE AND ITS MEASUREMENT

The uptake of 5-hydroxytryptamine by the platelet has been studied for over a decade. The principles of the measurement of the active uptake process are very simple. Furthermore, the analogies between platelets and serotonergic neurons have attracted the interest of scientists not primarily interested in the platelet, e.g., neurochemists and psychopharmacologists. However, many of the earlier investigations can be criticized on technical grounds. Tuomisto (32) has shown the importance of using low cell concentrations and short incubation time for assays, to ensure that substrate concentration does not change significantly during the experiment. Also, if incubation continues for more than a few minutes, the velocity of the uptake reaction declines from its initial rate. These principles have since been widely accepted and adopted in other studies (e.g., refs. 7,28). In outline, Tuomisto's method is as follows:

As in binding studies, platelet-rich plasma is obtained by low-speed centrifugation of EDTA-anticoagulated blood. The platelet count is adjusted to a predetermined level with autologous cell-free plasma. Small aliquots of diluted platelet-rich plasma incubated at 37°C in a relatively large volume of buffer containing a fixed concentration of [^{3}H]5-hydroxytryptamine and varying concentrations of the unlabeled amine. The maximal incubation time is 5 min. The reaction is stopped by rapid dilution of the assay mixture followed by filtration. The new radioactivity trapped on the filters is then measured in a liquid scintillation counter.

Using this technique, Tuomisto et al. (33) has estimated the initial velocity of the uptake reaction (V_{max}) at 35 to 50 pmoles/10^7/5 min. The K_m, a measure of the affinity of the uptake system for 5-hydroxytryptamine, was about 0.4 μM.

CLINICAL USES OF 5-HYDROXYTRYPTAMINE UPTAKE STUDIES

Contrary to earlier findings, it seems probable that platelets from depressed subjects have a lower V_{max} for 5-hydroxytryptamine uptake than those from normal controls (33). Significant reduction in uptake has also been shown in platelets from patients with Down's syndrome (4). Recently, disordered 5-hydroxytryptamine uptake has also been demonstrated in individuals with migraine and asthma (17). However, in the latter study there was considerable variability between subjects and some had apparently normal 5-hydroxytryptamine uptake. The results in a variety of other disorders, e.g., schizophrenia, have so far failed to show a divergence from normal (16).

An interesting application of uptake measurement has been to show the *in vivo* effect of an antidepressant drug, imipramine (33). Like other tricyclics, this compound inhibits 5-hydroxytryptamine and norepinephrine reuptake in brain synaptosome preparations. Platelets from patients treated with imipramine showed a definite increase in the K_m of the uptake process of 5-hydroxytryptamine. There was no appreciable change in V_{max} for this process. This indicates that the drug is an *in vivo* competitive uptake inhibitor in the platelets as it is *in vitro* in both platelets and brain synaptosomes.

KETANSERIN AND THE PLATELET

We have recently begun to study the interactions between human platelets and the selective 5-hydroxytryptamine antagonist, ketanserin. Experiments are still at an early stage, but the following observations may already be made:

1. Ketanserin is a potent inhibitor of 5-hydroxytryptamine-induced platelet aggregation. It is effective at nanomolar concentrations (Fig. 3).

2. Ketanserin is virtually inactive as an inhibitor of active 5-hydroxytryptamine uptake by the platelet.

3. Ketanserin has no effect on [³H]yohimbine binding to human platelets, even at micromolar concentrations. This is not unexpected, since ketanserin is believed to be primarily an α_1-blocker while yohimbine is a relatively selective α_2-antagonist.

We have not so far demonstrated that ketanserin affects [³H]5-hydroxytryptamine binding at the platelet high-affinity site. Possible reasons for this are discussed in the following section.

DISCUSSION

Technical Problems

Some problems still remain in establishing standardized binding techniques for platelet 5-hydroxytryptamine receptors. This is due to the large number of interactions possible between 5-hydroxytryptamine and the platelet: membrane binding, active and passive uptake, and release of 5-hydroxytryptamine can all take place simultaneously. This has several consequences:

1. 5-Hydroxytryptamine uptake is an extremely active process. Despite cooling to 0°C some uptake continues. This may obscure binding to site A of the low capacity high affinity receptor (23).

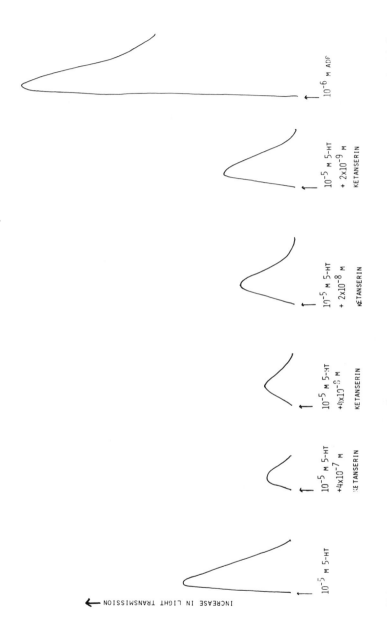

FIG. 3. Effect of ketanserin on 5-hydroxytryptamine (5-HT)-induced platelet aggregation. Increase in light transmitted indicates increased aggregation. Results from single experiment in normal subject.

2. The release of 5-hydroxytryptamine may also confound binding results. Cooling has some effect on platelet 5-hydroxytryptamine release but is very unlikely to stop it completely. Released 5-hydroxytryptamine interferes with binding by diluting radiolabeled ligand and by competing with the ligand for available binding sites (26).

3. As a consequence of performing incubations at low temperature, it is possible that properties attributed to receptors may be different from those existing at physiological temperatures (26).

For these reasons we have considered other possible ligands for the 5-hydroxytryptamine receptor. There are many other situations, e.g., dopamine and histamine receptors, where the natural compound is not used in the receptor characterization. In principle, the ligand should have at least as high an affinity for site A as 5-hydroxytryptamine itself, should not be taken up by the cell to a significant extent, even at 37°C, and should preferably be an agonist rather than an antagonist. The compound most likely to fulfill these requirements, of those currently available in radiolabeled form, is D-lysergic acid diethylamide (D-LSD). Laubscher et al. (14) have recently demonstrated a specific LSD binding site on rabbit platelets, but their work does not provide evidence that this site is identical with 5-hydroxytryptamine site A. We are at present examining LSD binding in human platelets, and performing preliminary experiments with other potential ligands.

Classification of Serotonergic Receptors

Peroutka and Snyder (21) have proposed that central serotonergic receptors may be divided into subtypes on the basis of physiological, pharmacological, and binding properties. Briefly, they state that $5-HT_1$ receptors are preferentially labeled by [³H]5-hydroxytryptamine, $5-HT_2$ receptors by [³H]spiperone, and that [³H]LSD labels both types equally. However, Yamamura (20) has suggested that [³H]5-hydroxytryptamine has equal affinity for all populations of central 5-hydroxytryptamine receptors, but two receptor types may be recognized on the basis of their affinity for [³H]spiperone. Leysen et al. (15) have shown that ketanserin is a very selective $5-HT_2$ antagonist on the basis of Snyder's classification. Ketanserin blocks 5-hydroxytryptamine-induced platelet aggregation, suggesting that the aggregation receptor (site A) can be classified as $5-HT_2$. Despite this, it is not yet clear if the platelet serotonergic receptors can be described in the same terms as central receptors. By analogy with such receptors, the platelet $5-HT_2$ receptor should have a high affinity with [³H]spiperone. Our experiments so far have failed to reveal a binding site for spiperone on the intact human platelet.

A recent related development has been the characterization of specific [³H]imipramine binding sites in human platelets (6,19), similar to those described in the rat brain. This may correspond to the 5-hydroxytryptamine uptake site, or may be closely related to it. A reduction in the number of [³H]imipramine sites has been described in depressed patients (5).

CONCLUSION

The role of 5-hydroxytryptamine in health and disease is still poorly understood, despite increased recent interest. The presence of specific serotonergic receptors on the platelet may allow some definition of, for instance, the role of 5-hydroxy-tryptamine in migraine (11). Other contributions indicate that 5-hydroxytryptamine may also be involved in the pathogenesis of cardiac failure and hypertension. Changes in platelet 5-hydroxytryptamine receptors in these conditions, with and without treatment, are of obvious interest both theoretically and in the development of more rational therapy. The introduction of selective and potent serotonergic antagonists may provide new approaches to the treatment of these and perhaps other unexpected disorders.

REFERENCES

1. Born, G. V. R., Dearnley, R., Foulks, J. G., and Sharp, D. E. (1978): Quantitation of the morphological reaction of platelets to aggregating agents and of its reversal by aggregation inhibitors. *J. Physiol. (Lond.)*, 280:193–212.
2. Born, G. V. R., Juengjarven, K., and Michael, F. (1972): Relative activities on and uptake by human blood platelets of 5-hydroxytryptamine and several analogues. *Br. J. Pharmacol.*, 44:117–123.
3. Boullin, D. J., Glenton, P. A. M., Molyneux, D., Peters, J. R., and Ruach, B. (1977): Binding of 5-hydroxytryptamine to human blood platelets. *Br. J. Pharmacol.*, 61:453P.
4. Boullin, D. J., and O'Brien, R. A. (1971): Abnormalities of 5-hydroxytryptamine uptake and binding by blood platelets from children with Down's syndrome. *J. Physiol. (Lond.)*, 212:287–297.
5. Briley, M. S., Langer, S. Z., Raisman, R., Sechter, D., and Zarifian, E. (1980): Tritiated imipramine binding sites are decreased in platelets of untreated depressed patients. *Science*, 209:303–305.
6. Briley, M. S., Raisman, R., and Langer, S. Z. (1979): Human platelets possess high-affinity binding sites for 3H-imipramine. *Eur. J. Pharmacol.*, 58:347–348.
7. Coppen, A., Ghose, K., Swade, C., and Wood, K. (1978): Effect of mianserin hydrochloride on peripheral uptake mechanisms for noradrenaline and 5-hydroxytryptamine in man. *Br. J. Clin. Pharmacol.*, 5:138–178.
8. Da Prada, M., Tranzer, J. P., and Pletscher, A. (1972): Storage of 5-hydroxytryptamine in human platelets. *Experientia*, 28:1328–1329.
9. Drummond, A. H., and Gordon, J. L. (1975): Specific binding sites for 5-hydroxytryptamine in rat blood platelets. *Biochem. J.*, 140:129–132.
10. Elliott, J. M., Peters, J. R., and Grahame-Smith, D. G. (1980): Oestrogen and progesterone change the binding characteristics of α-adrenergic and serotonin receptors in rabbit platelets. *Eur. J. Pharmacol.*, 66:21–30.
11. Hannington, E. (1978): Migraine: A blood disorder. *Lancet*, ii:501–502.
12. Kim, B. L., Steiner, M., and Baldini, M. G. (1980): Serotonin binding sites of human platelets. *Anal. Biochem.*, 106:92–98.
13. Laubscher, A., and Pletscher, A. (1979): Shape change and uptake of 5-hydroxytryptamine in human blood platelets: action of neuropsychiatric drugs. *Life Sci.*, 24:1833–1840.
14. Laubscher, A., Pletscher, A., and Noll, H. (1981): Interaction of D-LSD with blood platelets of rabbits: Shape change and specific binding. *J. Pharmacol. Exp. Ther.*, 216:385–389.
15. Leysen, J. E., Awouters, F., Kennis, L., Laduron, P. M., Vandenberk, J., and Janssen, F. A. J. (1981): Receptor binding profile of R41468, a novel antagonist at 5-HT$_2$ receptors. *Life Sci.*, 28:1015–1022.
16. Lucas, A. R., Warner, K., and Gottlieb, J. S. (1971): Biological studies in childhood schizophrenia: Serotonin uptake by platelets. *Biol. Psychiatry*, 3:123–128.
17. Malmgren, R., Olsson, P., Turnling, G., and Unge, G. (1980): The 5-hydroxytryptamine take-up mechanism in normal platelets and platelets from migraine and asthmatic patients. *Thromb. Res.*, 18:733–741.

18. Mustard, J. F., and Packham, M. A. (1975): Platelets, thrombosis and drugs. *Drugs*, 9:19–76.
19. Paul, S. M., Rehavi, M., Skulnick, P., and Goodwin, F. K. (1980): Demonstration of specific "high affinity" binding sites from [³H]imipramine on human platelets. *Life Sci.*, 26:953–959.
20. Pedigo, N. W., Yamamura, H. I., and Nelson, D. L. (1981): Discrimination of multiple [³H]5-hydroxytryptamine sites by the neuroleptic spiperone in rat brain. *J. Neurochem.*, 36:220–226.
21. Peroutka, S. J., and Snyder, S. H. (1979): Multiple serotonin receptors: Differential binding of [³H]5-hydroxytryptamine, [³H]lysergic acid diethylamide and [³H]spiroperidol. *Mol. Pharmacol.*, 16:687–699.
22. Peters, J. R., Elliott, J. M., and Grahame-Smith, D. G. (1979): Effect of oral contraception on platelet noradrenaline and 5-hydroxytryptamine receptors and aggregation. *Lancet*, ii:933–936.
23. Peters, J. R., and Grahame-Smith, D. G. (1980): Human platelet 5-HT receptors: Characterisation and functional association. *Eur. J. Pharmacol.*, 68:243–256.
24. Pletscher, A. (1978): Platelets as models for monoaminergic neurons. In: *Essays in Neurochemistry and Neuropharmacology*, Vol. 3, edited by M. B. H. Youdim. John Wiley, London.
25. Pletscher, A., and Laubscher, A. (1980): Use and limitations of platelets as models for neurons: Amine release and shape change. In: *Platelets: Cellular Response Mechanisms and Their Biological Significance*, edited by A. Rotman, F. A. Meyer, C. Gitler, and A. Silberberg. John Wiley, New York.
26. Shick, P. K., and McKeen, M-L. (1979): Serotonin binding in human platelets. *Biochem. Pharmacol.*, 28:2667–2669.
27. Sneddon, J. M. (1973): Blood platelets as a model for monoamine containing neurones. *Prog. Neurobiol.*, 1:153–198.
28. Stahl, S. M., and Meltzer, H. Y. (1978): A kinetic and pharmacologic analysis of 5-hydroxytryptamine transport by human platelets and platelet storage granules: Comparison with conetral serotonergic neurons. *J. Pharmacol. Exp. Ther.*, 205:118–132.
29. Talvenheimo, J., Nelson, P. J., and Rudnick, G. (1979): Mechanism of imipramine inhibition of platelet 5-hydroxytryptamine transport. *J. Biol. Chem.*, 245:6431–6435.
30. Thompson, J. H. (1971): Serotonin and the alimentary tract. *Res. Commun. Chem. Pathol. Pharmacol.*, 2:687–781.
31. Tranzer, J. P., Da Prada, M., and Pletscher, A. (1966): Ultrastructural localisation of 5-hydroxytryptamine in blood platelets. *Nature*, 212:1574–1575.
32. Tuomisto, J. (1974): A new modification for studying 5-HT uptake by blood platelets: A reevaluation of tricyclic antidepressants as uptake inhibitors. *J. Pharm. Pharmacol.*, 26:92–100.
33. Tuomisto, J., Tukiainen, E., and Ahlfors, U. G. (1979): Decreased uptake of 5-hydroxytryptamine in blood platelets in patients with endogenous depression. *Psychopharmacology*, 65:141–147.
34. Weissbach, H., Bogdanski, D. F., and Undenfriend, S. (1958): Binding of serotonin and other amines by blood platelets. *Arch. Biochem. Biophys.*, 73:492–499.

5-Hydroxytryptamine in Peripheral Reactions,
edited by Fred De Clerck and Paul M.
Vanhoutte. Raven Press, New York © 1982.

Detection of Platelet Activation *In Vivo*: Significance and Limitations of the Available Tests

*J. L. David and **F. De Clerck

*Hôpital de Bavière, Université de Liège, B-4200 Liège, Belgium; and
**Laboratory of Haematology, Janssen Pharmaceutica Research Laboratories,
B-2340 Beerse, Belgium

Ischemic episodes often are caused by arterial occlusions subsequent to thrombus or embolus formation initiated by aggregating platelets (33). Such platelet aggregation may be induced by several humoral or hemodynamic stimuli or by interactions with the vessel wall. The degree of platelet sensitivity to these stimuli of varying intensity and duration will further determine the extent of the platelet reactions such as adhesion, aggregation, and the release of platelet products including 5-hydroxytryptamine, adenine nucleotides, beta-thromboglobulin, platelet-factor-4, and thromboxane A_2 (10).

Recently several methods have been proposed in order to detect abnormal activation of the blood platelets *in vivo*. Among these, three are currently gaining large interest: (a) the assessment of the platelet aggregation index; (b) the radioimmunoassay of plasma beta-thromboglobulin and platelet-factor-4; and (c) the measurement of thromboxane B_2, the stable metabolite of thromboxane A_2. The relevance of these tests largely depends upon the rigid control of blood sampling and processing, in order to avoid *ex vivo* activation especially in pathologies possibly complicated by platelet hypersensitivity. In addition to technical pitfalls, the interpretation of the experimental results should take into account the fact that a local activation of platelets in a particular vascular bed such as the coronary circulation may be damped by metabolic or hemodynamic factors, and may not be apparent if determined in a systemic blood sample. The present chapter reviews some technical and interpretational aspects of these tests. For details on their application, in particular, clinical situations, the reader is referred to the appropriate literature.

PLATELET AGGREGATION INDEX

Methodology

Wu and Hoak (53) introduced a comparatively simple method to quantify circulating platelet aggregates. In essence the technique consists in the counting of the free platelets in two simultaneously obtained blood samples diluted either in a buffered formol-EDTA solution or in a buffered ethyldiaminetetraacetate (EDTA) solution, respectively. The latter solution will disperse aggregates while the former will fix them. The platelet aggregation index then is calculated as the ratio between free platelets in platelet-rich plasma prepared from the formol-EDTA solution versus those from the EDTA solution.

The lower the ratio or the index, the more platelet aggregates are present in the formol-treated blood sample. Although the platelet aggregation index in most studies is calculated from platelet counts in such platelet-rich plasmas, it is advisable to perform the counts in whole blood, since during centrifugation of diluted blood to the platelet-rich plasma, a population of formol-treated platelets may sediment together with the red blood cells, thus yielding abnormally low platelet aggregation indexes (34,35).

Nature and Origin of the Circulating Platelet Aggregates

The fact that the circulating aggregates must be dispersible by Ca^{2+}-chelation with EDTA limits the meaning of the original Wu and Hoak technique. This restriction implies that the aggregates in the former solution are not consolidated by fibrin, as platelet aggregates fragmented from a fibrin-rich thrombin tend to be. On the other hand, the cohesion of the formed aggregates should be strong enough to avoid disaggregation before fixation in the collecting fluid. Platelets, aggregated without subsequent fibrin consolidation, tend to disperse quickly by either metabolic or mechanical mechanisms (27). Therefore, the detection of a reduced platelet aggregation index according to Wu and Hoak should reflect a recent platelet activation occurring just before the blood sampling.

Unless they are formed locally in the punctured vein, the presence of platelet aggregates in systemic venous blood implies that they were stable enough to transit the pulmonary and peripheral capillary beds. In order to cope with the dispersibility of formed aggregates, sampling of the blood directly from the vascular bed where the platelet activation occurs is performed in some studies (29,38). However, the possibility exists that the induction of platelet aggregates is caused by a systemic rather than a localized activation process. Finally, whenever a low platelet aggregation index is detected, this may be due to a hyperreactivity of the platelets resulting in *ex vivo* aggregate formation favored (56) by stasis, turbulence, and contact with foreign surfaces upon blood sampling, rather than actually reflecting existing circulating aggregates *in vivo*.

Significance of the Platelet Aggregation Index

In patients with myocardial infarction and thromboembolic diseases, a positive correlation exists between a low platelet aggregation index and a shortened life span of the platelets (5,41). This suggests that the former parameter reflects *in vivo* activation of the platelets of sufficient duration and intensity to increase consumption and reduce survival. Although the correlation between the two parameters may reflect related or identical causes, the relative importance of exogenous stimuli causing platelet activation, and of endogenous changes in the platelet leading to hyperreactivity, cannot be dissociated. Similarly, a positive correlation exists between a low platelet aggregation index and an elevated plasma level of beta-thromboglobulin (6). Since the former parameters are not correlated with the *ex vivo* sensitivity of platelets to adenosine-5'-diphosphate (ADP), sustained stimulation *in vivo*, rather than intrinsic platelet hypersensitivity, seems to be responsible in this particular group of patients. However, artifacts producing elevated beta-thromboglobulin levels in plasma (36) and, on the other hand, reduction of the platelet reactivity by citrate-anticoagulation (18) as applied in these studies may limit the validity of the latter conclusion.

Platelet Reactivity

Several factors may affect the reactivity of the platelet and, hence, favor the formation of aggregates. First, plasma fibrinogen may be implicated. Indeed in patients with vascular as well as inflammatory diseases a positive correlation exists between the plasma fibrinogen level and the platelet aggregation index (26) reflecting the involvement of this protein as a co-factor for the platelet adhesion-aggregation reaction (1). Second, the reduced platelet aggregation index in patients with hyperlipoproteinemia (25) may reflect the impact of plasma lipids and platelet membrane lipid composition on platelet behavior (20). Third, environmental factors such as hypoxic metabolites, acid-base balance, PO_2-PCO_2 values, as well as interaction with red blood cells, may influence platelet reactivity (10,48).

When tested *ex vivo* using the turbidometric techniques on platelet-rich plasma, some of these factors are liable to change during the removal of red blood cells and platelet subpopulations by centrifugation (48,49); moreover, the age of the stored plasma sample, the type of anticoagulant used, pH-, oxygenation-, and temperature-control will affect platelet reactivity differently according to the agonist when studied with this technique (27,50). Therefore, it is imperative to study platelet reactivity in fresh, native blood, assessing preferentially those parameters (e.g., platelet aggregation index, beta-thromboglobulin release) used for the measurement of *in vivo* platelet activation (8).

Platelet Aggregation Index in Vascular Disease

The platelet aggregation index has been used mainly to study the occurrence of platelet activation in coronary artery disease. Most studies rely on the examination of a systemic blood sample obtained from an antecubital vein, implying that the platelet aggregates formed in the coronary vascular bed are sufficiently stable to be detectable peripherally. However, venous stasis or the consequences of cardiogenic shock might also be responsible for the lowered platelet aggregation index (47). According to Mehta (30) the platelet aggregation index tends to be lowered on the first day of a transmural myocardial infarction and is normalized on the seventh day thereafter. Similar changes are found in patients with anterior transmural infarction (29) suggesting that such a lesion will favor activation of the platelets. Others failed to detect significant changes in the platelet aggregation index subsequent to acute thrombotic events (35,40,45). However, a comparison between these studies suggests that the period after as well as during the incident may determine whether or not such a platelet abnormality is detectable.

"Vasospastic" angina seems to be determinant for the formation of platelet aggregates in the coronary vascular bed (7). Independent of the coronarographic aspect of the vascular bed, the platelet aggregation index in blood sampled from the coronary sinus is reduced during the crisis of spontaneous vasospastic angina; to the contrary, the aggregation index in systemic arterial blood is normal. Such a difference suggests the existence of a local activation phenomenon but does not exclude that the aggregates are mainly formed upon contact with the sampling catheter, rather than in the coronary vascular bed. A localized platelet sensitivation process indeed exists in coronary artery disease: In samples obtained from the coronary sinus, but not from the aorta of patients paced to tachycardia, the *ex vivo* platelet aggregability is increased (29).

The reduction of the platelet aggregation index in blood obtained by catheterization of coronary sinus of angina patients has been observed as well by Dalal (7). However, the persistence of a subnormal index in peripheral arterial blood in the latter patients suggests a stronger cohesion of the circulating aggregates during the angor crisis; again sensitization of the platelets rather than actual aggregate formation *in vivo* cannot be excluded. Moreover the systemic repercussions of stress or a transient defective ventricular function in such patients are difficult to analyze; they may explain the modification of the platelet aggregation index in venous peripheral blood in patients with unstable angina as reported by Schwartz et al. (45). The direct effect of a coronary spasm on the formation of platelet aggregates remains unknown: While no reduction of the platelet aggregation index was found during the injection of ergometrine (42), such a reduction has been found by others during the injection of this drug which does not induce platelet aggregation by itself (46). Although coronary vasospasm has been associated with platelet aggregate formation, the number of platelets in blood obtained from the coronary sinus does not differ from that sampled from a peripheral artery during a coronary vasospastic episode (38). These findings exclude platelet sequestration in the coronary vascular bed, expected to occur after the adhesion-aggregation process.

Therefore, the hypothesis claiming local formation of platelet aggregates during a coronary spasm is based upon experiments largely influenced by stimuli, and conditions favoring local sensitization of the platelets. The same restriction applies to the findings of a transiently reduced platelet aggregation index in venous peripheral blood obtained immediately after exercise from patients with coronary artery disease but not from normals (22). Such platelet aggregates may be formed in the coronary vascular bed or in the systemic circulation subsequent to hemodynamic and humoral changes caused by exercise. Again, the exercise stress in coronary patients may produce a transient sensitivation of the platelet resulting in aggregate formation which is precipitated by the blood sampling procedures.

BETA-THROMBOGLOBULIN AND PLATELET-FACTOR-4

Beta-thromboglobulin and platelet-factor-4 are two platelet-specific proteins stored in the alpha-granules; upon stimulation of the platelet they are released into the plasma (21). Increased plasma levels of the two proteins are believed to reflect an *in vivo* stimulation or destruction of the circulating platelets, as found mainly in various thromboembolic conditions.

Beta-Thromboglobulin

Characteristics

Beta-thromboglobulin (M.W. 36,000) is a protein composed of four identical subunits, containing each 81 amino acids. According to Niewiarowski et al. (32), beta-thromboglobulin results from the degradation of low affinity platelet-factor-4 by loss of a tetrapeptide at the level of the N-terminal side of each subunit. Beta-thromboglobulin and low affinity platelet-factor-4 have cross antigenicity. *In vivo* beta-thromboglobulin crosses the glomerulal filter barrier; its biological half-life in man is about 100 min (9). As evidenced by experiments performed on rats (3), human beta-thromboglobulin, or at least low affinity platelet-factor-4 is filtered in the glomeruli, reabsorbed by the tubular epithelial cells, and catabolized in the kidney.

Normal and Pathological Values

Normal values for beta-thromboglobulin in plasma are logarithmically distributed, most being below 20 ng/ml *(personal observation)*. Plasma beta-thromboglobulin levels are found increased in patients with various types of vascular diseases such as venous thrombosis, myocardial infarction, diabetes, Raynaud's disease, and preeclampsia (54). However the scatter of normal values as published is large, making a clear-cut dissociation from definite pathological values difficult. Nevertheless, the negative correlation between plasma levels of beta-thromboglobulin and the platelet survival time in various pathologies (5,12,13,35–37,54) supports the concept of *in vivo* liberation of beta-thromboglobulin.

As for the platelet aggregation index, platelet activation during blood sampling, especially in patients with hypersensitive platelets, may produce, *ex vivo*, abnormally high plasma levels of beta-thromboglobulin. The use of a suitable mixture of anticoagulant and antiaggregating substances during the collection of blood, as well as nearly total removal of platelets from the test plasma, is therefore imperative (36).

Nonthrombotic Elevation of Beta-Thromboglobulin

First, in patients with renal insufficiency the plasma levels of beta-thromboglobulin are elevated in parallel with those of creatinine and β_2-microglobulin due to a reduction of glomural filtration rate or renal catabolism of the protein (11,52). In the case of glomerulonephritis, superimposed thrombolic obstruction of the renal microcirculation may complicate the interpretation of the relative role of platelet activation and of renal processing (15,52).

Second, as demonstrated during extracorporeal circulation, a preferential release occurs of the content of the platelet alpha-granules containing beta-thromboglobulin as compared with that of the platelet dense bodies (17). Such a lability of the granules, rather than overt platelet activation, may be responsible for the basal levels of beta-thromboglobulin in normal man.

Platelet-Factor-4

Characteristics

Platelet-factor-4 (M.W. 30,000) is composed of 4 subunits containing two amino acids each. The protein is bound to proteoglycans (2), the dimensions of the resulting complex preventing glomerular filtration. *In vitro*, the platelet-factor-4 preferentially fixes to glycosamino-glycans on the surface of the endothelial cells from which it can be displaced, both *in vitro* and *in vivo*, by heparin (4). This preferential affinity may explain its comparatively short (10 min) biological half-life, and *in vivo* the sharp rise of its plasma level after the injection of heparin (9).

Normal and Pathological Values

Values for platelet-factor-4 in plasma from normal subjects range below 10 ng/ml *(personal observation)*. While *in vitro* stimulation of platelets produces an approximately parallel increase of both beta-thromboglobulin and platelet-factor-4 levels in the supernatant, the *ex vivo* plasma levels show a higher ratio for the two proteins, probably due to the faster clearance from the circulation of platelet-factor-4. The values reported for platelet-factor-4 in plasma of patients with various disorders show a large scatter, presumably due to differences in blood processing. For example, Green et al. (14) found elevated plasma levels of the protein in plasma after an exercise test in 11 out of 20 coronary patients with ECG changes, but only in 2 out of 20 such patients with normal ECGs. On the contrary, Mathis et al. (28) failed to detect such an elevation in patients with coronary vascular disease who were undergoing exercise tolerance tests; the necessity to remove all platelets from the plasma used for the radioimmunoassay of platelet-factor-4 by adequate centrifugation is stressed (36). Elevated values of platelet-factor-4 were reported by others (16,51) in acute myocardial infarction, and in patients with angina pectoris and diabetes. However, those findings should be reconsidered taking into account possible methodological artifacts. Indeed, an increased plasma level of platelet-factor-4 may well reflect *ex vivo* activation of the platelets due to their hypersensitivity, rather than an *in vivo* release reaction.

THROMBOXANE B$_2$

Thromboxane A$_2$ is synthesized through the fatty-acid cyclooxygenase pathway of arachidonic acid metabolism and released from the platelets subsequent to specific stimulation (31,44). Because of its fast turnover (31,44), dosage is performed of its chemically stable derivation thromboxane B_2. Increased levels of thromboxane B_2 in plasma, therefore, reflect another aspect of platelet activation *in vivo*. Thromboxane B_2 is rapidly cleared from the circulation (37), limiting its validity for the detection of a transient or local platelet activation process. The amounts of thromboxane B_2, generated locally in a particular vascular bed, e.g., the coronary tree, are rapidly diluted in the circulation yielding low and variable systemic values often below the detection limit of a radioimmunoassay. As for the estimation of beta-thromboglobulin and platelet-factor-4, strict precautions should be taken to avoid thromboxane formation during blood processing.

Levels in Coronary Artery Disease

Determination of thromboxane B_2 levels in plasma as an indication for *in vivo* activation of blood platelet in cardiovascular disease yielded contradictory results. Although elevated levels of thromboxane B_2 were detected in venous peripheral blood of patients with Prinzmetal's angina (23), no correlation was found between variations of such thromboxane B_2 levels and the occurrence of ischemic episodes in unstable angina (43). Levels of thromboxane B_2 in blood sampled simultaneously from the coronary sinus and from arteries have been compared repeatedly. The induction of tachycardia by endocardial stimulation in patients with pronounced coronary artery occlusion induced angor and a transient (<10 min) increase of thromboxane B_2, both in coronary venous and peripheral arterial blood (55). On the other hand, in patients with vasospastic angina, thromboxane B_2 was clearly elevated in coronary sinus but not in peripheral arterial blood; such a change occurred after the onset of ischemia (39). The intake of acetysalicylic acid and of indomethacin by these patients inhibited the production of thromboxane B_2 but did not prevent the anginal attack suggesting that this platelet-derived prostaglandin is not causing the coronary vasospasm. In a group of patients with unstable angina, Hirsch et al. (19) failed to detect significant changes in thromboxane B_2 levels in coronary sinus or aortic blood; nevertheless, the ratio between the levels in the coronary sinus and the aorta was increased. In this particular study, blood samples were obtained 24 and 96 hr after the ischemic attack. Therefore, it would seem that the platelet activation in the coronary bed persists after the disappearance of the ischemic episode possibly due to endothelial damage at the stenotic lesion of the spastic vascular segment (24).

As a whole, these data suggest that the elevation of thromboxane B_2 levels during various types of angina result from a local coronary rather than a systemic stimulation of the blood platelets. Nevertheless, activation of platelets upon contact with the sampling catheter in the coronary sinus may be involved especially in situations in which the platelets could be sensitized by a previous formation of thromboxane A_2 in the coronary vascular bed (43).

Again, as for the other tests for the detection of platelet activation, the technique of thromboxane B_2 measurement in plasma cannot dissociate true activation of the platelet in a specific vascular bed from that occurring during blood sampling, especially when the platelets themselves are hypersensitive.

REFERENCES

1. Bang, N. V., Heidenreich, R. O., and Trygstad, C. W. (1972): Plasma protein requirements for human platelet aggregation. *Ann. NY Acad. Sci.*, 201:280–289.
2. Barber, A. J., Käser-Glanzmann, R., Jakábová, M., and Lüscher, E. F. (1972): Characterization of chondroitin 4-sulfate proteoglycan carrier for heparin neutralizing activity (Platelet Factor 4) released from human blood platelets. *Biochem. Biophys. Acta*, 286:312–329.
3. Bastl, C. P., Musial, J., Guzzo, J., Berman, I., and Niewarouwski, S. (1981): Role of kidney in the catabolic clearance of human platelet antiherapin proteins from rat circulation. *Blood*, 57:233–238.
4. Busch, C., Dawes, J., Pepper, D. S., and Wasteson, A. (1980): Binding of platelet factor 4 to cultured human endothelial cells. *Thromb. Res.*, 19:129–137.
5. Cella, G., Zahavi, J., de Haas, H. A., and Kakkar, V. V. (1979): β-Thromboglobulin, platelet production time and platelet function in vascular disease. *Br. J. Haematol.*, 43:127–136.
6. Chen, Y. C., and Wu, K. K. (1980): A comparison of methods for the study of platelet hyperfunction in thromboembolic disorders. *Br. J. Haematol.*, 46:263–268.
7. Dalal, J. J., Sheridan, D. J., Bloom, A. L., and Henderson, A. H. (1980): Platelet aggregates and coronary spasm. *Lancet*, ii:1146–1147.
8. David, J. L., Raskinet, R., and Herion, F. (1980): Evaluation of platelet reactivity in native non-anticoagulated blood. VIIth International Conference on Thrombosis (Mediterranean League Against Thromboembolic Diseases), Monte Carlo, Abstract 149.
9. Dawes, J., Smith, R. C., and Pepper, D. S. (1978): The release, distribution and clearance of human β-thromboglobulin and platelet factor-4. *Thromb. Res.*, 12:851–861.
10. De Clerck, F., and David, J. L. (1981): Pharmacological control of platelet and red blood cell function in the microcirculation. *J. Cardiovasc. Pharmacol.*, 3:1388–1412.
11. Deppermann, D., Andrassy, K., Seelig, H., Ritz, E., and Post, D. (1980): Beta-thromboglobulin is elevated in renal failure without thrombosis. *Thromb. Res.*, 17:63–69.
12. Dougherty, Jr., J. H., Levy, D. E., and Weksler, B. B. (1977): Platelet activation in acute cerebral ischaemia (serial measurements of platelet function in cerebrovascular disease). *Lancet*, i:821–824.
13. Doyle, D. J., Chesterman, C. N., Cade, J. F., McGready, J. R., Rennie, G. C., and Morgan, F. J. (1980): Plasma concentrations of platelet-specific proteins correlated with platelet survival. *Blood*, 55:82–84.
14. Green, L. H., Seroppian, E., and Handin, R. I. (1980): Platelet activation during exercise-induced myocardial ischemia. *N. Engl. J. Med.*, 302:193–197.
15. Han, P., Turpic, A. G. G., and Genton, E. (1979): Plasma β-thromboglobulin: differentiation between intravascular and extravascular platelet destruction. *Blood*, 54:1122–1196.
16. Handin, R. I., McDonough, M., and Lesch, M. (1978): Elevation of platelet factor-4 in acute myocardial infarction: Measurements by radioimmunoassay. *J. Lab. Clin. Med.*, 91:340–349.
17. Harker, L. A., Malpass, T. W., Brauson, H. E., Hessel, E. A., and Slichter, S. J. (1980): Mechanism of abnormal bleeding in patients undergoing cardiopulmonary bypass; acquired transient patient dysfunction associated with selective α granule release. *Blood*, 56:824–834.
18. Heptinstall, S., and Taylor, P. M. (1979): The effects of citrate and extracellular calcium ions on the platelet release reaction induced by adenosine diphosphate and collagen. *Thromb. Haemost.*, 42:778–793.
19. Hirsh, P. D., Hillis, L. D., Cambell, W. B., Firth, B. G., and Willerson, J. T. (1981): Release of prostaglandins and thromboxane into the coronary circulation in patients with ischemic heart disease. *N. Engl. J. Med.*, 304:685–691.
20. Hornstra, G. (1980): Dietary fats and arterial thrombosis. *Thesis*. R.U.L. Maastricht, The Netherlands.
21. Kaplan, K. L., and Owen, J. (1981): Plasma levels of β-thromboglobulin and platelet factor-4 as indices of platelet activation *in vivo*. *Blood*, 57:199–202.
22. Kusupuris, A. G., Luchi, R. J., Waddel, C. C., and Miller, R. R. (1980): Production of circulating platelet aggregates by exercise in coronary patients. *Circulation*, 61:62–65.

23. Lewy, R. I., Smith, J. B., Silver, M. G., Sain, J., Waliwsky, P., and Wiener, L. (1979): Detection of thromboxane B_2 (TxB$_2$) in peripheral blood of patients with Prinzmetal's angina. *Clin. Res.*, 27:452A.
24. Lewy, R. I., Wiener, L., Walinsky, P., Zefer, A. M., Silver, M. J., and Smith, J. B. (1980): Thromboxane release during pacing induced angina pectoris; possible vasoconstrictor influence on the coronary vasculature. *Circulation*, 61:1165–1171.
25. Lowe, G. D. O., Drummond, M. M., Third, J. L. H. C., Bremmer, W. F., Forbes, C. D., Prentice, C. R. M., and Lawrie, T. D. V. (1979): Increased plasma fibrinogen and platelet-aggregates in type II hyperlipoproteinaemia. *Thromb. Haemost.*, 42:1503–1507.
26. Lowe, G. D. O., Reavey, M. M., Johnston, R. V., Forbes, C. D., and Prentice, C. R. M. (1979): Increased platelet aggregates in vascular and non-vascular illness: correlation with plasma fibrinogen and effect of ancrod. *Thromb. Res.*, 14:377–386.
27. Mustard, J. F., and Packham, M. A. (1970): Factors influencing platelet function—adhesion, release and aggregation. *Pharmacol. Rev.*, 22:97–187.
28. Mathis, P. C., Wohl, H., Wallack, S. R., and Engler, R. L. (1981): Lack of release of platelet factor-4 during exercise-induced myocardial ischemia. *N. Engl. J. Med.*, 304:1275–1278.
29. Mehta, J., Mehta, P., and Pepine, C. J. (1978): Platelet aggregation in aortic and coronary venous blood in patients with and without coronary disease. (3. Role of tachycardia stress and propranolol). *Circulation*, 58:881–886.
30. Mehta, P., and Mehta, J. (1979): Platelet function studies in coronary artery disease (V. Evidence for enhanced platelet microthrombus formation activity in acute myocardial infarction). *Am. J. Cardiol.*, 43:757–760.
31. Moncada, S., and Vane, J. R. (1979): Pharmacology and endogenous role of prostaglandin endoperoxides, thromboxane A_2 and prostacyclin. *Pharmacol. Rev.*, 30:293–331.
32. Niewiarowski, S., Walz, D. A., James, P., Rucinski, B., and Kueppers, F. (1980): Identification and separation of secreted platelet proteins by isoelectric focusing. Evidence that low-affinity platelet factor-4 is converted to β-thromboglobulin by limited proteolysis. *Blood*, 55:453–456.
33. Owren, P. A. (1973): Developments in thrombosis research. In: *Recent Advances in Thrombosis*, edited by L. Poller, pp. 1–16. Churchill Livingstone, Edinburgh.
34. Prazich, J. A., Rapaport, S. I., Samples, J. R., and Engler, R. (1977): Platelet aggregate ratios-standardization of technique and test results in patients with myocardial ischemia and patients with cerebrovascular disease. *Thromb. Haemost.*, 38:597–605.
35. Raper, C. G. L. (1978): Circulating platelet aggregates. *Thromb. Haemost.*, 39:537–538.
36. Rasi, V. (1980): β-Thromboglobulin in plasma. False high values caused by platelet enrichment of the top layer of plasma during centrifugation. *Thromb. Res.*, 15:543–552.
37. Roberts, L. J., Sweetman, B. J., and Oates, J. A. (1981): Metabolism of thromboxane B_2 in man. *J. Biol. Chem.*, 256:8384–8368.
38. Robertson, R. M., Robertson, D., Friesinger, G. C., Timmous, S., and Hawiger, J. (1980): Platelet aggregates in peripheral and coronary-sinus blood in patients with spontaneous coronary-artery spasm. *Lancet*, ii:829–831.
39. Robertson, R. M., Robertson, D., Roberts, L. J., Maas, R. L., Fitzgerald, G. A., Friesinger, G. C., and Oates, J. A. (1981): Thromboxane A_2 in vasotonic angina pectoris. *N. Engl. J. Med.*, 304:998–1003.
40. Rohrer, T. F., Pfister, B., Weber, C., Imhof, P. R., and Stucki, P. (1978): Validity of the Wu and Hoak method for the quantitative determination of platelet aggregation *in vivo*. *Blut*, 36:15–20.
41. Salem, H. H., Koutts, J., and Firkin, B. G. (1980): Circulating platelet aggregates in ischaemic heart disease and their correlation to platelet life span. *Thromb. Res.*, 17:707–711.
42. Salerno, J. A., Griguani, G., Previtali, M., Garuba, G., Chimienti, M., and Bobba, P. (1981): Platelet aggregates and malondialdehyde production by platelets during ergonovine-induced coronary spasm. *Lancet*, i:381–382.
43. Salzman, E. W., and Sobel, M. (1981): Thromboxane in ischemic heart disease. (To the Editor). *N. Engl. J. Med.*, 305:106.
44. Samuelson, B., Goldyne, M., Granström, E., Hamberg, M., Hammarström, S., and Malmsten, C. (1978): Prostaglandins and thromboxanes. *Annu. Rev. Biochem.*, 47:997–1029.
45. Schwartz, M. B., Hawiger, J., Timmonds, S., and Friesinger, G. C. (1980): Platelet aggregates in ischemic heart disease. *Thromb. Haemost.*, 43:185–188.
46. Sobel, M., Salzman, E. W., Davies, G. C., Handin, R. I., Sweeney, J., Ploetz, J., and Kurland, G. (1981): Circulating platelet products in unstable angina pectoris. *Circulation*, 63:300–306.

47. Swank, R. C., and Edwards, M. J. (1968): Microvascular occlusion by platelet emboli after transfusion and shock. *Microvasc. Res.*, 1:15–22.
48. Tang, S. S., and Frojmovic, M. M. (1977): The effects of pco_2 and pH in platelet shape change and aggregation for human and rabbit platelet-rich plasma. *Thromb. Res.*, 10:135–145.
49. Vainer, H. (1972): Separation of platelet populations from human and red blood. Method and application. In: *Platelet Function and Thrombosis. A Review of Methods*, edited by P. M. Mannucci, and S. Gorini, pp. 309–314. Plenum Press, New York.
50. Warlow, C., Corina, A., Ogston, D., and Douglas, A. J. (1974): The relationship between platelet aggregation and time interval after venepuncture. *Thromb. Diath. Haemorrh.*, 31:133–141.
51. White, G. C., II, and Marouf, A. A. (1981): Platelet factor-4 levels in patients with coronary artery disease. *J. Lab. Clin. Med.*, 97:369–378.
52. Woo, K. T., Junor, B. J. R., Salem, H., d'Apice, A. J. F., Whitworth, J. A., and Kincaid-Smith, P. (1980): Beta-thromboglobulin and platelet aggregates in glomerulonephritis. *Clin. Nephrol.*, 14:92–95.
53. Wu, K. K., and Hoak, J. C. (1974): A new method for the quantitative detection of platelet aggregates in patients with arterial insufficiency. *Lancet*, ii:924–926.
54. Zahavi, J., and Kakkar, V. V. (1980): β-Thromboglobulin—a specific marker of *in vivo* platelet release reaction. *Thromb. Haemost.*, 44:23–29.
55. Zelinger, A. B., Schick, E. C., and Ryan, T. J. (1981): Thromboxane in ischemic heart disease. (To the Editor.) *N. Engl. J. Med.*, 305:106–107.
56. Zucker, M. B. (1972): Proteolytic inhibitors, contact and other variables in the release reaction of human platelets. *Thromb. Diath. Haemorrh.*, 28:393–407.

5-Hydroxytryptamine in Peripheral Reactions,
edited by Fred De Clerck and Paul M.
Vanhoutte. Raven Press, New York © 1982.

Involvement of 5-Hydroxytryptamine in Peripheral Reactions: Historical Notes

F. Awouters

*Department of Pharmacology, Janssen Pharmaceutica Research Laboratories,
B-2340 Beerse, Belgium*

After thirty years of research the physiological role of the biogenic amine 5-hydroxytryptamine and its potential importance in pathology (5-HT, serotonin) is still debated (6–8,10,12). This is perhaps not too surprising, since the amine not only stimulates, or inhibits the function of a variety of smooth muscles and nerves, but also can induce heterogeneous responses, which differ not only between species, but also between animals of the same species, and even in successive tests in a given individual (6). In the periphery, 5-hydroxytryptamine affects mainly the cardiovascular, respiratory, and gastrointestinal systems (6). The present historical notes focus on a few early reports illustrating responses at the smooth muscle level.

SEROTONIN IS 5-HYDROXYTRYPTAMINE

A vasoconstricting agent that occurs in the serum of mammals was first described in 1868 (20). The vasoconstrictor and moderately hypertensive properties of serum and defibrinated blood have been observed repeatedly thereafter and the active principle, of which no chemical information was available, received various names such as "vaso-constrictine" (3), "adrenalin-like substance" (22), and "spätgift" (11). Much later the substance was obtained in crystalline form and renamed serotonin, as its source was serum and its activity one of causing vasoconstriction (27). Blood plasma hardly contained serotonin, but the product was set free during clotting of the blood in connection with the release reaction of platelets, which had already early been considered to be the likely source of all the vasoactive substance in blood (22). On the basis of color reactions and ultraviolet absorption spectrum, Rapport (26) obtained evidence for the presence of a 5-hydroxyindole nucleus in the crystalline material and proposed that serotonin corresponded chemically to 5-hydroxytryptamine. The first synthesis of 5-hydroxytryptamine was reported soon thereafter (15); the end product was obtained as the hydrochloride salt, which is a light-sensitive and hygroscopic product. Synthetic 5-hydroxytryptamine and the natural serotonin-creatinine complex obtained by Page and his colleagues (27) had indistinguishable vasoactive properties.

In the same period other laboratories had been working on biological material different from serum and the names of "thrombocytin" and "enteramine" clearly tell the source of the active principle they were studying. Particularly the work of Erspamer's laboratory on the specific "hormone" of the enterochromaffin cells from the gastrointestinal mucosa was a completely independent approach to the identification of a vasoactive amine. This work culminated in the recognition that serotonin and enteramine were identical (9).

Enterochromaffin cells belong to the amine precursor uptake decarboxylation (APUD) endocrine polypeptide cells (25). They are the major site of synthesis, storage, and release of 5-hydroxytryptamine in the periphery (ref. 7; H. Ahlman and A. Dahlström, *this volume*; J. M. Polak et al., *this volume*). The platelets actively take up (ref. 18; M. Schächter and D. G. Grahame-Smith, *this volume*) and probably remove rapidly any 5-hydroxytryptamine reaching the blood after being released by the enterochromaffin in cells. However, *in vivo* studies indicate that platelet uptake may not be fast enough to prevent removal of 5-hydroxytryptamine by other tissues, in particular the lungs (34). Free 5-hydroxytryptamine may be particularly important for the endothelial cells (P. D'Amore and D. Shepro, *this volume*); the amount of circulating 5-hydroxytryptamine can be increased in any vascular bed, especially when the platelets tend to aggregate (J. David and F. De Clerck, *this volume*).

In the rat and the mouse, mast cells are another rich source of 5-hydroxytryptamine. Normal rat peritoneal mast cells contain 630 to 700 μg 5-hydroxytryptamine per ml cells (2). When a specific mast cell activator, compound 48/80, is used to perfuse rat tissues, considerably more histamine than 5-hydroxytryptamine is released (3), but, on the other hand, 5-hydroxytryptamine is much more potent as mediator of vascular injury than histamine in this species (30). Released 5-hydroxytryptamine by mast cells has important pathological consequences (F. Awouters et al., *this volume*).

PHARMACOLOGICAL ACTIONS OF 5-HYDROXYTRYPTAMINE

The availability of pure, synthetic 5-hydroxytryptamine resulted in an almost explosive expansion of studies of its pharmacological effects. The following actions have been reported in 1952 (28) and may be considered typical. Among isolated tissues the sheep carotid artery was particularly sensitive to 5-hydroxytryptamine, but also the guinea pig jejunum and the rat uterus contracted in the presence of low concentrations of the amine. In cats, low doses of intraarterially injected 5-hydroxytryptamine contracted the nictitating membrane, released epinephrine, and decreased the flow in perfused hind limbs. A systemic pressor action in the anesthetized cat was obtained by intravenous injection of 10 to 40 μg, which also affected the uterus and the bronchi.

Several of these observations are consistent with a vasoconstrictor action of 5-hydroxytryptamine. However, a number of studies performed in other conditions and other species indicate that the frequent absence of a monophasic pressor response to 5-hydroxytryptamine is due to important compensating mechanisms, to varying initial vascular tone, or to organ and species differences (see ref. 8). In the rat, e.g., the typical cardiovascular response to low doses of 5-hydroxytryptamine is triphasic (31): a transient small decrease in blood pressure, followed by a small increase above normal, and finally by a prolonged marked hypotension; the latter is the usual response when 5-hydroxytryptamine is infused. After pithing the animals or treating them with a ganglion blocker, 5-hydroxytryptamine causes only an increase in blood pressure (31). The vascular effects of 5-hydroxytryptamine exhibit marked regional differences as regards both the intensity and the type of response (21,23). Upon infusion of various doses of 5-hydroxytryptamine, skin vascular resistance of the innervated canine forelimb increases, whereas skeletal muscle vascular resistance either remains unchanged or decreases (21). In the dog, no increase in capillary permeability is observed with infusion of 5-hydroxytryptamine in marked contrast to the effect of histamine and to that of 5-hydroxytryptamine in other species, such as the rat.

When exogenous or endogenous 5-hydroxytryptamine causes predominant veno-constriction with reduced tissue blood flow, pronounced changes in organ function may follow. The changes can be complex in organs of which not only the vascular smooth muscle is sensitive to 5-hydroxytryptamine. In the lung, 5-hydroxytrypt-amine produces both vasoconstriction and bronchoconstriction (5). Relatively small doses of 5-hydroxytryptamine constrict the pulmonary precapillary vessels espe-cially; larger doses constrict the pulmonary veins as well (33). Other experiments with lung lobe preparations of the dog did not confirm a primary vascular action of 5-hydroxytryptamine. Intravenous administration of small amounts of 5-hydroxy-tryptamine causes a decrease in lobe volume without elevation of bronchial pressure or expulsion of fluid; this can be attributed to direct constriction of the bronchial and bronchiolar musculature, which compresses lung capillaries, thereby decreasing the pulmonary blood flow (29). The pharmacological action of 5-hydroxytryptamine on the bronchi of the dog, is rather weak generally (see ref. 8), particularly in comparison to the guinea pig which rapidly responds with dyspnea and convulsions to inhalation of 5-hydroxytryptamine (17).

In the gastrointestinal tract the effects of the amine are of great interest because of the presence of the enterochromaffin cells and the high sensitivity of the vascular beds as well as of gastric and small intestinal smooth muscle to 5-hydroxytryptamine (see ref. 35). Small doses of 5-hydroxytryptamine given by intravenous infusion stimulate intestinal motility of the dog and higher doses inhibit gastric acid secretion (16). Similarly, lysergic acid diethylamide (LSD), known at that time as a potent 5-hydroxytryptamine antagonist in various tests (4), markedly potentiated the stim-ulatory action of 5-hydroxytryptamine on the intestinal motility. Also in other respects, such as the pressor action in dogs, LSD exerted 5-hydroxytryptamine-like activities (32).

5-HYDROXYTRYPTAMINE ANTAGONISTS

Numerous isolated tissues are very sensitive to 5-hydroxytryptamine. Most of those generally are also sensitive to other agents, which offers the opportunity for *in vitro* study of the specificity of the blocking activity of a putative serotonergic antagonist (14). *In vivo* responses to 5-hydroxytryptamine are less easily reproducible, but at least the 5-hydroxytryptamine-induced paw-edema in the rat (30) is a simple test that has been used extensively to study serotonergic antagonists. The list of methods collected by Gyermek (14) includes 26 tests on isolated organs, 33 *in vivo* tests, and a great number of indirect methods. An impressive list of compounds which show 5-hydroxytryptamine antagonistic properties, therefore, is available (13,14,19,24). Several of these compounds are still used in experimental work, but only two, methysergide and cyproheptadine, are known as 5-hydroxytryptamine antagonists with established clinical applications (6). Cyproheptadine is used mainly in the treatment of allergic conditions, for which its primary histamine H_1 antagonistic properties probably are most relevant (6). Methysergide is used mainly in the prophylactic treatment of migraine but is also, as cyproheptadine, of some benefit in postgastrectomy dumping syndrome and in the intestinal hypermotility of carcinoid syndrome. The use in the two latter conditions can be linked to the role of 5-hydroxytryptamine, whereas a number of side-effects of methysergide may be due to its structural similarity to 5-hydroxytryptamine (6).

The two examples of clinically useful 5-hydroxytryptamine antagonists may indicate sufficiently that there is still much room for the development of compounds which specifically block 5-hydroxytryptamine-induced responses at low doses and do not have intrinsic 5-hydroxytryptamine-like actions at all. For a more final study of the role of 5-hydroxytryptamine in peripheral reactions they preferably should not cross the blood-brain barrier, to avoid the additional complications of interference with central serotonergic regulation.

REFERENCES

1. Battelli, F. (1905): Recherches sur les vaso-constrictines des sérums sanguins. *J. Physiol. Pathol. Gen.*, 7:625–638.
2. Benditt, E. P., Wong, R. L., Arase, M., and Roeper, E. (1955): 5-Hydroxytryptamine in mast cells. *Proc. Soc. Exp. Biol. Med.*, 90:303–304.
3. Bhattacharya, B. K., and Lewis, G. P. (1956): The release of 5-hydroxytryptamine by histamine liberators. *Br. J. Pharmacol.*, 11:202–208.
4. Cerletti, A., and Konzett, H. (1956): Spezifische Hemmung von 5-Oxytryptamin-Effekten durch Lysergsäurediäthylamid und ähnliche Körper. *Naunyn Schmiedebergs Arch. Pharmacol.*, 228:146–148.
5. Comroe, J. H., Van Lingen, B., Stroud, R. C., and Roncoroni, A. (1953): Reflex and direct cardiopulmonary effects of 5-HO-tryptamine (serotonin). *Am. J. Physiol.*, 173:379–389.
6. Douglas, W. W. (1980): Histamine and 5-hydroxytryptamine (serotonin) and their antagonists. In: *The Pharmacological Basis of Therapeutics*, 6th ed., edited by A. Goodman, L. S. Goodman, and A. Gilman, pp. 609–646. MacMillan, New York.
7. Erspamer, V. (1954): Pharmacology of indolealkylamines. *Pharmacol. Rev.*, 6:425–487.
8. Erspamer, V. (1966): Peripheral physiological and pharmacological actions of indolealkylamines. In: *Handbook of Experimental Pharmacology*, Vol. 19, edited by O. Eichler and A. Farah, pp. 245–359. Springer Verlag, Berlin.

9. Erspamer, V., and Asero, B. (1952): Identification of enteramine, the specific hormone of the enterochromaffin cell system as 5-hydroxytryptamine. *Nature*, 169:800–801.
10. Essman, W. B. (editor) (1977–1978): *Serotonin in Health and Disease*, Vol. 5. Spectrum, New York.
11. Freund, H. (1920): Ueber die pharmakologischen Wirkungen des defibrinierten Blutes. *Arch. Exp. Pathol. Pharmakol.*, 86:266–280.
12. Garattini, S., and Valzelli, L. (1965): *Serotonin*. Elsevier, Amsterdam.
13. Green, A. F., Garland, L. G., and Hodson, H. F. (1979): Antagonists of histamine, 5-hydroxytryptamine and SRS-A. In: *Handbook of Experimental Pharmacology*, Vol. 50/II, Anti-inflammatory drugs, edited by J. R. Vane and S. H. Ferreira, pp. 415–466. Springer-Verlag, Berlin.
14. Gyermek, L. (1966): Drugs which antagonize 5-hydroxytryptamine and related indolealkylamines. In: *Handbook of Experimental Pharmacology*, Vol. 19, edited by O. Eichler and A. Farah, pp. 471–528. Springer-Verlag, Berlin.
15. Hamlin, K. E., and Fischer, F. E. (1951): The synthesis of 5-hydroxytryptamine. *J. Am. Chem. Soc.*, 73:5007–5008.
16. Haverback, B. J., Hogben, C. A. M., Moran, N. C., and Terry, L. L. (1957): Effect of serotonin (5-hydroxytryptamine) and related compounds on gastric secretion and intestinal motility in the dog. *Gastroenterology*, 32:1058–1065.
17. Herxheimer, H. (1955): The 5-hydroxytryptamine shock in the guinea pig. *J. Physiol.*, 128:435–445.
18. Humphrey, J. H., and Toh, C. C. (1954): Absorption of serotonin (5-hydroxytryptamine) and histamine by dog platelets. *J. Physiol.*, 124:300–304.
19. Jacob, J. (1960): Les antagonistes des actions périphériques de la 5-hydroxytryptamine. Examples d'antagonismes. *Actual. Pharmacol.*, 13:131–160.
20. Ludwig, C., and Schmidt, A. (1868): Das Verhalten der Gase, welche mit dem Blut durch den Reissbaren säugetiermuskel Strömen. *Arb. a. d. Physiol. Anstalt Leipzig*, 3:12.
21. Merrill, G. F., Kline, R. L., Haddy, F. J., and Grega, G. J. (1974): Effects of locally infused serotonin on canine forelimb weight and segmental vascular resistances. *J. Pharmacol. Exp. Ther.*, 189:140–148.
22. O'Connor, J. M. (1912): Über den Adrenalingehalt des Blutes. *Arch. Exp. Pathol. Pharmakol.*, 67:195–232.
23. Page, I. H. (1957): Cardiovascular actions of serotonin (5-hydroxytryptamine). In: *5-Hydroxytryptamine*, edited by G. P. Lewis, pp. 93–108. Pergamon Press, London.
24. Page, I. H. (1958): Serotonin (5-hydroxytryptamine): The last four years. *Physiol. Rev.*, 38:277–335.
25. Pearse, A. G. E., Polak, J. M., Bloom, S. R., Adams, C., Dryburgh, J. R., and Brown, J. C. (1974): Enterochromaffin cells of the mammalian small intestine as the source of motilin. *Virchows Arch. (Cell Pathol.)*, 16:111–120.
26. Rapport, M. M. (1949): Serum vasoconstrictor (serotonin). V. The presence of creatinine in the complex. A proposed structure of the vasoconstrictor principle. *J. Biol. Chem.*, 180:961–969.
27. Rapport, M. M., Green, A. A., and Page, I. H. (1948): Crystalline serotonin. *Science*, 108:329–330.
28. Reid, G., and Rand, M. (1952): Pharmacological actions of synthetic 5-hydroxytryptamine (serotonin, thrombocytin). *Nature*, 169:800–801.
29. Rodbard, S., and Kira, S. (1972): Lobar, airway, and pulmonary vascular effects of serotonin. *Angiology*, 23:188–197.
30. Rowley, D. A., and Benditt, E. P. (1956): 5-Hydroxytryptamine and histamine as mediators of vascular injury produced by agents which damage mast cells in rats. *J. Exp. Med.*, 103:399–411.
31. Salmoiraghi, G. C., Page, I. H., and McCubbin, J. W. (1956): Cardiovascular and respiratory response to intravenous serotonin in rats. *J. Pharmacol.*, 118:477–481.
32. Shaw, E., and Woolley, D. W. (1956): Some serotonin-like activates of lysergic acid diethylamide. *Science*, 124:121–122.
33. Shepherd, J. J., Donald, D. E., Linder, R., and Swan, H. J. C. (1959): Effect of small doses of 5-hydroxytryptamine (serotonin) on pulmonary circulation in the closed-chest dog. *Am. J. Physiol.*, 197:963–967.
34. Thomas, D. P., and Vane, J. R. (1967): 5-Hydroxytryptamine in the circulation of the dog. *Nature*, 216:335–338.
35. Thompson, J. H. (1971): Serotonin and the alimentary tract. *Res. Commun. Chem. Pathol. Pharmacol.*, 2:687–781.

5-Hydroxytryptamine in Peripheral Reactions,
edited by Fred De Clerck and Paul M.
Vanhoutte. Raven Press, New York © 1982.

Serotonergic Amplification Mechanisms in Vascular Tissues

J. M. Van Nueten

*Department of Pharmacology, Janssen Pharmaceutica Research Laboratories,
B-2340 Beerse, Belgium*

The physiological role of 5-hydroxytryptamine has been a matter of debate for several decades (11,12,16). Levels of endogenous 5-hydroxytryptamine may be important in interfering with physiological functions and may induce some pathological events, for instance, when the release of the amine from platelets aggregating at endothelial lesions is exaggerated (ref. 20; P. M. Vanhoutte, *this volume*).

DIRECT EFFECTS OF 5-HYDROXYTRYPTAMINE

5-Hydroxytryptamine displays complex properties on vascular tissues, producing constriction in some blood vessels (e.g., venules) while dilating others (e.g., arterioles). Thus, in a given vascular bed, the net effect of 5-hydroxytryptamine is determined by the balance between these actions. This is illustrated when studying the response of a perfused vascular bed to the amine. Figure 1 shows that the vasoconstrictor effect of 5-hydroxytryptamine on the arterially perfused stomach of the guinea pig is inhibited in a dose-dependent way by ketanserin, a novel 5-HT$_2$ receptor antagonist (20). Abolition of the vasoconstrictor effect by the highest doses of the antagonist unmasked a dilator response to 5-hydroxytryptamine (P. M. Vanhoutte, *this volume*).

INDIRECT (AMPLIFYING) EFFECTS OF 5-HYDROXYTRYPTAMINE

The action of 5-hydroxytryptamine on blood vessels is even more complex, in that it also displays indirect effects. At the beginning of this century (1,2) the effect of combining drugs had already been described by Bürgi (1): "In combining drugs with the same end-effect, the resulting activity is additive, when the sites of action of the component are identical, and superadditive if these sites are different." The latter activity has been called potentiation. This term is also used for the enhancement seen with uptake inhibitors or with enzymatic degradation inhibitors. Since the indirect superadditive effect of 5-hydroxytryptamine is not due to inhibition of the disposition of norepinephrine, the name "amplifying effect" seems more appropriate than "potentiation."

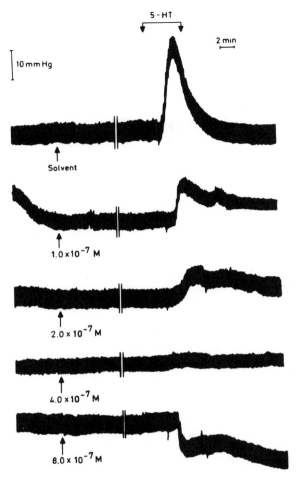

FIG. 1. Perfusion pressure recording in the isolated arterially perfused stomach of the guinea pig. Effect of infusion of 5-hydroxytryptamine (5-HT: 1.25×10^{-8} g/5 min) in control solution (solvent) and in the presence of increasing concentrations *(arrows)* of ketanserin (R 41 468). Ketanserin caused a dose-dependent depression of the vasoconstrictor response. The abolition by ketanserin (8×10^{-7} M) of the vasoconstrictor responses to 5-HT unmasked a dilator response to the amine. (Data from ref. 19, with permission.)

Earlier observations have shown the interaction between 5-hydroxytryptamine and other vasoactive substances, such as epinephrine, norepinephrine, vasopressin, histamine, and angiotensin II on vascular and nonvascular tissues. For example, in the intact organism (e.g., in rats), 5-hydroxytryptamine amplified blood pressure increase induced by epinephrine (15). The amplifying effects of 5-hydroxytryptamine in isolated blood vessels have been studied in detail by de la Lande et al. (6,7) who showed that 5-hydroxytryptamine markedly enhanced the vasoconstrictor effects of norepinephrine. Similar results have been obtained in the human (17), where the norepinephrine-induced decrease in forearm blood flow is enhanced by virtually inactive doses of 5-hydroxytryptamine (Fig. 2).

INHIBITION BY KETANSERIN OF THE AMPLIFYING EFFECTS OF 5-HYDROXYTRYPTAMINE

Since ketanserin is devoid of agonistic effect, in contrast with a number of other serotonergic antagonists (20), it will not produce additive effects as shown with partial agonists (8,9) and, thus, is an appropriate tool to study the amplifying effects of 5-hydroxytryptamine.

In a study on isolated rat caudal artery strips (20), the arteries were made to contract alternatively every 10 min with low concentrations of 5-hydroxytryptamine or, after a washout period, with norepinephrine. Then the same concentration of 5-hydroxytryptamine was introduced followed, without washout, by norepinephrine at a lower concentration so that the total molarity of monoamines equalled that when norepinephrine alone was given the first time. The further contraction caused by norepinephrine in presence of 5-hydroxytryptamine was larger than that obtained before, which suggests that not an additive, but an amplifying effect is involved. This effect is reproducible and is inhibited by ketanserin at concentrations which antagonize the direct effect of 5-hydroxytryptamine but not the contractile response to norepinephrine (Fig. 3). 5-Hydroxytryptamine also amplifies the contractile responses of blood vessels obtained with a variety of other nonadrenergic vasoconstrictor agonists (3,10,13,14). Ketanserin antagonized the amplifying effect of 5-hydroxytryptamine on the contractions of various blood vessels in response to nonadrenergic substances such as angiotensin II, histamine, and prostaglandins (Fig. 4) (18). These findings suggest that the amplifying effects of 5-hydroxytryptamine on vascular tissues are linked to its interaction with $5-HT_2$ receptors in these tissues.

Ketanserin reduces arterial blood pressure in spontaneously hypertensive rats (19) and in hypertensive patients (5). Since norepinephrine- and angiotensin II-induced constriction of the arterioles can be an important factor in blood pressure regulation, inhibition by ketanserin of the amplifying effects of 5-hydroxytryptamine on vascular responses to these neurohumoral mediators may explain, in part, the antihypertensive properties of the compound. This might be particularly important if

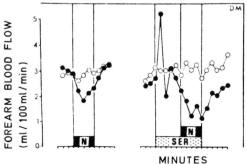

FIG. 2. The effect of intraarterial norepinephrine (N = 50 ng/min for 4 min) on human forearm blood flow (*solid circle* = infused forearm; *open circle* = control forearm) when given by itself *(left)* and then during the last 4 min of a 9-min intraarterial infusion of 5-hydroxytryptamine (SER = 500 ng/min, *right*). 5-Hydroxytryptamine augmented the vasoconstrictor effect of norepinephrine. (Data from ref. 17, with permission.)

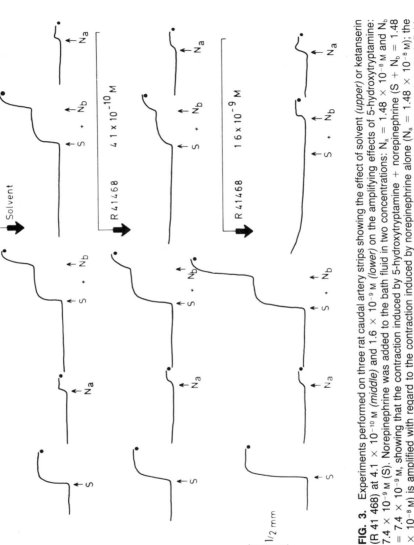

FIG. 3. Experiments performed on three rat caudal artery strips showing the effect of solvent *(upper)* or ketanserin (R 41 468) at 4.1×10^{-10} M *(middle)* and 1.6×10^{-9} M *(lower)* on the amplifying effects of 5-hydroxytryptamine: 7.4×10^{-9} M (S). Norepinephrine was added to the bath fluid in two concentrations: $N_a = 1.48 \times 10^{-8}$ M and $N_b = 7.4 \times 10^{-9}$ M (S), showing that the contraction induced by 5-hydroxytryptamine + norepinephrine (S + $N_b = 1.48 \times 10^{-8}$ M) is amplified with regard to the contraction induced by norepinephrine alone ($N_a = 1.48 \times 10^{-8}$ M); the total molar concentration of the agonists being equal in both cases. ● = washing by replacement of the bath fluid. Ketanserin in concentrations which did not affect the contractile responses to norepinephrine, abolished the amplifying effect of 5-hydroxytryptamine on alpha-adrenergic activation. (Data from ref. 19, with permission.)

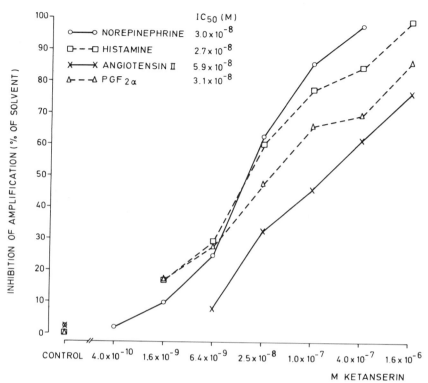

FIG. 4. Experiments performed on the rabbit femoral artery showing the effect of ketanserin on the amplifying effect of 5-hydroxytryptamine on contraction induced by norepinephrine (1.8 × 10^{-9} M), histamine (2.2 × 10^{-7} M), angiotensin II (1.5 × 10^{-10} M), and prostaglandin $F_{2\alpha}$ (4.5 × 10^{-7} M). Ketanserin inhibited in a similar dose-related way the amplifying effects of 5-hydroxy-tryptamine on alpha-adrenergic and nonadrenergic activities.

the levels of 5-hydroxytryptamine in the vicinity of the vascular smooth muscle cells are augmented in the hypertensive blood vessel wall (18).

CONCLUSIONS

Although the role of 5-hydroxytryptamine in blood flow regulation is still debated, endogenously released 5-hydroxytryptamine may interfere with the normal functions of the vascular wall and of the blood platelets. Stimulation of serotonergic receptors may initiate a chain of events that culminate in important responses; the strong amplifying property of 5-hydroxytryptamine makes it likely that it contributes, by exaggerating the constrictor effects of other neurohumoral mediators, to abnormal tissue responses. The availability of selective 5-HT$_2$ serotonergic antagonists without agonistic properties, such as ketanserin, provides a tool for further investigation of this potential role of 5-hydroxytryptamine. Thus, the therapeutic effects of low doses of ketanserin could be related to the inhibition of the amplifying effects of

5-hydroxytryptamine; the latter may be of particular importance since the concentrations of 5-hydroxytryptamine which cause amplification correspond to the concentrations of the monoamine, or its metabolites, found in human plasma (4).

REFERENCES

1. Bürgi, E. (1912a): Über wirkungspotenzierende Momente in Arzneigemischen. *Med. Klin.*, 50:2037–2040.
2. Bürgi, E. (1912b): Über wirkungspotenzierende Momente in Arzneigemischen. *Med. Klin.*, 51:2073–2075.
3. Bevan, J. A., Duckles, S. P., and Lee, T. J.-F. (1975): Histamine potentiation of nerve- and drug-induced responses of a rabbit cerebral artery. *Circ. Res.*, 36:647–653.
4. Crawford, N. (1963): Plasma-free serotonin (5-hydroxytryptamine). *Clin. Chim. Acta*, 8:39–45.
5. De Cree, J., Leempoels, J., De Cock, W., Geukens, H., and Verhaegen, H. (1981): The antihypertensive effects of a pure and selective serotonin-receptor blocking agent (R 41 468) in elderly patients. *Angiology*, 32:137–144.
6. de la Lande, I. S., Cannell, V. A., and Waterson, J. G. (1966): The interaction of serotonin and noradrenaline on the perfused artery. *Br. J. Pharm. Pharmacol.*, 28:255–272.
7. de la Lande, I. S., Frewin, D., Waterson, J., and Cannell, V. (1967): Factors influencing supersensitivity to noradrenaline in the isolated perfused artery, comparative effects of cocaine, denervation, and serotonin. *Circ. Res.*, 20(Suppl. III):177–189.
8. Edvinsson, L., Hardebo, J. E., and Owman, C. (1978): Pharmacological analysis of 5-hydroxytryptamine receptors in isolated intracranial and extracranial vessels of cat and man. *Circ. Res.*, 42:143–151.
9. Fozard, J. R. (1973): Drug interactions on an isolated artery. In: *Background to Migraine*, edited by J. N. Cumings, pp. 150–169. William Heinemann, London.
10. Fozard, J. R. (1977): The mechanism by which migraine prophylactic drugs modify vascular reactivity *in vitro*. In: *Headache: New Vistas*, pp. 259–278. Biomedical Press, Florence, Italy.
11. Gaddum, J. H., and Picarelli, Z. P. (1957): Two kinds of tryptamine receptors. *Br. J. Pharmacol.*, 12:323–328.
12. Gyermek, L. (1961): 5-Hydroxytryptamine antagonists. *Pharmacol. Rev.*, 13:399–439.
13. Hurwitz, R., Campbell, R. W., Gordon, P., and Haddy, F. J. (1961): Interaction of serotonin with vasoconstrictor agents in the vascular bed of the denervated dog forelimb. *J. Pharmacol. Exp. Ther.*, 133:57–62.
14. Khairallah, P. A., Page, I. H., and Turker, R. K. (1967): Some properties of prostaglandin E action on muscle. *Arch. Int. Pharmacodyn. Ther.*, 169:328–341.
15. Lecomte, J. (1953): Sensibilisation à l'adrénaline par la 5-hydroxytryptamine. *Arch. Int. Physiol.*, 61:84–85.
16. Page, I. H. (1958): Cardiovascular actions of serotonin (5-hydroxytryptamine). In: *5-Hydroxytryptamine*, edited by G. P. Lewis, pp. 93–108. Pergamon Press, London.
17. Scroop, G. C., and Walsh, J. A. (1968): Interactions between angiotensin, noradrenaline and serotonin on the peripheral blood vessels in man. *Aust. J. Exp. Biol. Med. Sci.*, 46:573–580.
18. Van Nueten, J. M., Janssen, P. A. J., De Ridder, W., and Vanhoutte, P. M. (1982): Interaction between 5-hydroxytryptamine and other vasoconstrictor substances in the isolated femoral artery of the rabbit; Effect of ketanserin (R 41 468). *Eur. J. Pharmacol.*, 77:281–287.
19. Van Nueten, J. M., Janssen, P. A. J., Van Beek, J., Xhonneux, R., Verbeuren, T. J., and Vanhoutte, P. M. (1981): Vascular effects of ketanserin (R 41 468), a novel antagonist of 5-HT$_2$ serotonergic receptors. *J. Pharmacol. Exp. Ther.*, 218:217–230.
20. Van Nueten, J. M., and Vanhoutte, P. M. (1981): Selectivity of calcium-antagonism and serotonin-antagonism with respect to venous and arterial tissues. *Angiology*, 32:476–484.

5-Hydroxytryptamine in Peripheral Reactions, edited by Fred De Clerck and Paul M. Vanhoutte. Raven Press, New York © 1982.

Serotonergic Amplification Mechanisms in Blood Platelets

*F. De Clerck, **J. L. David, and *P. A. J. Janssen

*Janssen Pharmaceutica Research Laboratories, B-2340 Beerse, Belgium; and **Hôpital de Bavière, Université de Liège, B-4200 Liège, Belgium

5-Hydroxytryptamine activates platelets of various mammalian species including man (14). In contrast to cat, pig, and sheep platelets, human platelets of most normal individuals respond to 5-hydroxytryptamine with a shape change and only a weak, reversible aggregation (2,7). However, depending upon the concentration and the time interval between its addition and that of another agonist, 5-hydroxytryptamine amplifies the human platelet aggregation induced by adenosine-5'-diphosphate (ADP), collagen, epinephrine, or norepinephrine (1,2); moreover, when platelets first are sensitized with norepinephrine or lysolecithin, 5-hydroxytryptamine itself induces irreversible aggregation (1,4).

Platelet activation by 5-hydroxytryptamine is inhibited by numerous compounds of various chemical classes (14); in receptor binding studies on brain tissue most of these serotonergic antagonists bind to both 5-HT$_1$ and 5-HT$_2$ receptors (23); therefore conclusions about the type of 5-hydroxytryptamine receptor involved in platelet activation, on the basis of pharmacological dissection, are difficult to draw. In an attempt to clarify the involvement of the type of 5-hydroxytryptamine receptor in the complex sequence of induction-transmission-extrusion reactions of platelet activation, we applied the selective 5-HT$_2$ receptor antagonist ketanserin (23) to platelet function studies.

METHODS

Blood Sampling and Preparation of Platelet-Rich Plasma

The collection of human and rat citrated venous blood (Na$_3$-citrate 2H$_2$O, pH 7.35, 0.313%), the preparation of platelet-rich plasma and of platelet-poor plasma by centrifugation was performed as previously described (12,13). Platelet number was adapted to 350,000/µl in human platelet-rich plasma, and to 500,000/µl in rat platelet-rich plasma by appropriate dilution with autologous platelet-poor plasma. Plasma samples were gassed with a mixture of 5% CO$_2$-95% O$_2$ (30) and were stored at room temperature (20–22°C) in sealed plastic tubes.

Platelet Aggregation

The turbidimetric measurement of platelet aggregation was performed as previously described (12) using a Chronolog-Dual Channel Aggregometer. The rate and extent of aggregation were assessed by measuring the slopes (mm/2 min) and the maxima of turbidity tracings (mm) (15), 100% T corresponding to 250 mm.

Release of β-Thromboglobulin and Platelet-Factor-4

After 5 min of aggregation, 0.1 ml of a release-inhibiting cocktail containing ethyldiaminetetraacetate (EDTA) 0.03%, adenosine 1 mM, and prostaglandin E_1 (PGE_1) 1 μM in acid-citrate-dextrose (ACD) was added to 0.5 ml of the reaction mixture containing human platelet-rich plasma. The sample was immediately cooled on ice, and was centrifuged (10,000 g × 5 min) to platelet-free plasma. Platelet-free plasma was kept frozen at −25°C until testing. Total release was induced by freezing and thawing twice appropriate platelet-rich plasma samples. The levels of β-thromboglobulin and platelet-factor-4 in platelet-free plasma were assayed by radioimmunoassay (10). Results are expressed as ng/ml of plasma.

Production of Thromboxane B_2

After 5 min of aggregation, 0.1 ml of a prostaglandin biosynthesis-inhibiting cocktail containing EDTA 0.7% and suprofen 5 × 10^{-5} M in NaCl 0.15 M was added to 0.5 ml of the reaction mixture containing human platelet-rich plasma. Thereafter platelet-free plasma was prepared as for the estimation of β-thromboglobulin and platelet-factor-4. The amount of thromboxane B_2 generated was assayed by a radioimmunoassay, using a thromboxane B_2 [^{3}H] radioimmunoassay kit (New England Nuclear). Results are expressed as pg/0.1 ml of plasma.

Uptake of [^{14}C]5-Hydroxytryptamine by Human Platelets

The determination of the active uptake of [^{14}C]5-hydroxytryptamine (The Radiochemical Centre, Amersham) by human platelets in plasma or buffer solutions was performed as previously described (11). In order to assess possible compound-induced release of [^{14}C]5-hydroxytryptamine, the uptake of the monoamine (1.72 × 10^{-7}M) by human platelet-rich plasma was allowed to proceed for 60 min at 37°C before the addition of the compound. Platelet-bound radioactivity was assessed after a further incubation of 10 min (11).

Retraction of Platelet-Rich Plasma Clots

Retraction of rat platelet-rich plasma clots was evaluated using thromboelastography (T.E.G. Digital 501, Probio DMS) (8). In the cups, 0.02 ml of platelet-rich plasma (500,000 platelets/μl), 0.05 ml of tris-hydroxymethylamino methane (Tris) 0.1 M pH 7.35 and 1 to 10 μl of solvent or compound solution were pre-warmed for 5 min at 37°C before the addition of 0.05 ml of $CaCl_2$ 0.05 M and of 0.05 ml of thrombin (Topostasine®, Roche) 2 N.I.H. U/ml.

Malondialdehyde Formation by Human Platelets

Malondialdehyde formation by human platelets stimulated with thrombin 20 N.I.H. U/ml, as an indicator for prostaglandin biosynthesis, was evaluated spectrofluorimetrically using a modification of the method of McMillan (26). Results are expressed as nM malondialdehyde/2 × 10^8 platelets/30 min.

Statistical Analysis

The data are expressed as means ± SEM derived from n-experiments as indicated. Statistical evaluation of the results was performed using the Student's t-test. P-values smaller or equal to 0.05 were considered as being significant. The concentration causing 50% inhibition of the original response (IC_{50}) was determined by probit analysis (17).

RESULTS

5-Hydroxytryptamine-Induced Platelet Aggregation

In vitro, ketanserin inhibits in a concentration-dependent way the reversible aggregation induced by 5-hydroxytryptamine in human platelet-rich plasma, the compound being equipotent to cyproheptadine. Methysergide is less active than ketanserin and cyproheptadine (Fig. 1).

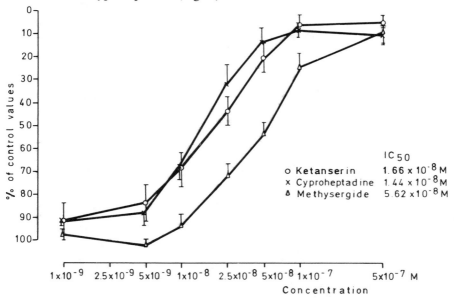

FIG. 1. Concentration-dependent inhibition (and IC_{50}-values) of 5-hydroxytryptamine-induced human platelet aggregation by ketanserin (R 41 468), cyproheptadine, and methysergide *in vitro*. Mean ± SEM (n = 3 to 7) percent inhibition of slopes of aggregation versus solvent values.

The oral administration of 40 mg of ketanserin to 5 volunteers produces complete inhibition of 5-hydroxytryptamine-induced platelet aggregation in platelet-rich plasma obtained 2.30 hr after medication; ADP-induced platelet aggregation is not significantly affected (Table 1).

Amplification of Human Platelet Aggregation by 5-Hydroxytryptamine

When added to stirred human platelet-rich plasma, 3 sec beforehand, 5-hydroxytryptamine amplifies the platelet aggregation induced by threshold concentrations of collagen, ADP, epinephrine, or norepinephrine. The monoamine exerts this effect from concentrations of 1×10^{-7} M on up to 1×10^{-5} M, maximal amplification being reached from 1×10^{-6} M on. As shown for the combination of 5-hydroxytryptamine with ADP (Fig. 2) or with collagen, the maximal extent of aggregation is more enhanced than the rate of the reaction. At a constant concentration, 5-hydroxytryptamine amplifies the platelet response to various concentrations of the other agonists, e.g., collagen; the amplification effect is more pronounced on responses induced by a threshold concentration of collagen than in those due to a strongly aggregating concentration of the agonist.

In vitro, ketanserin inhibits the serotonergic amplification of platelet aggregation induced by collagen (Fig. 3), ADP, epinephrine, or norepinephrine. As shown for the aggregation induced by combined 5-hydroxytryptamine and collagen challenge, the compound reduces in a concentration-dependent way the amplified platelet response to the level of the reaction to the potentiated agonist alone (Fig. 4). In contrast to ketanserin, the inhibition of prostaglandin synthesis with suprofen at 1×10^{-4} M reduces the serotonergic amplification of collagen-induced but not of ADP-induced platelet aggregation.

TABLE 1. *Effect of oral treatment with ketanserin on human platelet aggregation induced by 5-hydroxytryptamine (5-HT), ADP, or the combination 5-HT/ADP*

Volunteer[b]	Human platelet aggregation[a]					
	Before			After[c]		
	5-HT[d]	ADP[e]	5-HT + ADP	5-HT	ADP	5-HT + ADP
J.B.	13	48	74	0	46	55
J.S.	5	30	105	0	25	47
E.D.	5	44	81	0	45	55
J.C.	10	41	75	0	47	65
H.S.	7	30	78	0	23	60
	8 ± 1.5^{f}	38.6 ± 3.6^{f}	82.6 ± 5.7^{f}	$0^{f,g}$	37.2 ± 5.4^{f}	$56.4 \pm 2.9^{f,g}$

[a]Maximum of aggregation in mm (250 mm = 100% T).
[b]Fasting volunteers treated orally with 40 mg of ketanserin.
[c]Blood sampled 2.30 hr post medication.
[d]5-Hydroxytryptamine 2×10^{-6} M.
[e]ADP 5×10^{-7} M.
[f]Mean ± SEM.
[g]$P < 0.05$ versus before (Student t-test).

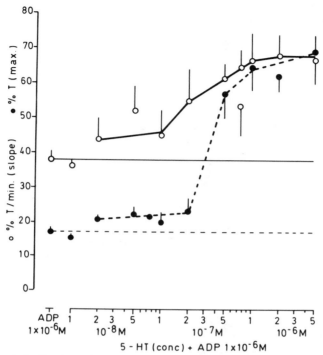

FIG. 2. Concentration-dependent amplification by 5-hydroxytryptamine (5-HT) of human platelet aggregation induced by ADP (1×10^{-6} M). *Solid circle:* maxima of aggregation (% T); *open circle:* slopes of aggregation (% T/min). Mean $\pm$ SEM of 3 to 5 experiments.

After oral administration of 40 mg of ketanserin to human volunteers both the 5-hydroxytryptamine-induced and the amplified response to ADP are inhibited without effect on that to ADP alone (Table 1). When human platelets are presensitized by incubation with a nonaggregating concentration of a partial thromboplastin reagent (Thrombofax®, Ortho Pharmaceutica), the subsequent addition of 5-hydroxytryptamine induces aggregation, the intensity and profile of which depends upon the concentration of the monoamine (Fig. 5). Ketanserin at 1×10^{-7} M abolishes the 5-hydroxytryptamine-induced irreversible aggregation of presensitized platelets.

Release and/or Synthesis of Platelet-Specific Proteins and of Thromboxane B_2

Low concentrations of collagen and of 5-hydroxytryptamine produced a weak aggregation reaction and do not induce the release of platelet-specific proteins exceeding the platelet-rich plasma-baseline values. When combined, they produced a marked release of β-thromboglobulin and platelet-factor-4 in proportion to the extent of aggregation. In these conditions ketanserin at 1×10^{-7} M reduces both the extent of the amplified aggregation reaction and of the release markers to the levels obtained with collagen alone (Table 2).

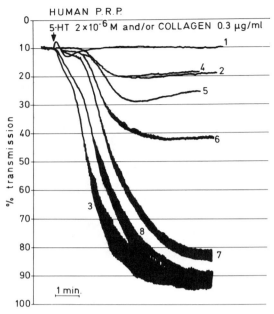

FIG. 3. Inhibition by ketanserin (R 41 468) of the amplification by 5-hydroxytryptamine (2 × 10⁻⁶ M) of human platelet aggregation induced by threshold concentrations of collagen 0.3 µg/ml. Superimposed tracing obtained on the same platelet-rich plasma (P.R.P.). Meaning of numbers: 1. 5-hydroxytryptamine (5-HT); 2. collagen (coll.); 3. 5-HT + coll.; 4. 5-HT + coll. + ketanserin 5 × 10⁻⁷ M; 5. 5-HT + coll. + ketanserin 1 × 10⁻⁷ M; 6. 5-HT + coll. + ketanserin 7.5 × 10⁻⁸ M; 7. 5-HT + coll. + ketanserin 5 × 10⁻⁸ M; 8. 5-HT + coll. + ketanserin 1 × 10⁻⁸ M.

In contrast to β-thromboglobulin and platelet-factor-4, thromboxane B_2 is produced in substantial amounts by threshold concentrations of collagen producing a weak aggregation reaction only. 5-Hydroxytryptamine has no such effect. However, amplification by the monoamine of the aggregation reaction to collagen results in a two-fold increase of thromboxane B_2 synthesis. Ketanserin at 1×10^{-7} M reduces the extent of prostaglandin biosynthesis to that obtained with collagen alone (Table 3).

Uptake of [¹⁴C]5-Hydroxytryptamine by Human Platelets

In contrast to imipramine, ketanserin up to 5×10^{-6} M does not affect the initial velocity nor the maximal extent of the uptake of [¹⁴C]5-hydroxytryptamine, at concentrations of 1.72, 0.86, or 0.43 $\times$ 10⁻⁷ M during 10 sec to 5 min by human platelets suspended in plasma or buffer solutions. At concentrations exceeding 5×10^{-6} M, ketanserin, in a concentration-dependent way, reduces the initial velocity (10, 20, 30, 60 sec) but not the maximal extent (5 min) of [¹⁴C]5-hydroxytryptamine uptake by human platelets in platelet-rich plasma (Table 4). The addition of ketanserin, 1×10^{-4} M, to platelets in platelet-rich plasma, prelabeled with

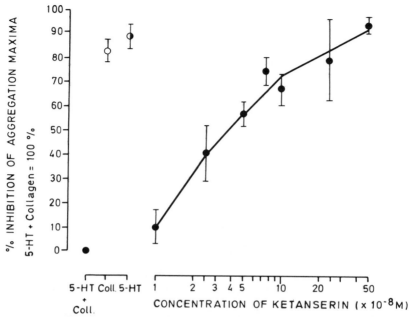

FIG. 4. Concentration-dependent inhibition by ketanserin (R 41 468) of the amplification by 5-hydroxytryptamine (2×10^{-6} M) of human platelet aggregation induced by collagen (0.75 µg/ml). Mean ± SEM ($n = 3$ to 6) percent inhibition on the maxima of aggregation versus the combination 5-hydroxytryptamine (5-HT) + collagen *(coll.)*.

[^{14}C]5-hydroxytryptamine, does not induce loss of cell-bound radioactivity during an additional incubation period of 10 min at 37°C.

General Platelet Function Tests

Ketanserin at 1×10^{-4} M does not affect human platelet aggregation induced by ADP 1 to 5×10^{-6} M, collagen 0.3 to 2 µg/ml, nor the maximal extent of aggregation induced by epinephrine 1×10^{-5} M, or Thrombofax® 10 to 20% V/V. The slight reduction of the rate of aggregation of epinephrine- or Thrombofax®-induced aggregation and of the second phase of ADP-induced aggregation is lost on reduction of the concentration of ketanserin from 1×10^{-4} M to 5×10^{-6} M. At concentrations of 1×10^{-5} M and 1×10^{-4} M, respectively, ketanserin does not affect the production of malondialdehyde from thrombin-stimulated platelets nor the thromboelastographic behavior of rat platelet-rich plasma coagulated with thrombin.

DISCUSSION

Our present results show that ketanserin, a selective 5-HT$_2$ receptor antagonist as characterized in receptor-binding studies in brain tissues (23), inhibits in a

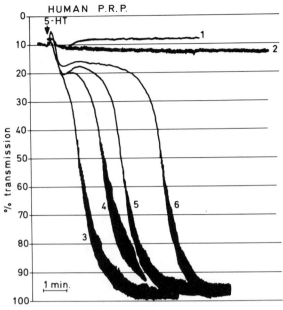

FIG. 5. Concentration-dependent aggregation by 5-hydroxytryptamine (5-HT) of human plate-lets presensitized with Thrombofax® (10 % V/V). Superimposed tracings obtained on the same platelet-rich plasma. Meaning of numbers: 1. 5-HT 2×10^{-6} M; 2. Thrombofax 10%; 3. Thrombofax + 5-HT 5×10^{-6} M; 4. Thrombofax + 5-HT 2×10^{-6} M; 5. Thrombofax + 5-HT 1×10^{-6} M; 6. Thrombofax + 5-HT 5×10^{-7} M.

TABLE 2. *Inhibition by ketanserin of the human platelet release reaction induced by serotonergic (5-HT) amplification of collagen-stimulated aggregation in platelet-rich plasma (P.R.P)*

Treatment	Parameter[a]		
	Aggregation[b]	PF-4[c]	β-TG[c]
P.R.P. base line	0	149.5 ± 9.2	251 ± 61.8
Collagen 2 μg/ml	213 ± 16.1	629 ± 71	>500 (1,506)[d]
Collagen 0.5–1 μg/ml	9 ± 5.6	134.1 ± 14.8	278 ± 26.9
5-HT 2×10^{-6} M + collagen 0.5–1 μg/ml	195 ± 11.5	587.5 ± 46.8	>500 (1,051.7)[d]
Ketanserin 1×10^{-7} M + 5-HT + collagen	7.5 ± 4.3	186.2 ± 21.6	348 ± 93.4

[a]Mean ± SEM of 2 to 4 experiments.
[b]Maximum of aggregation in mm.
[c]Platelet proteins, in ng/ml, released in 5 min. PF-4 = platelet-factor-4; β-TG = β-thromboglobulin.
[d]Extrapolated values; maximal capacity of the radioimmunoassay = 500 ng/ml.

TABLE 3. *Inhibition by ketanserin of the human platelet thromboxane B_2 production induced by serotonergic (5-HT) amplification of collagen-stimulated aggregation in platelet-rich plasma (P.R.P.)*

| Treatment | Parameter[a] | |
	Aggregation[b]	TXB$_2$[c]
P.R.P. base line	0	80 ± 30
Thrombin 20 U/ml	—	>12,500
Collagen 2 μg/ml	183.5 ± 13.5	4,500
Collagen 0.5 μg/ml	10.5 ± 1.5	1,750
5-HT 2 × 10^{-6} M	6.1 ± 0.09	48.5 ± 3.5
5-HT 2 × 10^{-6} M + collagen 0.5 μg/ml	134.2 ± 11.3	3,050 ± 263
Ketanserin 1 × 10^{-7} M + 5-HT + collagen	27.6 ± 6.7	2,066 ± 235

[a]Mean ± SEM of 2 to 4 experiments.
[b]Maximum of aggregation in mm.
[c]Thromboxane B_2 in pg/0.1 ml, released in 5 min.

TABLE 4. *Effect of various compounds on the active uptake of 5-hydroxytryptamine by human platelets in plasma*

Compounds[a]	Inhibition of serotonin uptake (IC$_{50}$)[b]
Ketanserin	>10^{-4} M
Cyproheptadine	>10^{-4} M
Methysergide	>10^{-4} M
Imipramine	2 × 10^{-8} M (2.59–1.55 × 10^{-8} M)

[a]Compounds preincubated for 5 min at 37°C with platelet-rich plasma containing 350,000 platelets/μl ($n = 4$).
[b]IC$_{50}$ and 95% confidence limits versus solvent for the uptake of [^{14}C]5-hydroxytryptamine at 1.72 × 10^{-7} M for 5 min at 37°C.

concentration-dependent way the activation of human platelets induced and amplified by 5-hydroxytryptamine both *in vitro* and *ex vivo* after oral administration to volunteers. At concentrations up to 500 times in excess of the IC$_{50}$ for 5-hydroxytryptamine-induced reactions, ketanserin does not affect the human platelet aggregation induced by ADP, epinephrine, collagen, or Thrombofax®, the prostaglandin biosynthesis of thrombin-stimulated human platelets nor the contractile capacity of rat platelet-rich plasma clots formed with thrombin. In contrast to imipramine, the initial velocity and the saturation of active uptake of 5-hydroxytryptamine by human platelets suspended in plasma or buffer are not affected by ketanserin at concentrations below 5 × 10^{-6} M.

Since the consequences of receptor-agonist interaction leading to the typical platelet response are similar to some extent for various agonists (20,22,24), the present evidence strongly suggests a specific interaction of ketanserin with serotonergic receptors on the platelet rather than an effect on later biochemical pathways involved in platelet activation.

Previously, it was assumed that platelet receptors for 5-hydroxytryptamine resemble the pharmacologically defined D-receptors described in intestinal smooth muscles (21,27); indeed, sheep platelet aggregation induced by 5-hydroxytryptamine is selectively inhibited by lysergic acid diethylamide (LSD) and by phenoxybenzamine, but not by morphine or cocaine, and only weakly by atropine (27). Recently receptors for 5-hydroxytryptamine have been reclassified into 5-HT$_1$, labeled with [^{3}H]5-hydroxytryptamine in rat brain tissues and 5-HT$_2$, labeled with [^{3}H]spiperone in the frontal cortex in receptor binding studies (23,31); these receptors are different from the pharmacological D- and M-types since morphine is inactive in both 5-HT$_1$- and 5-HT$_2$-receptor binding models and phenoxybenzamine is only weakly active (23). Baumgartner (2,3) formulated the hypothesis that 5-hydroxytryptamine would activate human platelets by combining with membrane receptors identical to those involved in the active uptake of the monoamine. Platelet shape changes and/or aggregation induced by 5-hydroxytryptamine are inhibited by numerous compounds from various chemical classes including ergot alkaloids and derivatives, cyproheptadine, mianserin, cinanserin, the adrenolytic compound phenoxybenzamine, neuroleptics like spiperone, metitepine, chlorpromazine, butaclamol, and tricyclic antidepressants (11). In receptor binding studies all previously studied serotonergic antagonists behave as mixed 5-HT$_1$- and 5-HT$_2$-receptor ligands (23) making definite conclusions about the type of 5-hydroxytryptamine receptor involved in human platelet function difficult. Our present findings of potent and selective inhibition of 5-hydroxytryptamine-induced and -amplified human and cat platelet reactions by ketanserin suggest the presence of functional 5-HT$_2$-receptor on the platelet; in addition to other evidence (6,28,29) our results show that these functional receptors are different from those involved in the uptake of the monoamine since ketanserin at concentrations which block its effect does not reduce the active uptake of 5-hydroxytryptamine by human platelets.

In human platelet-rich plasma, 5-hydroxytryptamine induces the platelet shape change and a weak reversible aggregation only; irreversible aggregation occurs in a limited number of individuals and in patients treated with chlorpromazine (4,7,35). However, the monoamine largely amplifies the human platelet aggregation response to various agonists including ADP, epinephrine, norepinephrine, and collagen and induces itself strong aggregation of human platelets, sensitized with norepinephrine or lysolecithin (1–4,28). Similar amplification effects have been observed on platelets from the rat, guinea pig, rabbit, cat, dog, pig, horse, and primate monkeys (3,9,25,32,33). In agreement with earlier findings (2) we found that the serotonergic amplification effect on human platelets is observed with concentrations of 5-hydroxytryptamine from 1×10^{-7} M (17.6 ng/ml) on up to 1×10^{-5} M (1,760 ng/ml), which cover the normal range of 5-hydroxytryptamine levels present in human blood (19). In the case of combination of 5-hydroxytryptamine with ADP or collagen, the amplification by the monoamine is more pronounced on the maximal extent than on the initial rate of aggregation. The amplification of 5-hydroxytryptamine, when added to platelet-rich plasma beforehand, results in a platelet response typical for the potentiated agonist; as shown for the combination of the monoamine with collagen, such a serotonergic amplification results in the release of platelet specific proteins and of excessive formation of thromboxane B$_2$ of comparable intensity as obtained with high concentrations of collagen alone; in contrast with thrombin (34), threshold concentrations of collagen, producing only a weak aggregation response, already generate substantial amounts of thromboxane B_2. Such serotonergic amplification of collagen-induced reactions is inhibited by the cyclooxygenase inhibitor suprofen, suggesting the involvement of the arachidonate pathway of aggregation (12,34); however, serotonergic amplification of ADP-induced aggregation is not affected by suprofen.

The amplification of aggregation by 5-hydroxytryptamine and the direct aggregation induced by 5-hydroxytryptamine in presensitized human platelets is inhibited by ketanserin, regardless of the nature of the agonist combined with the monoamine. Taking into account the fact that ketanserin does not inhibit 5-hydroxytryptamine-independent platelet reactions, this evidence suggests that 5-hydroxytryptamine initiates an early event in platelet activation common to, or operative in, the three pathways of platelet aggregation (34). According to Detwiler et al. (16) and Lüscher et al. (24), the mobilization of Ca^{2+} from intracellular stores following membrane perturbance is a primary event in the various stages of platelet activation by several agonists. Such a mechanism could be involved in 5-hydroxytryptamine-induced and -amplified platelet reactions. On the other hand, since platelets swell when exposed to 5-hydroxytryptamine, the combination of the monoamine with its receptors may induce conformational changes in the platelet surface thereby unmasking receptors for other agonists and, hence, amplifications of the platelet response, as postulated for ADP (3,5,18).

ACKNOWLEDGMENTS

The authors would like to thank Betty Wouters, Yves Somers, Lambert Leijssen, and François Herion for their valuable assistance at various stages of this study.

Blood was kindly donated by research members of Janssen Pharmaceutica. This study was partly supported by a grant from the I. W. O. N. L.

REFERENCES

1. Ball, S. E., Bouillin, D. J., and Glenton, P. A. M. (1977): Interactions between noradrenaline and 5-hydroxytryptamine involving platelet aggregation. *J. Physiol.*, 272:98P–99P.
2. Baumgartner, H. R., and Born, G. V. R. (1968): Effects of 5-hydroxytryptamine on platelet aggregation. *Nature*, 218:137–141.
3. Baumgartner, H. R., and Born, G. V. R. (1969): The relation between the 5-hydroxytryptamine content and aggregation of rabbit platelets. *J. Physiol.*, 201:397–408.
4. Besterman, E. M. M., and Gillet, M. P. T. (1973): Influence of lysolecithin on platelet aggregation initiated by 5-hydroxytryptamine. *Nature*, 241:223–224.
5. Born, G. V. R. (1965): Uptake of adenosine diphosphate by human blood platelets. *Nature*, 206:1121–1122.
6. Born, G. V. R., Jwengjaroen, K., and Michal, F. (1972): Relative activities on and uptake by human blood platelets of 5-hydroxytryptamine and several analogues. *Br. J. Pharmacol.*, 44:117–139.
7. Bouillin, D. J., Woods, H. F., Grimes, R. P. J., Grahame-Smith, D. G., Wiles, D., Gelder, M. G., and Kolakowska, T. (1975): Increased platelet aggregation responses to 5-hydroxytryptamine in patients taking chlorpromazine. *Br. J. Clin. Pharmacol.*, 2:29–35.
8. Caen, J., Larrieu, M. J., and Samama, M. (1968): *l'Hémostase. Méthodes d'Exploration et Diagnostique Pratique*, pp. 98–107. l'Expansion Scientifique, Paris.

9. Calkins, J., Lane, K. P., Lossasso, G., and Thurber, L. E. (1974): Comparative study of platelet aggregation in various species. *J. Med.*, 5:292–296.
10. David, J. L., Herion, F., and Closset, J. (1981): *(in preparation).*
11. De Clerck, F., and Reneman, R. S. (1973): Effect of lidoflazine (R 7904) on uptake and release of serotonin by human platelets *in vitro*. *Naunyn Schmiedebergs Arch. Pharmacol.*, 278:261–269.
12. De Clerck, F., Vermylen, J., and Reneman, R. (1975): Effects of suprofen, an inhibitor of prostaglandin biosynthesis on platelet function, plasma coagulation and fibrinolysis. I. *In vitro* experiments. *Arch. Int. Pharmacodyn. Ther.*, 216:263–279.
13. De Clerck, F., Goossens, J., and Beerens, M. (1976): Lack of platelet Factor-3 activation after incubation of platelet-rich plasma with kaolin in the rat. *Experientia*, 32:1602–1603.
14. De Clerck, F., and David, J. L. (1981): Pharmacological control of platelet and red blood cell function in the microcirculation. *J. Cardiovasc. Pharmacol.*, 3:1388–1412.
15. De Gaetano, G., Van den Bussche, A., and Vermylen, J. (1972): Étude de l'agrégation plaquettaire par le Thrombofax. *Experientia*, 28:1117–1128.
16. Detwiler, T. L., Charo, I. F., and Feinman, R. D. (1978): Evidence that calcium regulates platelet function. *Thromb. Haemost.*, 40:207–211.
17. Finney, D. J. (1962): In: *Probit Analysis*, pp. 236–254. Cambridge University Press, Cambridge.
18. Evans, R. J., and Gordon, J. L. (1974): Refractoriness in blood platelets: effect of prior exposure to aggregating agents on subsequent aggregation responses. *Br. J. Pharmacol.*, 51:123P.
19. Geeraerts, F., Schimpfessel, L., and Crokaert, R. (1974): A simple routine-method to preserve and determine blood serotonin. *Experientia*, 30:837–838.
20. Gerrard, J. M., White, J. G., and Peterson, D. A. (1978): The platelet dense tubular system: Its relationship to prostaglandin biosynthesis and calcium fluid. *Thromb. Haemost.*, 40:224–231.
21. Gyermek, L. (1961): 5-Hydroxytryptamine antagonists. *Pharmacol. Rev.*, 13:399–439.
22. Haslam, R. J., Davidson, M. M. L., Desjardins, J. V., Fox, J. E. P., and Lyndham, J. A. (1979): Factors affecting the formation and actions of cyclic AMP in blood platelets. In: *Advances in Pharmacology and Therapeutics, Vol. 4, Prostaglandins-Immunopharmacology*, edited by B. B. Vargaftig, pp. 75–85. Pergamon Press, Oxford.
23. Leysen, J. E., Awouters, F., Kennis, L., Laduron, P. M., Vandenberk, J., and Janssen, P. A. J. (1981): Receptor binding profile of R 41 468, a novel antagonist at 5-HT$_2$ receptors. *Life Sci.*, 28(9):1015–1022.
24. Lüscher, E. F., Massini, P., and Käser-Glanzmann, R. (1979): The role of calcium ions in the regulation of platelet function and their pharmacological control. In: *Advances in Pharmacology and Therapeutics, Vol. 4, Prostaglandins-Immunopharmacology*, edited by B. B. Vargaftig, pp. 87–95. Pergamon Press, Oxford.
25. Mason, R. G., and Read, M. S. (1967): Platelet response to six agglutinating agents: Species similarities and differences. *Exp. Mol. Pathol.*, 6:370–381.
26. McMillan, R. M., Macintyre, D. E., and Gordon, J. L. (1977): Simple, sensitive fluorimetric assay for malondialdehyde production by blood platelets. *Thromb. Res.*, 11:425–428.
27. Michal, F. (1969): D-Receptors for serotonin in blood platelets. *Nature*, 221:1253–1254.
28. Michal, F., and Motamed, M. (1975): Time-dependent potentiation and inhibition by 5-hydroxytryptamine of platelet aggregation induced by ADP. *Br. J. Pharmacol.*, 54:221P–222P.
29. Peeters, J. R., and Graham-Smith, D. (1980): Human platelet 5-HT receptors: Characterization and functional association. *Eur. J. Pharmacol.*, 68:243–256.
30. Rogers, A. B. (1972): The effect of pH on platelet aggregation induced by epinephrine and ADP. *Proc. Soc. Exp. Biol. Med.*, 139:1100–1103.
31. Snyder, S. H., and Goodman, R. R. (1980): Multiple neurotransmitter receptors. *J. Neurochem.*, 35:5–15.
32. Takano, S., and Suzuki, T. (1978): The comparison between ADP-induced aggregation and noradrenaline plus 5-hydroxytryptamine-induced aggregation. *Fukushima J. Med. Sci.*, 25:1–7.
33. Tschopp, T. B. (1970): Aggregation of cat platelets *in vitro*. *Thromb. Diath. Haemorrh.*, 23:601–620.
34. Vargaftig, B. B., Chignard, M., and Benveniste, J. (1981): Present concepts on the mechanisms of platelet aggregation. *Biochem. Pharmacol.*, 30:263–271.
35. White, J. G. (1970): A biphasic response of platelets to serotonin. *Scand. J. Haematol.*, 7:145–151.

5-Hydroxytryptamine in Peripheral Reactions,
edited by Fred De Clerck and Paul M.
Vanhoutte. Raven Press, New York © 1982.

Cardiovascular Effects of Prostacyclin

A. G. Herman

University of Antwerp, Department of Experimental Pharmacology,
B2610 Wilrijk, Belgium

PROSTAGLANDINS

Biosynthesis

Prostaglandins are unsaturated fatty acids containing a twenty carbon skeleton and consisting of a cyclopentane ring with two lateral chains. They are "essential" in that their precursors have to be present in sufficient quantities in the food. The essential precursor of the prostaglandins of the 2 series, which is thought to be the most important series in man is linoleic acid, a fatty acid with 18 carbon atoms and 2 double bonds.

Once absorbed, this compound is modified by a process of desaturation and chain elongation into arachidonic acid (61), a 20 carbon fatty acid with 4 double bonds, which is the final substrate for the synthesis of the prostaglandins of the 2 series and a number of hydroxy fatty acids as well as the leukotrienes (see later). The main bulk of the absorbed arachidonic acid, derived from the linoleic acid or from the dietary absorption of arachidonic acid itself, does not remain in the circulation but is transported, bound to plasma albumins, to several tissues where it is incorporated in mono-, di-, and triglycerides, cholesterol esters and, mostly, in the phospholipid fraction of the cell membranes, usually in the 2-position of the glycerol moiety. Since prostaglandin synthesis will not take place for as long as the fatty acid precursor remains esterified in the phospholipids, it must become available in the free acid form to serve as a substrate. As soon as the integrity of the phospholipid-bilayer in the membrane is disturbed, cellular phospholipids by now become available to phospholipases which are able to free arachidonic acid. Although it is still not exactly known by which mechanisms the activity of the phospholipases is turned on, a whole range of different stimuli (e.g., mechanical, chemical, hormonal, immunological) are able to modify the release of arachidonic acid.

The main enzyme involved in the liberation of the substrate is the phospholipase A_2 (27,47) which cleaves arachidonic acid from its 2-position, although evidence has been accumulating that it also can be released by the combined action of phospholipase C and a diglyceride lipase (5,6).

Once arachidonic acid has been freed, it can be metabolized by two enzyme systems, i.e., the cyclooxygenase and/or the lipoxygenase. The cyclooxygenase (Fig. 1) transforms arachidonic acid into the prostaglandin endoperoxides PGG_2 and PGH_2 (33,34) which are unstable in aqueous solution (half-life approximately 5 min at 37°C) and which are broken down either enzymatically or nonenzymatically to the stable prostaglandins, PGE_2, $PGF_{2\alpha}$ and PGD_2, a 17-carbon hydroxy acid (12-hydroxy-5-8,10-heptadecatrienoic acid or HHT) and malondialdehyde.

These prostaglandin endoperoxides play a pivotal role in the arachidonic acid metabolism from which different prostaglandins can be formed. Several factors are involved in the determination which prostaglandin will predominantly be formed by a certain tissue, e.g., the amount of substrate available (19,31), the presence of certain co-factors such as glutathione, l-epinephrine, hydroquinone (28,63) or Cu^{2+} ions (50) or the tissue-specificity as such. The latter is best illustrated by what is happening at the level of the platelet-vessel wall interaction. Indeed, platelets transform the prostaglandin endoperoxides into the unstable compound thromboxane A_2 (half-life of about 30 sec at 37°C) (35) by an enzyme called thromboxane synthetase (56). Thromboxane A_2 is a potent inducer of platelet aggregation and is a powerful constrictor of the vascular smooth muscle cells. On the contrary, the vessel wall and, in particular, the endothelial cells (38,53), do not possess a thromboxane synthetase, but they transform the prostaglandin endoperoxides into another labile substance, prostacyclin or PGI_2 (half-life of about 7 min at 37°C, pH 7.5) by an enzyme called prostacyclin synthetase (52). Prostacyclin has effects which are opposite to those of thromboxane A_2, i.e., it is a very potent antiaggregating and vasodilator substance.

Whereas the cyclooxygenase seems to be present in the membranes of all cells, with the exception of the erythrocytes, the lipoxygenase has so far only been detected in platelets, lungs, and white cells. This enzyme transforms arachidonic acid in the platelets into the hydroxy acid 12L-hydroxy-5,8,10,14-eicosatetraenoic acid or 12-HETE (34), whereas in the leukocytes it gives rise not only to hydroxy acids such as 5-HETE and 5,12 DHETE but also to a recently discovered new class of substances called "leukotrienes" (11) (Fig. 2). Leukotriene C_4 (containing glutathione) and leukotriene D_4 (containing cysteinyl-glycine) appear to be responsible for the biological activity of the earlier discovered "slow reacting substance of anaphylaxis" or SRS-A (18,54).

Metabolism

Prostaglandins or other arachidonic acid metabolites are not stored in the cell, but are synthesized *de novo*. They are avidly taken up and metabolized by the lung and the liver which remove 80 to 95% of the prostaglandins on first pass (26,71). The main enzymes involved in their breakdown are the 15-hydroxyprostaglandin dehydrogenase, which has the highest activity in the lung, spleen, and kidney (1), and a $\Delta 13$ reductase which is abundant in the spleen, liver, kidney, adrenals, and the small intestine (1). Most of the metabolites have less (or no) activity as compared

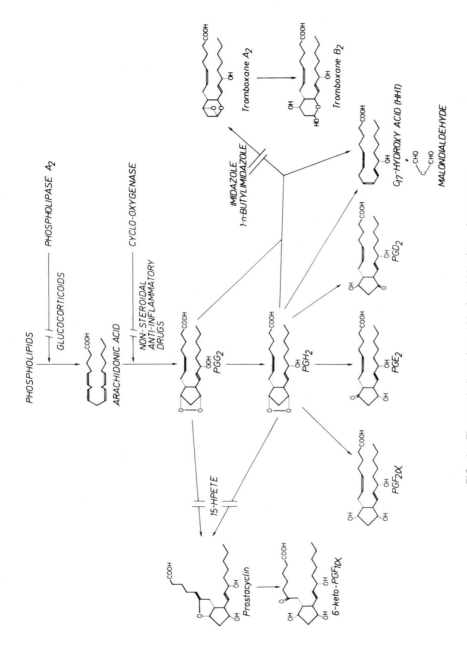

FIG. 1. The metabolism of arachidonic acid by the cyclooxygenase.

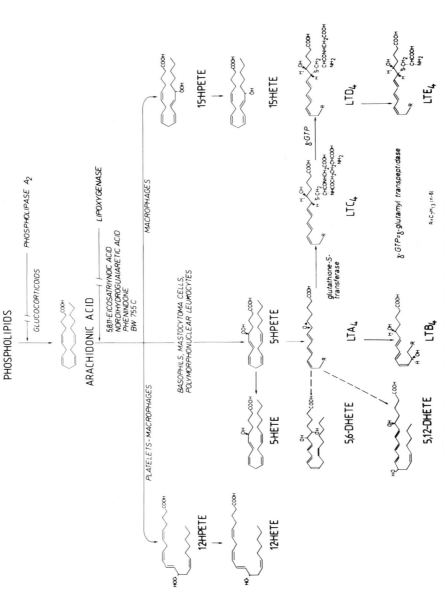

FIG. 2. The metabolism of arachidonic acid by the lipoxygenase.

to the parent compound and are mostly excreted via the kidney or the bile (64,65). Prostacyclin seems to be an exception since it is not removed by the lung and, apart from an important nonenzymic breakdown to 6-keto-PGF$_{1\alpha}$, it appears that the liver is the main site of its metabolism, presumably by the 15-hydroxyprostaglandin dehydrogenase and by β- and ω-oxidation as with the other prostaglandins (24,67). The very efficient removal mechanisms result in very low concentrations of these substances in the arterial circulation (pg per ml range).

Inhibition of Biosynthesis

The release of arachidonic acid from the phospholipids by the activity of the phospholipases, in particular phospholipase A$_2$, can be blocked by the corticosteroids (32), most likely via the synthesis of a specific peptide, called "macrocortin", which has antiphospholipase activity (7). Aspirin and other nonsteroidal antiinflammatory drugs specifically inhibit the cyclooxygenase thereby preventing the formation of the prostaglandin endoperoxides and their metabolites PGE$_2$, PGF$_{2\alpha}$, PGD$_2$, thromboxane A$_2$, HHT, and prostacyclin (72). The mechanism by which the nonsteroidal antiinflammatory drugs inhibit the cyclooxygenase can vary. Aspirin acetylates a serine residue at the active site of the enzyme (62) thereby irreversibly inactivating the cyclooxygenase; prostaglandins can only be formed again as new enzyme is synthesized. The other nonsteroidal antiinflammatory drugs have a different mode of action, although they all prevent the initial oxygen uptake. It should be realized that by inhibiting the cyclooxygenase in certain tissues, the pathway of metabolism of the arachidonic acid will be shifted in favor of the lipoxygenase which could result in an increased production of, e.g., the leukotrienes. Such a mechanism could explain the occurrence of an asthmatic attack in certain patients after the administration of aspirin or another nonsteroidal antiinflammatory substance, since in humans SRS-A is thought to play an important role in the etiopathology of asthma (58).

Since some of the lipoxygenase products are not only involved in asthma, but have also been shown to have chemokinetic and chemotactic activity and to accumulate at some inflammatory sites (29,46), it may be therapeutically advantageous to inhibit this enzyme in certain pathological conditions. Although highly specific inhibitors are so far not yet known, a series of pyrazolidone derivatives such as BW 755C or 3-amino-1-[m-(trifluoromethyl)-phenyl]-2-pyrazoline (41) and phenindone (8) have been found to block the cyclooxygenase as well as the lipoxygenase.

The formation of the potent aggregating and vasoconstricting thromboxane A$_2$ can specifically be inhibited by substances such as imidazole (51) and 1-n-butylimidazole (9). In clinical conditions in which there is hyperreactivity of the platelets, the administration of specific thromboxane synthetase inhibitors could be beneficial by a double mechanism: Indeed, not only the formation of thromboxane A$_2$ would be abolished but the metabolism of the prostaglandin endoperoxides (their mutual precursors) would be redirected towards the formation of the antiaggregating prostacyclin. Such a redirection of pathway has recently been shown to occur in humans after the administration of the specific thromboxane inhibitor UK-37, 248-01 (73).

Although specific inhibitors of the prostacyclin synthetase will probably have no broad therapeutic spectrum of application, some of them, such as 15-hydroperoxy arachidonic acid and hydroperoxy derivatives of other fatty acids, may have pathological relevance. Indeed some of these inhibitors have been identified in atherosclerotic plaques (36) and it could well be that their presence in those plaques are responsible for the impairment of the formation of prostacyclin which could result in an increased incidence of, e.g., arterial thrombosis. Although the clinical importance of inhibitors of the enzymes involved in the metabolism of the prostaglandins is as yet unknown, the anti-ulcer agent carbenoxolone has been claimed to exert its beneficial effect in the treatment of gastric ulcer by inhibiting the gastric 15-hydroxyprostaglandin dehydrogenase, thereby giving rise to higher tissue levels of the cytoprotective prostaglandins (59).

CARDIOVASCULAR EFFECTS OF PROSTACYCLIN

In Vitro

Prostacyclin relaxes a series of vascular strips including bovine coronary arteries (22,55), rabbit celiac and mesenteric arteries (13), human and baboon cerebral arteries (12), lamb ductus arteriosus (17), the human umbilical artery (60), and the dog saphenous vein (39). On the contrary, some vascular smooth muscle cells are, although rather weakly, contracted by prostacyclin, e.g., porcine coronary arteries (23), and some strips of human saphenous and rat venous tissue (49). Langendorf perfused hearts of rabbits (20,55), rats (20), and guinea pigs (66), as well as perfused rabbit kidneys (55) convert arachidonic acid mainly to prostacyclin and the latter is a potent vasodilator in this preparation. Prostacyclin has no direct cardiostimulatory activity since it does not affect the electrically driven cat papillary muscle (48).

In Vivo

Prostacyclin produces in most species, including man, a dose-dependent fall in blood pressure which is mainly due to its arteriolar vasodilator effect (2,3,68). Since it is not inactivated by the lung, prostacyclin is equipotent as a vasodilator when given either intraarterially or intravenously (3).

Intravenous infusions of prostacyclin in man, starting from 2 ng/kg/min on, is followed by a lowering of the diastolic blood pressure with little effect on the systolic blood pressure, an increase in heart rate, a decrease in the preejection time, a rise in venous oxygen pressure, and a decrease in pulmonary vascular resistance (57,69). Stroke volume, cardiac output, mean right atrial pressure, and left ventricular end-diastolic pressure showed no significant changes (69). The chronotropic and inotropic stimulation of the heart is reflexogenic in origin, which is also the case for the bradycardia occasionally observed in man (68) and in dogs (14,44); vagotomy and atropine block the latter effect in the animal experiments.

The vasodilator effects of prostacyclin are most likely responsible for the lowering of the diastolic blood pressure and the appearance of erythema of the face (facial flushing) and palms, increase in skin temperature, venous blood arterialization, and the occasionally experienced headache (57). Facial flushing and headache disappears within 5 to 10 min after the end of the prostacyclin infusion. Intracoronary injection of prostacyclin (0.05–0.5 μg) in the open chest dog increases the coronary blood flow and reduces the coronary vascular resistance without affecting aortic pressure or heart rate, although higher doses have systemic effects (21). PGE$_1$ (0.1–0.5 μg) also dilates the coronary vessels, has a longer lasting effect, and is 1 to 4 times more potent than prostacyclin, whereas PGE$_2$ is less potent than prostacyclin. Inhibition of the cyclooxygenase by indomethacin or meclofanamate reduces the coronary flow in these animals and potentiates the coronary dilatory effects of prostacyclin but not of PGE$_2$ (21). The observation that prolonged coronary vaso-dilatation can be obtained by dripping prostacyclin directly upon the epicardial surface (21) is interesting in the light of the findings by Herman and colleagues (15,37) that pericardial tissue produces high amounts of prostacyclin and that high levels of 6-keto-PGF$_{1\alpha}$ can be detected in pericardial fluid. It could well be that prostacyclin, continuously generated by the pericardial tissue, contributes to the regulation of the blood flow in the epicardium so that, in case the heart frequency increases, a concomitant rise in the formation of prostacyclin helps to keep the blood flow adequate in the outer layers of the myocardium.

Prostacyclin reduces the pulmonary artery pressure in man (70) as well as in the dog (45). Intravenous infusion of prostacyclin in the dog reduces renal vascular resistance and increases blood flow and urinary excretion of sodium, potassium, and chloride ions (10,42); in the anesthetized rat, prostacyclin decreases renal vascular resistance in contrast to the effect of PGE$_2$ which markedly increases the resistance in this species (4). Intrarenal infusion of prostacyclin in the dog induces the release of renin (30) and increases the arterial concentration of angiotensin II (43). In the femoral and mesenteric vascular bed of the dog, prostacyclin is a strong vasodilator (25). At the level of the microcirculation, prostacyclin applied system-ically or locally onto the hamster cheek pouch, causes an increase in the diameter of the precapillary arterioles, and is more potent than PGE$_1$, PGE$_2$, or bradykinin. The postcapillary venules in this preparation do not respond by dilatation to pros-tacyclin or any of the other prostaglandins (40). Intradermal injection of prostacyclin in the rabbit dorsal skin increases the blood flow and potentiates the plasma exu-dation by bradykinin and other vascular permeability-increasing mediators (74).

Although PGE$_2$ is less abundant than prostacyclin in the ductus arteriosus, it is thought to be functionally the most important prostaglandin formed in that vessel. Prostacyclin may contribute to ductus patency by complementing the action of PGE$_2$ on the vascular smooth muscle cells and preventing mechanical obstruction by the platelets (16).

REFERENCES

1. Änggard, E., and Samuelsson, B. (1966): Purification and properties of a 15-hydroxyprostaglandin dehydrogenase from swine lung. *Arkh. Kemi.*, 25:293–300.

2. Armstrong, J. M., Chapple, D. J., Dusting, G. J., Hughes, R., Moncada, S., and Vane, J. R. (1977): Cardiovascular actions of prostacyclin (PGI₂) in chloralose anaesthetized dogs. *Br. J. Pharmacol.*, 61:136P.

3. Armstrong, J. M., Lattimer, N., Moncada, S., and Vane, J. R. (1978): Comparison of the vasodepressor effects of prostacyclin and 6-oxo-prostaglandin $F_{1\alpha}$ with those of prostaglandin E_2 in rats and rabbits. *Br. J. Pharmacol.*, 62:125–130.

4. Baer, P. G., and McGiff, J. (1979): Comparison of effects of prostaglandins E_2 and I_2 on rat renal vascular resistance. *Eur. J. Pharmacol.*, 54:359–363.

5. Bell, R. L., Kennerly, D. A., Stanford, N., and Majerus, P. W. (1979): Diglyceride lipase: A pathway for arachidonate release from human platelets. In: *Advances in Prostaglandin and Thromboxane Research Vol. 8*, edited by B. Samuelsson, P. Ramwell, and R. Paoletti, pp. 219–224. Raven Press, New York.

6. Billah, M. M., Lapetina, E. G., and Cuatrecasas, P. (1979): Phosphatidylinositol-specific phospholipase C of platelets: Association with 1,2-diacylglycerol-kinase and inhibition by cyclic AMP. *Biochem. Biophys. Commun.*, 90:92–98.

7. Blackwell, G. J., Carnuccio, R., Di Rosa, M., Flower, R. J., Parente, L., and Persico, P. (1980): Macrocortin: A polypeptide causing the anti-phospholipase effect of glucocorticoids. *Nature*, 287:147–149.

8. Blackwell, G. J., and Flower, R. J. (1978): 1-Phenyl-3-pyrazolidone: An inhibitor of cyclo-oxygenase and lipoxygenase pathways in lungs and platelets. *Prostaglandins*, 16:417–425.

9. Blackwell, G. J., Flower, R. J., Russel-Smith, N., Salmon, J. A., Thorogood, P. B., and Vane, J. R. (1978): 1-*n*-Butylimidazole: A potent and selective inhibitor of "thromboxane synthetase." *Br. J. Pharmacol.*, 64:435P.

10. Bolger, P. M., Eisner, G. M., Ramwell, P. M., Slotkoff, L. M., and Corey, E. J. (1978): Renal actions of prostacyclin. *Nature*, 271:467–469.

11. Borgeat, P., and Samuelsson, B. (1979): Metabolism of arachidonic acid in polymorphonuclear leukocytes: Structure analysis of novel hydroxylated compounds. *J. Biol. Chem.*, 254:7865–7869.

12. Boullin, D. J., Bunting, S., Blaso, W. P., Hunt, T. M., and Moncada, S. (1979): Responses of human and baboon arteries to prostaglandin endoperoxides and biologically generated and synthetic prostacyclin: Their relevance to cerebral arterial spasm in man. *Br. J. Clin. Pharmacol.*, 7:139–147.

13. Bunting, S., Gryglewski, R., Moncada, S., and Vane, J. R. (1976): Arterial walls generate from prostaglandin endoperoxides a substance (prostaglandin X) which relaxes strips of mesenteric and coeliac arteries and inhibits platelet aggregation. *Prostaglandins*, 12:897–914.

14. Chapple, D. J., Dusting, G. J., Hughes, R., and Vane, J. R. (1978): A vagal reflex contributes to the hypotensive effect of prostacyclin (PGI₂) in anaesthetized dogs. *J. Physiol.*, 281:43–44P.

15. Claeys, M., Van Hove, C., Duchateau, A., and Herman, A. G. (1980): GC/MS measurement of 6-oxo-PGF₁α in biological fluids. In: *Prostaglandins, Prostacyclin, and Thromboxanes Measurements*, edited by J. M. Boeynaems and A. G. Herman, pp. 105–120. Martinus Nijhoff Publishers, The Hague.

16. Coceani, F., Bishai, I., Bodack, E., White, E. P., and Olley, P. M. (1979): On the evidence implicating PGE₂ rather than prostacyclin in the patency of the fetal ductus arteriosus. In: *Prostacyclin*, edited by J. R. Vane and S. Bergström, pp. 247–251. Raven Press, New York.

17. Coceani, F., Bishai, I., White, E., Bodach, E., and Olley, P. M. (1978): Action of prostaglandins, endoperoxides, and thromboxanes on the lamb ductus arteriosus. *Am. J. Physiol.*, 234:H117–H122.

18. Corey, E. J., Clark, D. A., Goto, G., Marfat, A., Mioskowski, C., Samuelsson, B., and Hammarström, S. (1980): Stereospecific total synthesis of a slow reacting substance of anaphylaxis, leukotriene C-1. *J. Am. Chem. Soc.*, 102:1436–1439.

19. Cottee, F., Flower, R. J., Moncada, S., Salmon, J. A., and Vane, J. R. (1977): Synthesis of 6-keto-PGF₁α by ram seminal vesicle microsomes. *Prostaglandins*, 14:413–423.

20. De Deckere, E. A. M., Nugteren, D. H., and Ten Hoor, F. (1977): Prostacyclin is the major prostaglandin released from the isolated, perfused rabbit and rat heart. *Nature*, 268:160–163.

21. Dusting, G. J., Chapple, D. J., Hughes, R., Moncada, S., and Vane, J. R. (1979): Prostacyclin (PGI₂) induces coronary vasodilatation in anaesthetized dogs. *Cardiovasc. Res.*, 12:720–730.

22. Dusting, G. J., Moncada, S., and Vane, J. R. (1977): Prostacyclin (PGX) is the endogenous metabolite responsible for relaxation of coronary arteries induced by arachidonic acid. *Prostaglandins*, 13:3–15.

23. Dusting, G. J., Moncada, S., and Vane, J. R. (1977): Prostacyclin is a weak contractor of coronary arteries of the pig. *Eur. J. Pharmacol.*, 45:301–304.
24. Dusting, G. J., Moncada, S., and Vane, J. R. (1978): Recirculation of prostacyclin (PGI₂) in the dog. *Br. J. Pharmacol.*, 64:315–320.
25. Dusting, G. J., Moncada, S., and Vane, J. R. (1978): Vascular actions of arachidonic acid and its metabolites in perfused mesenteric and femoral beds of the dog. *Eur. J. Pharmacol.*, 49:65–72.
26. Ferreira, S. H., and Vane, J. R. (1967): Prostaglandins: Their disappearance from and release into the circulation. *Nature*, 216:868–873.
27. Flower, R. J., and Blackwell, G. J. (1976): The importance of phospholipase A₂ in prostaglandin biosynthesis. *Biochem. Pharmacol.*, 25:285–291.
28. Flower, R. J., Cheung, H. S., and Cushman, D. W. (1973): Quantitative determination of prostaglandins and malondialdehyde formed by the arachidonate oxygenase (prostaglandin synthetase) system of bovine seminal vesicle. *Prostaglandins*, 4:325–341.
29. Ford-Hutchinson, A. W., Bray, M. A., Doig, M. V., Shipley, M. E., and Smith, M. J. H. (1980): Leukotriene B, a potent chemokinetic and aggregating substance released from polymorphonuclear leukocytes. *Nature*, 286:264–265.
30. Gerber, J. G., Branch, R. A., Nies, A. S., Gerkens, J. F., Shand, D. G., Hollifield, J., and Oates, J. A. (1978): Prostaglandins and renin release: II. Assessment of renin secretion following infusion of PGI₂, E₂ and D₂ into the renal artery of anesthetized dogs. *Prostaglandins*, 15:81–88.
31. Gryglewski, R. J., Korbut, R., Ocetkiewicz, A., Splawinski, J., Wojtaszek, B., and Swis, J. (1978): Lungs as a generator of prostacyclin-hypothesis on physiological significance. *Naunyn Schmiedebergs Arch. Pharmacol.*, 304:45–50.
32. Gryglewski, R. J., Panczenko, B., Korbut, R., Grodzinska, L., and Ocetkiewicz, A. (1975): Corticosteroids inhibit prostaglandin release from perfused mesenteric blood vessels of rabbit and from perfused lungs of sensitized guinea-pig. *Prostaglandins*, 10:343–355.
33. Hamberg, M., and Samuelsson, B. (1973): Detection and isolation of an endoperoxide intermediate in prostaglandin biosynthesis. *Proc. Natl. Acad. Sci. USA*, 70:899–903.
34. Hamberg, M., and Samuelsson, B. (1974): Prostaglandin endoperoxides. Novel transformation of arachidonic acid in human platelets. *Proc. Natl. Acad. Sci. USA*, 71:3400–3404.
35. Hamberg, M., Svensson, J., and Samuelsson, B. (1975): Thromboxanes: A new group of biologically active compounds derived from prostaglandin endoperoxides. *Proc. Natl. Acad. Sci. USA*, 78:2994–2998.
36. Harland, W. A., Gilbert, J. D., and Brooks, C. J. W. (1973): Lipids of human atheroma. VIII. Oxidised derivatives of cholesterol linoleate. *Biochim. Biophys. Acta*, 316:378–385.
37. Herman, A. G., Claeys, M., Moncada, S., and Vane, J. R. (1977): Biosynthesis of prostacyclin (PGI₂) and 12L-hydroxy-5,8,10,14-eicosatetraenoic acid (HETE) by pericardium, pleura, peritoneum and aorta of the rabbit. *Prostaglandins*, 18:439–452.
38. Herman, A. G., Moncada, S., and Vane, J. R. (1977): Formation of prostacyclin (PGI₂) by different layers of the arterial wall. *Arch. Int. Pharmacodyn.*, 227:162–163.
39. Herman, A. G., Verbeuren, T. J., Moncada, S., and Vanhoutte, P. M. (1978): Effect of prostacyclin on myogenic activity and adrenergic interaction in canine isolated veins. *Prostaglandins*, 16:911–921.
40. Higgs, G. A., Cardinal, D. C., Moncada, S., and Vane, J. R. (1979): Microcirculatory effects of prostacyclin (PGI₂) in the hamster cheek pouch. *Microvasc. Res.*, 18:245–254.
41. Higgs, G. A., Flower, R. J., and Vane, J. R. (1979): A new approach to anti-inflammatory drugs. *Biochem. Pharmacol.*, 28:1959–1961.
42. Hill, T. W. K., and Moncada, S. (1979): The renal haemodynamic and excretory actions of prostacyclin and 6-oxo-PGF₁ₐ in anaesthetized dogs. *Prostaglandins*, 17:87–98.
43. Hill, T. W. K., Moncada, S., and Vane, J. R. (1978): Stimulation of renin release by prostacyclin (PGI₂) in anaesthetized dogs. *7th International Congress of Pharmacology*, Paris, Abstract 869, p. 343.
44. Hintze, T. H., Kaley, G., Martin, E. G., and Messina, E. J. (1978): PGI₂ induces bradycardia in the dog. *Prostaglandins*, 15:712.
45. Kadowitz, P. J., Chapnick, B. M., Feigen, L. P., Hyman, A. L., Nelson, P. K., and Spannhake, E. W. (1978): Pulmonary and systemic vasodilator effects of the newly-discovered prostaglandin I₂. *J. Appl. Physiol.*, 45:408–413.
46. Klickstein, L. B., Shapleigh, T., and Goetzl, E. J. (1980): Unique products of the oxygenation of arachidonic acid in synovial fluid in rheumatoid arthritis and spondylarthritis. *Arthritis Rheum.*, 23:704–705.

47. Kunze, H., and Vogt, W. (1971): Significance of phospholipase A for prostaglandin formation. *Ann. NY Acad. Sci.*, 180:123–125.
48. Lefer, A. M., Ogletree, M. L., Smith, J. B., Silver, M. J., Nicolau, K. C., Barnette, W. E., and Gasic, G. P. (1978): Prostacyclin: A potentially valuable agent for preserving myocardial tissue in acute myocardial ischemia. *Science*, 200:52–54.
49. Levy, S. V. (1978): Contractile responses of prostacyclin (PGI₂) of isolated human saphenous and rat venous tissue. *Prostaglandins*, 16:93–97.
50. Maddox, I. J. (1973): The role of copper in prostaglandin synthesis. *Biochim. Biophys. Acta*, 306:74–81.
51. Moncada, S., Bunting, S., Mullane, K. M., Thorogood, P., and Vane, J. R. (1977): Imidazole: A selective potent antagonist of thromboxane synthetase. *Prostaglandins*, 13:611–618.
52. Moncada, S., Gryglewski, R. J., Bunting, S., and Vane, J. R. (1976): An enzyme isolated from arteries transforms prostaglandin endoperoxides to an unstable substance that inhibits platelet aggregation. *Nature*, 263:663–665.
53. Moncada, S., Herman, A. G., Higgs, E. A., and Vane, J. R. (1977): Differential formation of prostacyclin (PGX or PGI₂) by layers of the arterial wall. An explanation for the anti-thrombotic properties of vascular endothelium. *Thromb. Res.*, 11:323–344.
54. Murphy, R. C., Hammarström, S., and Samuelsson, B. (1979): Leukotriene C: A slow reacting substance from murine mastocytoma cells. *Proc. Natl. Acad. Sci. USA*, 76:4275–4279.
55. Needleman, P., Bronson, S. D., Sycke, A., Sivakoff, M., and Nicolaou, K. C. J. (1978): Cardiac and renal prostaglandin I₂. Biosynthesis and biological effects in isolated perfused rabbit tissues. *J. Clin. Invest.*, 61:839–849.
56. Needleman, P. S., Moncada, S., Bunting, S., Vane, J. R., Hamberg, M., and Samuelsson, B. (1976): Identification of an enzyme in platelet microsomes which generates thromboxane A₂ from prostaglandin endoperoxides. *Nature*, 261:558–560.
57. O'Grady, J., Warrington, S., Moti, M. J., Bunting, S., Flower, R., Fowle, A. S. E., Higgs, E. A., and Moncada, S. (1979): Effects of intravenous prostacyclin infusions in healthy volunteers—some preliminary observations. In: *Prostacyclin*, edited by J. R. Vane and S. Bergström, pp. 409–417. Raven Press, New York.
58. Orange, R. P., and Austen, K. F. (1969): Slow-reacting substance of anaphylaxis. *Adv. Immunol.*, 10:105–144.
59. Peskar, B. M., Holland, A., and Peskar, B. A. (1976): Effect of carbenoxolone on prostaglandin synthesis and degradation. *J. Pharm. Pharmacol.*, 28:146–148.
60. Pomerantz, K., Sintetos, A., and Ramwell, P. (1978): The effect of prostacyclin on the human umbilical artery. *Prostaglandins*, 15:1035–1044.
61. Ramwell, P. W., Leovey, E. M. K., and Sintetos, A. L. (1977): Regulation of the arachidonic acid cascade. *Biol. Reprod.*, 16:245–248.
62. Roth, G. J., Stanford, N., and Majerus, P. W. (1975): Acetylation of prostaglandin synthetase by aspirin. *Proc. Natl. Acad. Sci. USA*, 72:3073–3076.
63. Salmon, J. A., Smith, D. R., Flower, R. J., Moncada, S., and Vane, J. R. (1978): Further studies on the enzymic conversion of prostaglandin endoperoxides into prostacyclin by porcine aorta microsomes. *Biochim. Biophys. Acta*, 523:250–262.
64. Samuelsson, B. (1964): Synthesis of tritium-labeled prostaglandin E₁ and studies on its distribution and excretion in the rat. *J. Biol. Chem.*, 239:4091–4096.
65. Samuelsson, B., Granström, E., Gréen, K., and Hamberg, M. (1971): Metabolism of prostaglandins. *Ann. NY Acad. Sci.*, 180:138–161.
66. Schrör, K., Moncada, S., Ubatuba, F. B., and Vane, J. R. (1978): Transformation of arachidonic acid and prostaglandin endoperoxides by the guinea pig heart. Formation of RCS and prostacyclin. *Eur. J. Pharmacol.*, 47:103–114.
67. Sun, F. F., McGuire, J. C., and Taylor, B. M. (1978): Metabolism of prostacyclin (PGI₂). *Prostaglandins*, 15:724.
68. Szczeklik, A., and Gryglewski, J. R. (1979): Actions of prostacyclin in man. In: *Prostacyclin*, edited by J. R. Vane, and S. Bergström, pp. 393–407. Raven Press, New York.
69. Szczeklik, J., Szczeklik, A., and Nizankowski, R. (1980): Haemodynamic changes induced by prostacyclin in man. *Br. Heart J.*, 44:254–258.
70. Szczeklik, J., Szczeklik, A., and Nizankowski, R. (1980): Prostacyclin for pulmonary hypertension. *Lancet*, i:1076.
71. Vane, J. R. (1969): The release and fate of vasoactive hormones in the circulation. *Br. J. Pharmacol.*, 35:209–242.

72. Vane, J. R. (1971): Inhibition of prostaglandin synthesis as a mechanism of action for aspirin-like drugs. *Nature (New Biol.)*, 231:232–235.
73. Vermylen, J., Carreras, L. O., Van Schaeren, J., Defreyn, G., Machin, S. J., and Verstraete, M. (1981): Thromboxane synthetase inhibition as antithrombotic strategy. *Lancet*, i:1073–1075.
74. Williams, T. J. (1979): Prostaglandin E_2, prostaglandin I_2 and the vascular changes in inflammation. *Br. J. Pharmacol.*, 65:517–524.

5-Hydroxytryptamine in Peripheral Reactions,
edited by Fred De Clerck and Paul M.
Vanhoutte. Raven Press, New York © 1982.

Pharmacological Manipulation of Prostacyclin Release and Activity

Jos Vermylen and Luis O. Carreras

*Center for Thrombosis and Vascular Research, Department of Medical Research,
University of Leuven, Campus Gasthuisberg, B-3000 Leuven, Belgium*

The normal vascular endothelium behaves as an antithrombotic surface. Among several mechanisms involved in this property, the production of prostacyclin (PGI_2) seems to play a central role (13).

Prostacyclin, discovered in 1976 (57), is the most potent natural inhibitor of platelet aggregation described so far, and is also a powerful vasodilator (63). It is synthesized, as all bienoic prostaglandins, from free arachidonic acid released from phospholipids of the cell membrane. Arachidonic acid then is transformed by cyclo-oxygenase into cyclic endoperoxides, which are further converted by prostacyclin-synthetase into prostacyclin (60). This is the major product of arachidonic acid metabolism in vascular endothelium (84) and also in vascular smooth muscle cells (4,5,24,59). In addition, many other tissues may form this substance (64), as well as endothelial cells in culture (50,53,100,102). Prostacyclin is not stored by endothelial cells but immediately released after synthesis in response to stimuli (97). It is an unstable prostaglandin, being rapidly and spontaneously transformed *in vitro* into the stable degradation product 6-keto-prostaglandin $F_{1\alpha}$ (6-keto $PGF_{1\alpha}$) (60). It can also be enzymatically converted by 15-hydroxyprostaglandin dehydrogenase into 15-keto-PGI_2. By the combined action of both mechanisms 6,15-di-keto-prostaglandin $F_{1\alpha}$ is formed. In the presence of Δ_{13} reductase 15-keto-PGI_2 can be further converted into 13,14-dihydro-6,15-di-keto-prostaglandin $F_{1\alpha}$ (89).

In this chapter we will briefly deal with the mechanisms involved in the regulation of prostacyclin synthesis by the vessel wall in physiological conditions, and the possible ways to manipulate prostacyclin production and degradation using pharmacological agents and dietary means will be discussed.

STIMULATION OF PROSTACYCLIN RELEASE AND ACTIVITY

Several investigators, mainly working with endothelial cells in culture and measuring the release of 6-keto-$PGF_{1\alpha}$, have demonstrated that PGI_2 production may be provoked by a wide variety of chemical agents and physical stimuli (Fig. 1). Indeed, simply rocking or vibrating endothelial cells (100) or vascular rings (60) and pulsatile flow (90) induce the synthesis of PGI_2, a finding suggesting that blood

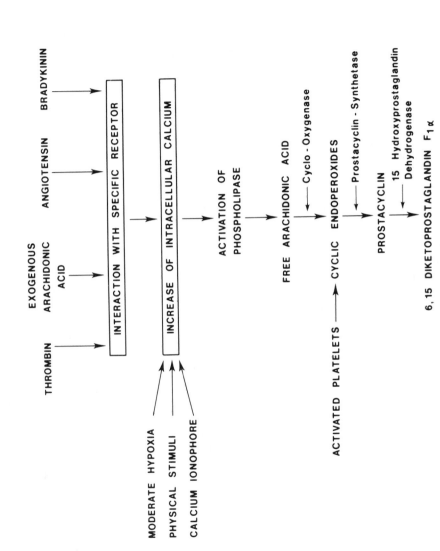

FIG. 1. Possible pathways for prostacyclin production by the endothelial cell.

flow could stimulate PGI_2 production *in vivo* (97). Exogenous arachidonic acid (the substrate for the production of PGI_2) and the intermediate cyclic endoperoxide PGH_2 stimulate prostacyclin release by endothelial cells (8,49,102). Exogenously added arachidonic acid probably stimulates PGI_2 synthesis in part by inducing the release of arachidonic acid bound to membrane phospholipids (99). In contrast, exogenous cyclic endoperoxides can easily be converted by endothelial cell prostacyclin-syn-thetase into prostacyclin (49). Some controversy still exists with regard to the primary source of cyclic endoperoxides for the production of PGI_2 *in vivo*. Moncada and co-workers (57) have demonstrated that vessel microsomes can utilize endo-peroxides but not arachidonic acid to synthetize PGI_2. In addition, they have shown that fresh vascular tissue can produce PGI_2 from both substrates, but is far more effective in utilizing cyclic endoperoxides (12), and that indomethacin-treated vessel microsomes or vascular rings generate PGI_2 when incubated with platelets (12,13,29). In view of these observations, they have suggested a biochemical cooperation between platelets and vessel wall in which activated platelets adhering to the dam-aged vessel wall could release endoperoxides that endothelial cells could further transform into PGI_2, thus preventing thrombus formation (62,63). This hypothesis has been confirmed *in vitro* by Marcus et al. (51), who demonstrated that cultured human endothelial cells treated with aspirin can utilize platelet-derived endoperox-ides for PGI_2 formation to a significant extent. However, this mechanism has been questioned by others (4,38,69), and it remains to be elucidated whether it takes place *in vivo* in physiological conditions. On the other hand, selective inhibition of platelet thromboxane-synthetase could result in reorientation of the metabolism of the cyclic endoperoxides (56,66,70), leading not only to a reduced formation of thromboxane A_2 but also to an enhanced release of cyclic endoperoxides, from which the vessel wall synthesizes PGI_2, as mentioned above. This concept has been verified *in vitro* using platelets preincubated with a thromboxane-synthetase inhibitor and cultured endothelial cells (4) or blood vessel microsomes (69). We have recently demonstrated that this also happens *in vivo* in man after administration of a selective thromboxane-synthetase inhibitor (93). In this case we found that the reduced formation of thromboxane B_2, the stable metabolite of thromboxane A_2, was as-sociated with a parallel rise in the levels of plasma 6-keto-$PGF_{1\alpha}$. In addition, in a family with congenital partial thromboxane-synthetase deficiency of platelets we also observed that the reduced serum levels of thromboxane B_2 were associated with increased plasma levels of 6-keto-$PGF_{1\alpha}$ (18). These studies suggest that, at least in this particular situation where the main metabolic pathway for transformation of endoperoxides by platelets is blocked, the vessel wall can utilize platelet-derived cyclic endoperoxides to generate PGI_2 *in vivo*. Furthermore, endoperoxides released by leukocytes have also been proposed as a possible substrate for PGI_2 generation by the vessel wall (64).

The production of PGI_2 by human endothelial cells is stimulated by thrombin (8,34,99) and trypsin (99). The enzymatic active site of thrombin must be present to obtain this effect (3,99). Specific thrombin receptors are present on the endothelial surface (3), which become resistant to further stimulation after challenge with this enzyme until new receptors are synthesized (17). However, the cells remain sensitive to other stimuli of PGI_2 production (17,99). The thrombin-induced production of prostacyclin by normal endothelial cells adjacent to an injured area could limit platelet deposition and localize thrombus formation (99).

Other stimuli capable of inducing PGI_2 synthesis by vascular endothelium include bradykinin (34), angiotensin II (65), and moderate hypoxia (42). All these agents, as well as the proteolytic enzymes thrombin and trypsin, probably induce the release of endogenous arachidonic acid by activating phospholipase A_2, a calcium-dependent enzyme (8,97). Furthermore, calcium ionophore A 23187, which induces mobilization of intracellular calcium (43,77), also is a powerful stimulator of PGI_2 generation by endothelial cells (8,99).

The production of PGI_2 by the vessel wall can also be stimulated by some pharmacological agents. Of particular interest is the recent demonstration that plasma from normal volunteers after ingestion of Bay g 6575 (now given the generic name nafazatrom), a compound with marked antithrombotic activity in experimental models (85), increases PGI_2 release from the vessel wall, as compared with the plasma from the same volunteers before the intake of the drug (92). We have also observed significantly increased release of PGI_2-like material by fresh aortic rings from normal and diabetic rats during chronic treatment with this compound (16). Dipyridamole has been reported to increase PGI_2 synthesis by rat stomach fundus homogenates and the microsomal fraction of pig aorta (7). This effect was obtained *in vitro* with high concentrations of the drug and was not observed by others (91). It has, however, recently been demonstrated that, even if dipyridamole at a concentration of 10 μg/ml is not able to stimulate PGI_2 production by human endothelial cells in culture, it can increase such production when endothelial cells are challenged with arachidonic acid or thrombin in the presence of the drug (97). On the other hand, dipyridamole, as a phosphodiesterase inhibitor, potentiates the antiaggregating effect of PGI_2 by slowing the breakdown of the raised platelet cyclic adenosine monophosphate (AMP) level induced by this substance (61).

It has also been reported that nitroglycerin, another vasodilator agent, at concentrations reached in plasma during treatment with the drug (0.1–10 ng/ml), enhances PGI_2 production by cultured human endothelial cells (48,97). It has been suggested that the increased production of PGI_2 induced by this drug could improve myocardial ischemia by causing peripheral vasodilatation and decreasing cardiac work. In addition, it could inhibit platelet aggregation and thromboxane A_2 generation, thus decreasing coronary artery vasospasm (48). Isoprenaline and nicotinic acid have been reported to increase PGI_2 synthesis by isolated perfused rabbit heart (42).

Suloctidil has also been suggested to increase PGI_2 release by the vessel wall (45); this effect was, however, not observed by other investigators (94). We have not been able to find a significant increase in the stimulatory activity of plasma on PGI_2 production by "repeatedly washed" rings of rat aorta after ingestion of suloctidil by normal volunteers *(not published)*.

Finally, the biological activity of PGI_2 can be enhanced by substances that interfere with its degradation. Most of the *in vivo* catabolism of PGI_2 is probably via 15-hydroxyprostaglandin dehydrogenase, giving 15-keto-PGI_2 as the first degradation product (89). The 15-hydroxyprostaglandin dehydrogenase present in the vascular wall may degrade PGI_2 *in situ* before its release into the circulation. Several drugs have been reported to be inhibitors of 15-hydroxyprostaglandin dehydrogenase from diverse tissues (32). These include furosemide and ethacrynic acid, theophylline, phloretin phosphate, xylocaine, probenecid, and several nonsteroidal antiinflammatory agents, which are weak inhibitors of the enzyme. The possible effect of these drugs on PGI_2 metabolism in blood vessels has not yet been completely elucidated.

INHIBITION OF PROSTACYCLIN RELEASE AND ACTIVITY

The production of prostacyclin by the vessel wall may be reduced by inhibition of one of the three enzymatic steps involved in the biosynthesis of this substance.

1. Phospholipase A_2 is the first enzyme of this pathway, responsible for the release of free arachidonic acid from membrane phospholipids. PGI_2 increases the intracellular cyclic AMP level of vascular endothelium (8,37,55). It has been shown that cyclic AMP inhibits phospholipase A_2 activity in platelets, thus preventing the release of arachidonic acid and its transformation into prostaglandins (46). If this reaction also holds for endothelial cells, PGI_2 could diminish its own synthesis by a negative feedback (37,97). However, the high activity of phosphodiesterase in vascular endothelium could rapidly lower the cyclic AMP level increased by PGI_2 and thus protect against this feedback mechanism (8,37). Glucocorticoids can inhibit phospholipase A_2, thus preventing the release of arachidonic acid and its subsequent transformation into prostaglandins and leukotrienes which are important mediators of the inflammatory process. Glucocorticoids seem to exert this effect by inducing the synthesis of a phospholipase A_2 inhibitory protein (33). Blajchman and co-workers (6) have recently demonstrated that hydrocortisone treatment can indeed reduce prostacyclin formation by the vessel wall in rabbits. They have also shown that this treatment is able to shorten the bleeding time of thrombocytopenic animals. Since PGI_2 also is a powerful vasodilator, it is possible that the inhibition of its generation by the vessel wall could have reduced bleeding in this condition. This demonstration gives support to the well-known clinical impression that corticosteroids often reduce the bleeding tendency in thrombocytopenic patients, even when the platelet count remains unchanged. Other agents capable of inhibiting phospholipase A_2 activity include mepacrine and phentermine, local anesthetics, and several serine protease inhibitors (27).

2. The second step in the generation of PGI_2 consists of the enzymatic conversion of arachidonic acid into cyclic endoperoxides by cyclooxygenase. This enzyme can be blocked by aspirin and nonsteroidal antiinflammatory drugs. Acetylsalicylic acid irreversibly acetylates the active site of platelet cyclooxygenase (14). As platelets are unable to synthesize new proteins, the inactivation of this enzyme after *in vivo*

exposure to acetylsalicylic acid persists for the lifetime of platelets. In view of this capacity to block platelet thromboxane A_2 generation, acetylsalicylic acid has been extensively used as an antithrombotic agent. However, this drug can also inhibit the vessel wall cyclooxygenase, thus blocking the production of PGI_2, a substance potentially protective against platelet deposition, and could in this way promote thrombosis (63). In view of the high sensitivity of platelet cyclooxygenase to acetylsalicylic acid, considerable effort has been directed to ascertain whether, at certain doses of the drug, this enzyme could be selectively inhibited in platelets but not in other tissues, particularly in the vessel wall. In support of this possibility, it was demonstrated that cyclooxygenase in cultured smooth muscle cells from human aorta and in skin fibroblasts is more resistant to inactivation by acetylsalicylic acid than the platelet enzyme (5). In contrast, Jaffe and Weksler (39) have recently demonstrated that cyclooxygenase from human endothelial cells in culture is as sensitive to acetylsalicylic acid as the enzyme in platelets. Nevertheless, the inhibition was shorter lasting than in platelets, and PGI_2 production in endothelial cells returned to control levels within 35 hr after exposure to acetylsalicylic acid. It was shown that recovery of endothelial cell cyclooxygenase was due to renewed synthesis of the enzyme.

Considerable controversy still exists with regard to the possible selective inhibition of platelet cyclooxygenase by low dose acetylsalicylic acid in man. Of particular interest is the demonstration of O'Grady and Moncada (74) that the bleeding time is increased in humans 2 hr after ingestion of a single low dose of acetylsalicylic (0.3 g), whereas a high dose (3.9 g) had no effect. The authors consider that the prolongation of the bleeding time induced by low dose acetylsalicylic acid is due to an alteration of the thromboxane A_2/prostacyclin balance, a possible mechanism of control of platelet aggregability *in vivo* (44,62). In favor of this hypothesis, they have also demonstrated that the bleeding time becomes prolonged 24 to 72 hr after ingestion of the high dose of acetylsalicylic acid, at a time when the vessel wall cyclooxygenase activity could have recovered (1). These results have been confirmed by some investigators (79), but not by others (20,28). On the other hand, Masotti and co-workers (52) have shown that 3.5 mg/kg body weight (b.w.) is the dose of acetylsalicylic acid most likely to produce a consistent inhibition of platelet aggregation and only a slight inhibition of PGI_2 synthesis in humans. However, these findings have not been confirmed by others (75), and considerable between-person differences in the response to acetylsalicylic acid may exist (35,73). Moreover, Preston et al. (78) have recently reported a marked inhibition of PGI_2 production by vein segments from normal human volunteers 2 to 6 hr after the ingestion of 150 to 300 mg acetylsalicylic acid. Hanley et al. (31) have shown that the production of PGI_2 by human venous tissue was strongly inhibited 14 hr after the ingestion of 80 mg acetylsalicylic acid, while the effect of 300 mg was still evident 48 hr after ingestion. In addition, Villa et al. (95) have demonstrated that rat venous tissues are almost as sensitive to acetylsalicylic acid as platelets, arteries being more resistant. In contrast, Buchanan et al. (9) have found that the inhibitory effect of acetylsalicylic acid on the production of prostacyclin lasts longer in rabbit arteries than in veins, suggesting that turnover of cyclooxygenase is more rapid in veins.

In spite of theoretical considerations on the possible thrombogenic effect of high dose acetylsalicylic acid, this has so far only been confirmed *in vivo* in an experimental model of venous thrombosis in rabbits after intravenous infusion with 200 mg/kg b.w. of this drug (41). However, it has recently been demonstrated that platelet accumulation onto injured carotid arteries of rabbits is enhanced with acetylsalicylic acid at a dose of 10 mg/kg (10). In contrast, acetylsalicylic acid at doses up to 200 mg/kg failed to increase experimentally-induced venous and arterial thrombus formation in rats (82). In addition, Pareti et al. (76) have recently reported a patient with a congenital deficiency of cyclooxygenase in both platelets and vessel wall and presenting with a mild bleeding disorder instead of a thrombotic tendency.

Finally, it should be kept in mind that almost all the clinical trials conducted until now, and in which acetylsalicylic acid was shown to be effective as an antithrombotic agent, have been performed using relatively high doses of the drug (54). Moreover, it has recently been demonstrated that acetylsalicylic acid at high doses not only prevents thromboxane A_2 formation, but also interferes with platelet function independently of the prostaglandin pathway (11). Compounds that selectively inhibit platelet thromboxane-synthetase and simultaneously enhance vascular PGI_2 formation, as previously mentioned, would certainly constitute a more rational approach to antithrombotic therapy, and would solve the dilemma of the acetylsalicylic acid effect on the thromboxane A_2-prostacyclin balance.

3. Prostacyclin-synthetase, the terminal enzyme involved in the synthesis of PGI_2, can be inhibited by several lipid peroxides such as 15-hydroperoxy-arachidonic acid (29,58,84). Lipid peroxidation has been reported in hyperlipidemia accompanying atherosclerosis, and the inhibition of prostacyclin formation by lipid peroxides has been proposed as the biochemical basis for the increased tendency to thrombosis observed during atherosclerosis (60,63). Moreover, a decreased synthesis of PGI_2 by atherosclerotic vessels has been demonstrated (2,19,47). In addition, it has been shown that the cholesterol carrying low density lipoproteins (LDL), and cholesterol itself, may also inhibit PGI_2 synthesis, whereas high density lipoproteins (HDL) protect against this inhibitory effect (26,72,97). On the other hand, free oxygen radicals may inactivate prostacyclin-synthetase from endothelial cell microsomes (96) and also the biological activity of prostacyclin (98). Free oxygen radicals are produced during transformation of endoperoxides into prostacyclin, and the generation of these substances has been proposed as an autoinactivating process. However, the intact endothelium is considerably more resistant than the isolated enzyme to the inhibitory effect of free oxygen radicals on PGI_2 synthesis (97). Among pharmacological agents, tranylcypromine is an inhibitor of prostacyclin synthetase, an effect only obtained at high concentrations of the compound (29).

Finally, β-thromboglobulin, a protein released from the α-granules during platelet activation, has been reported to suppress prostacyclin production by endothelial cells (36), a phenomenon that could locally promote platelet aggregation.

Heparin may interfere with the biological activity of prostacyclin. Saba et al. (83) have recently reported that heparin neutralizes *in vitro* the inhibitory effect of PGI_2 on platelet aggregation and inhibits the PGI_2-induced enhancement of platelet cyclic AMP levels. The described mechanism appears to involve a direct interaction in which heparin neutralizes the inhibitory effect of PGI_2 on platelet aggregation but does not lose its anticoagulant activity. Eldor and Weksler (25) also reported that heparin antagonizes PGI_2 inhibition of platelet aggregation. However, these authors were unable to demonstrate a direct neutralization of PGI_2 by heparin (23); and they have attributed their findings to the opposing effects of PGI_2 and heparin on platelet adenylate cyclase (81). The above mentioned mechanisms may explain the potentiation of platelet aggregation by heparin and some cases of heparin-related thrombocytopenia and thrombosis (15). It should be stressed here that heparin is not a homogeneous substance, and that binding and activation of platelets by heparin has mainly been seen with heparin preparations of higher molecular weight.

DIETARY MANIPULATION OF PROSTACYCLIN SYNTHESIS

Arachidonic acid, the substrate for PGI_2 production, can be obtained from the diet as such, or synthesized from dietary linoleic acid through processes of desaturation and elongation (27). Changes in intake of polyunsaturated fatty acids, that would modify prostaglandin synthesis in a way that could help prevent thrombosis, have been proposed. The first approach to this problem, before the discovery of prostacyclin, was to propose the dietary use of dihomo-γ-linolenic acid, the precursor of the monoenoic series of prostaglandins (103). In this case the cyclic endoperoxides formed (PGG_1 and PGH_1) do not promote platelet aggregation; moreover, if platelets could synthesize PGE_1, platelet aggregation would be inhibited. In spite of this, PGG_1 and PGH_1 are not substrates for the production of prostacyclin (64), and it has recently been reported that the addition of dihomo-γ-linolenic acid (71), as well as other fatty acids (88), to the incubation medium reduces the release of prostacyclin from endothelial cells in culture.

More recently, the dietary use of eicosapentaenoic acid, the precursor of the trienoic series of prostaglandins, has been suggested for the same purpose (22). This suggestion was based on the observation that Eskimos, who present a low incidence of myocardial infarction and a moderate tendency to bleed, use a diet that has a high eicosapentaenoic and low arachidonic acid content (21). In these conditions thromboxane A_3 is synthesized, and this compound is less proaggregatory than thromboxane A_2 (30,67,80,87). In addition, it has recently been demonstrated that the cyclic endoperoxide PGH_3 is very rapidly transformed into PGD_3, which potently inhibits platelet aggregation (68,101). On the other hand, the cyclic endoperoxides of this series could also be transformed by the vessel wall into PGI_3 (Δ_{17}-prostacyclin) (30,67). This compound has been synthesized and has antiaggregating properties and potency similar to PGI_2 (40). In view of these findings, it has been suggested that the use of eicosapentaenoic acid could offer a dietary protection against thrombosis (21,22,86). However, it has recently been demonstrated that this fatty acid is a poor substrate for cyclooxygenase (67) and for the generation of PGI_2-like activity (90). In consequence, more experimental and clinical work will be necessary to determine the most rational approach to dietary control of thrombus formation in man.

ACKNOWLEDGMENTS

This work was supported in part by the Belgian Fonds voor Geneeskundig Wetenschappelijk Onderzoek. Dr. L. O. Carreras is the recipient of a grant from the "Consejo Nacional de Investigaciones Científicas y Técnicas de la República Argentina."

REFERENCES

1. Amezcua, J. L., O'Grady, J., Salmon, J. A., and Moncada, S. (1979): Prolonged paradoxical effect of aspirin on platelet behaviour and bleeding time in man. *Thromb. Res.*, 16:69–79.
2. Angelo, V. D., Villa, S., Myskiewiec, M., Donati, M. B., and de Gaetano, G. (1978): Defective fibrinolytic and prostacyclin-like activity in human atheromatous plaques. *Thromb. Diath. Haemorrh.*, 39:535–536.
3. Awbrey, B. J., Hoak, J. C., and Owen, W. G. (1979): Binding of human thrombin to cultured human endothelial cells. *J. Biol. Chem.*, 254:4092–4095.
4. Baenziger, N. L., Becherer, P. R., and Majerus, P. W. (1979): Characterization of prostacyclin synthesis in cultured human arterial smooth muscle cells, venous endothelial cells and skin fibroblasts. *Cell*, 16:967–974.
5. Baenziger, N. L., Dillender, M. J., and Majerus, P. W. (1977): Cultured human skin fibroblasts and arterial cells produce a labile platelet-inhibitory prostaglandin. *Biochem. Biophys. Res. Commun.*, 78:294–301.
6. Blajchman, M. A., Senyi, A. F., Hirsh, J., Surya, Y., Buchanan, M., and Mustard, J. F. (1979): Shortening of the bleeding time in rabbits by hydrocortisone caused by inhibition of prostacyclin generation by the vessel wall. *J. Clin. Invest.*, 63:1026–1035.
7. Blass, K. E., Block, H. U., Förster, W., and Pönicke, K. (1980): Dipyridamole: A potent stimulator of prostacyclin (PGI_2) biosynthesis. *Br. J. Pharmacol.*, 68:71–73.
8. Brotherton, A. F., and Hoak, J. C. (1980): Role of Ca^{++} ions and cyclic AMP in the regulation of PGI_2 release from the vascular endothelium. *Circulation*, 62, Part III:165(Abstract).
9. Buchanan, M. R., Dejana, E., Cazenave, J. P., Richardson, M., Mustard, J. F., and Hirsh, J. (1980): Differences in inhibition of PGI_2 production by aspirin in rabbit artery and vein segments. *Thromb. Res.*, 20:447–460.
10. Buchanan, M. R., Dejana, E., Gent, M., Mustard, J. F., and Hirsh, J. (1981): Enhanced platelet accumulation onto injured carotid arteries in rabbits after aspirin treatment. *J. Clin. Invest.*, 67:503–508.
11. Buchanan, M. R., and Hirsh, J. (1980): The inhibitory effect of aspirin on platelet function independent of acetylation of cyclo-oxygenase. *Circulation*, 62(Suppl. III):108(Abstract).
12. Bunting, S., Gryglewski, R., Moncada, S., and Vane, J. R. (1976): Arterial walls generate from prostaglandin endoperoxides a substance (prostaglandin X) which relaxes strips of mesenteric and coeliac arteries and inhibits platelet aggregation. *Prostaglandins*, 12:897–913.
13. Bunting, S., Moncada, S., and Vane, J. R. (1977): Antithrombotic properties of vascular endothelium. *Lancet*, 2:1075–1076.
14. Burch, J. W., Stanford, N., and Majerus, P. W. (1978): Inhibition of platelet prostaglandin synthetase by oral aspirin. *J. Clin. Invest.*, 61:314–319.
15. Carreras, L. O. (1980): Thrombosis and thrombocytopenia induced by heparin. In: *Clinical Usage of Heparin. Present and Future Trends*, edited by M. Verstraete and S. J. Machin. *Scand. J. Haematol.*, 25(Suppl. 36):64–80.
16. Carreras, L. O., Chamone, D. A. F., Klerckx, P., and Vermylen, J. (1980): Decreased vascular prostacyclin (PGI_2) in diabetic rats. Stimulation of PGI_2 release in normal and diabetic rats by the antithrombotic compound Bay g 6575. *Thromb. Res.*, 19:663–670.

17. Czervionke, R. L., Hoak, J. C., and Fry, G. L. (1978): Effect of aspirin on thrombin-induced adherence of platelets to cultured cells from the blood vessel wall. *J. Clin. Invest.*, 62:847–856.
18. Defreyn, G., Machin, S. J., Carreras, L. O., Vergara Dauden, M., Chamone, D. A. F., and Vermylen, J. (1981): Familial bleeding tendency with partial platelet thromboxane synthetase deficiency. Reorientation of cyclic endoperoxide metabolism. *Br. J. Haematol.*, 49:29–41.
19. Dembinska-Kiec, A., Gryglewska, T., Zmuda, A., and Gryglewski, R. J. (1977): The generation of prostacyclin by arteries and by the coronary vascular bed is reduced in experimental atherosclerosis in rabbit. *Prostaglandins*, 14:1025–1034.
20. Dybdahl, J. H., Daae, L. N. W., Eika, C., Godal, H. C., and Larsen, S. (1981): Acetylsalicylic acid-induced prolongation of bleeding time in healthy men. *Scand. J. Haematol.*, 26:50–56.
21. Dyerberg, J., and Bang, H. O. (1979): Haemostatic function and platelet polyunsaturated fatty acids in eskimos. *Lancet*, 2:433–435.
22. Dyerberg, J., Bang, H. O., Stoffersen, E., Moncada, S., and Vane, J. R. (1978): Eicosapentaenoic acid and prevention of thrombosis and atherosclerosis? *Lancet*, 2:117–119.
23. Eldor, A., Allan, G., and Weksler, B. B. (1980): Heparin-prostacyclin interactions: Heparin does not modify the prostacyclin induced relaxation of coronary vasculature. *Thromb. Res.*, 19:719–723.
24. Eldor, A., Falcone, D. J., Hajjar, D. P., Minick, C. R., and Weksler, B. B. (1981): Recovery of prostacyclin production by de-endothelialized rabbit aorta. Critical role of neointimal smooth muscle cells. *J. Clin. Invest.*, 67:735–741.
25. Eldor, A., and Weksler, B. B. (1979): Heparin and dextran sulfate antagonize PGI_2 inhibition of platelet aggregation. *Thromb. Res.*, 16:617–628.
26. Evensen, S. A. (1979): Injury to cultured endothelial cells: The role of lipoproteins and thromboactive agents. *Hemostasis*, 8:203–210.
27. Garattini, S., Di Minno, G., and de Gaetano, G. (1980): Modulation of arachidonic acid metabolism: Dietary and pharmacological perspectives. In: *Hemostasis, Prostaglandins, and Renal Disease*, edited by G. Remuzzi, G. Mecca, and G. de Gaetano, pp. 217–233. Raven Press, New York.
28. Godal, H. C., Eika, C., Dybdahl, J. H., Daae, L., and Larsen, S. (1979): Aspirin and bleeding time. *Lancet*, 1:1236.
29. Gryglewski, R. J., Bunting, S., Moncada, S., Flower, R. J., and Vane, J. R. (1976): Arterial walls are protected against deposition of platelet thrombi by a substance (prostaglandin X) which they make from prostaglandin endoperoxides. *Prostaglandins*, 12:685–714.
30. Gryglewski, R. J., Salmon, J. A., Ubatuba, F. B., Weatherly, B. C., Moncada, S., and Vane, J. R. (1979): Effects of all *cis*-5,8,11,14,17 eicosapentaenoic acid and PGH_3 on platelet aggregation. *Prostaglandins*, 18:453–478.
31. Hanley, S. P., Bevan, J., Cockbill, S. R., and Heptinstall, S. (1981): Differential inhibition by low-dose aspirin of human venous prostacyclin synthesis and platelet thromboxane synthesis. *Lancet*, 1:969–971.
32. Hansen, H. S. (1976): 15-Hydroxyprostaglandin dehydrogenase. A review. *Prostaglandins*, 12:647–676.
33. Hirata, F., Schiffmann, E., Venkatasubramanian, K., Salomon, D., and Axelrod, J. (1980): A phospholipase A_2 inhibitory protein in rabbit neutrophils induced by glucocorticoids. *Proc. Natl. Acad. Sci. USA*, 77:2533–2536.
34. Hong, S. L. (1980): Effect of bradykinin and thrombin on prostacyclin synthesis in endothelial cells from calf and pig aorta and human umbilical cord vein. *Thromb. Res.*, 18:787–799.
35. Hoogendijk, E. M. G., and ten Cate, J. W. (1980): Aspirin and platelets. *Lancet*, 1:93–94.
36. Hope, W., Martin, T. J., Chesterman, C. N., and Morgan, F. J. (1979): Human beta thromboglobulin inhibits PGI_2 production and binds to a specific site on bovine aortic endothelial cells. *Nature*, 282:210–212.
37. Hopkins, N. K., and Gorman, R. R. (1981): Regulation of endothelial cell cyclic nucleotide metabolism by prostacyclin. *J. Clin. Invest.*, 67:540–546.
38. Hornstra, G., Haddeman, E., and Don, J. A. (1979): Blood platelets do not provide endoperoxides for vascular prostacyclin production. *Nature*, 279:66–68.
39. Jaffe, E. A., and Weksler, B. B. (1979): Recovery of endothelial cell prostacyclin production after inhibition by low doses of aspirin. *J. Clin. Invest.*, 63:532–535.
40. Johnson, R. A., Lincoln, F. H., Nidy, E. G., Schneider, W. P., Thompson, J. L., and Axen, U. (1978): Synthesis and characterization of prostacyclin, 6-ketoprostaglandin $F_{1\alpha}$, prostaglandin I_1, and prostaglandin I_3. *J. Am. Chem. Soc.*, 100:7690–7705.

41. Kelton, J. G., Hirsh, J., Carter, C. J., and Buchanan, M. R. (1978): Thrombogenic effect of high-dose aspirin in rabbits. Relationship to inhibition of vessel wall synthesis of prostaglandin I_2-like activity. *J. Clin. Invest.*, 62:892–895.
42. Kirstein, A. (1979): Cardiac prostacyclin release: Stimulation by hypoxia and various agents. *Scand. J. Haematol.*, 23(Suppl. 34):105–111.
43. Knapp, H. R., Oelz, O., Roberts, L. J., Sweetman, B. J., Oates, J. O., and Reed, P. W. (1977): Ionophores stimulate prostaglandin and thromboxane biosynthesis. *Proc. Natl. Acad. Sci. USA*, 74:4251–4255.
44. Korbut, R., and Moncada, S. (1978): Prostacyclin (PGI_2) and thromboxane A_2 interaction *in vivo*. Regulation by aspirin and relationship with antithrombotic therapy. *Thromb. Res.*, 13:489–500.
45. Lansen, J., Biagi, G., Niebes, P., Gordon, J., and Roncucci, R. (1979): Effect of suloctidil on PGI_2 production and inhibition of platelet aggregation. *Thromb. Haemost.*, 42:368(Abstract).
46. Lapetina, E. G., Schmitges, C. G., Chandrabose, K., and Cuatrecasas, P. (1977): cAMP and PGX inhibit membrane phospholipase activity in platelets. *Biochem. Biophys. Res. Commun.*, 76:828–835.
47. Larrue, J., Rigaud, M., Daret, D., Demond, J., Durand, J., and Bricaud, H. (1980): Prostacyclin production by cultured smooth muscle cells from atherosclerotic rabbit aorta. *Nature*, 285:480–482.
48. Levin, R. I., Jaffe, E. A., Weksler, B. B., and Tack-Goldman, K. (1981): Nitroglycerin stimulates synthesis of prostacyclin by cultured human endothelial cells. *J. Clin. Invest.*, 67:762–769.
49. Marcus, A. J., Weksler, B. B., and Jaffe, E. A. (1978): Enzymatic conversion of prostaglandin endoperoxide H_2 and arachidonic acid to prostacyclin by cultured human endothelial cells. *J. Biol. Chem.*, 253:7138–7141.
50. Marcus, A. J., Weksler, B. B., and Jaffe, E. A. (1979): Synthesis of prostacyclin by cultured human endothelial cells. In: *Prostacyclin*, edited by J. R. Vane and S. Bergström, pp. 65–73. Raven Press, New York.
51. Marcus, A. J., Weksler, B. B., Jaffe, E. A., and Broekman, M. J. (1980): Synthesis of prostacyclin from platelet-derived endoperoxides by cultured human endothelial cells. *J. Clin. Invest.*, 66:979–986.
52. Masotti, G., Galanti, G., Poggesi, L., Abbate, R., and Neri Serneri, G. G. (1979): Differential inhibition of prostacyclin production and platelet aggregation by aspirin. *Lancet*, 2:1213–1216.
53. McIntyre, D. E., Pearson, J. D., and Gordon, J. L. (1978): Localization and stimulation of prostacyclin production in vascular cells. *Nature*, 271:549–551.
54. McKenna, R., Galante, J., Bachmann, F., Wallace, D. L., Kaushal, S. P., and Meredith, P. (1980): Prevention of venous thromboembolism after total knee replacement by high-dose aspirin or intermittent calf and thigh compression. *Br. Med. J.*, 280:514–517.
55. Miller, O. V., Aiken, J. W., Hemker, D. P., Shebuski, R. J., and Gorman, R. R. (1979): Prostacyclin stimulation of dog arterial cyclic AMP levels. *Prostaglandins*, 18:915–925.
56. Moncada, S., Bunting, S., Mullane, K., Thorogood, P., Vane, J. R., Ray, A., and Needleman, P. (1977): Imidazole: A selective inhibitor of thromboxane synthetase. *Prostaglandins*, 13:611–618.
57. Moncada, S., Gryglewski, R. J., Bunting, S., and Vane, J. R. (1976): An enzyme isolated from arteries transforms prostaglandin endoperoxides to an unstable substance that inhibits platelet aggregation. *Nature*, 263:663–665.
58. Moncada, S., Gryglewski, R. J., Bunting, S., and Vane J. R. (1976): A lipid peroxide inhibits the enzyme in blood vessel microsomes that generates from prostaglandin endoperoxides the substance (prostaglandin X) which prevents platelet aggregation. *Prostaglandins*, 12:715–733.
59. Moncada, S., Herman, A. G., Higgs, E. A., and Vane, J. R. (1977): Differential formation of prostacyclin (PGX or PGI_2) by layers of the arterial wall. An explanation for the antithrombotic properties of vascular endothelium. *Thromb. Res.*, 11:323–344.
60. Moncada, S., Higgs, E. A., and Vane, J. R. (1977): Human arterial and venous tissues generate prostacyclin (prostaglandin X), a potent inhibitor of platelet aggregation. *Lancet*, 1:18–20.
61. Moncada, S., and Korbut, R. (1978): Dipyridamole and other phosphodiesterase inhibitors act as antithrombotic agents by potentiating endogenous prostacyclin. *Lancet*, 1:1286–1289.
62. Moncada, S., and Vane, J. R. (1978): Unstable metabolites of arachidonic acid and their role in haemostasis and thrombosis. *Br. Med. Bull.*, 34:129–135.
63. Moncada, S., and Vane, J. R. (1979): Arachidonic acid metabolites and the interactions between platelets and blood-vessel walls. *N. Engl. J. Med.*, 300:1142–1147.

64. Moncada, S., and Vane, J. R. (1979): Pharmacology and endogenous roles of prostaglandin endoperoxides, thromboxane A₂, and prostacyclin. *Pharmacol. Rev.*, 30:293–331.

65. Needleman, P., Bronson, S. D., Wyche, A., Sivakoff, M., and Nicolaou, K. D. (1978): Cardiac and renal prostaglandin I₂: Biosynthesis and biological effects in isolated perfused rabbit tissues. *J. Clin. Invest.*, 61:839–849.

66. Needleman, P., Raz, A., Ferrendelli, J. A., and Minkes, M. (1977): Application of imidazole as a selective inhibitor of thromboxane synthetase in human platelets. *Proc. Natl. Acad. Sci. USA*, 74:1716–1720.

67. Needleman, P., Raz, A., Minkes, M. S., Ferrendelli, J. A., and Sprecher, H. (1979): Triene prostaglandins: Prostacyclin and thromboxane biosynthesis and unique biological properties. *Proc. Natl. Acad. Sci. USA*, 76:944–948.

68. Needleman, P., Sprecher, H., Whitaker, M. O., and Wyche, A. (1980): Mechanism underlying the inhibition of platelet aggregation by eicosapentaenoic acid and its metabolites. In: *Advances in Prostaglandin and Thromboxane Research*, Vol. 6, edited by B. Samuelsson, P. W. Ramwell, and R. Paoletti, pp. 61–68. Raven Press, New York.

69. Needleman, P., Wyche, A., and Raz, A. (1979): Platelet and blood vessel arachidonate metabolism and interactions. *J. Clin. Invest.*, 63:345–349.

70. Nijkamp, R. P., Moncada, S., White, H. L., and Vane, J. R. (1977): Diversion of prostaglandin endoperoxide metabolism by selective inhibition of thromboxane A₂ biosynthesis in lung, spleen or platelets. *Eur. J. Pharmacol*, 44:179–186.

71. Nordoy, A., Svensson, B., and Hoak, J. C. (1979): The effects of albumin bound fatty acids on the platelet inhibitory function of human endothelial cells. *Eur. J. Clin. Invest.*, 9:5–10.

72. Nordoy, A., Svensson, B., Wiebe, D., and Hoak, J. C. (1978): Lipoproteins and the inhibitory effect of human endothelial cells on platelet function. *Circ. Res.*, 43:527–534.

73. O'Brien, J. R. (1980): Platelets and the vessel wall: how much aspirin? *Lancet*, 1:372–373.

74. O'Grady, J., and Moncada, S. (1978): Aspirin, a paradoxical effect on bleeding time. *Lancet*, 2:780.

75. Pareti, F. I., D'Angelo, A., Mannucci, P. M., and Smith, J. B. (1980): Platelets and the vessel wall: How much aspirin? *Lancet*, 1:371–372.

76. Pareti, F. I., Mannucci, P. M., D'Angelo, A., Smith, J. B., Sautebin, L., and Galli, G. (1980): Congenital deficiency of thromboxane and prostacyclin. *Lancet*, 1:898–901.

77. Pickett, W. C., Jesse, R. L., and Cohen, P. (1977): Initiation of phospholipase A₂ activity in human platelets by the calcium ion ionophore A 23187. *Biochim. Biophys. Acta*, 486:209–213.

78. Preston, F. E., Whipps, S., Jackson, C. A., French, A. J., Wyld, P. J., and Stoddard, C. J. (1981): Inhibition of prostacyclin and platelet thromboxane A₂ after low-dose aspirin. *N. Engl. J. Med.*, 304:76–79.

79. Rajah, S. M., and Penny, S. (1978): Aspirin and bleeding time. *Lancet*, 2:1104.

80. Raz, A., Minkes, M. S., and Needleman, P. (1977): Endoperoxides and thromboxanes. Structural determinants for platelet aggregation and vasoconstriction. *Biochim. Biophys. Acta*, 488:305–311.

81. Reches, A., Eldor, A., and Salomon, Y. (1979): Heparin inhibits PGE₁-sensitive adenylate cyclase and antagonizes PGE₁ antiaggregating effect in human platelets. *J. Lab. Clin. Med.*, 93:638–644.

82. Reyers, I., Mussoni, L., Donati, M. B., and de Gaetano, G. (1980): Failure of aspirin at different doses to modify experimental thrombosis in rats. *Thromb. Res.*, 18:669–674.

83. Saba, H. I., Saba, S. R., Blackburn, C. A., Hartmann, R. C., and Mason, R. G. (1979): Heparin neutralization of PGI₂: Effects upon platelets. *Science*, 205:499–501.

84. Salmon, J. A., Smith, D. R., Flower, R. J., Moncada, S., and Vane, J. R. (1978): Further studies on the enzymatic conversion of prostaglandin endoperoxide into prostacyclin by porcine aorta microsomes. *Biochim. Biophys. Acta*, 523:250–262.

85. Seuter, F., Busse, W. D., Meng, K., Hoffmeister, F., Moller, E., and Horstmann, H. (1979): The antithrombotic activity of Bay g 6575. *Arzneim. Forsch.*, 29:54–59.

86. Siess, W., Roth, P., Scherer, B., Kurzmann, I., Böhlig, B., and Weber, P. C. (1980): Platelet-membrane fatty acids, platelet aggregation, and thromboxane formation during a mackerel diet. *Lancet*, 1:441–444.

87. Smith, D. R., Weatherly, B. C., Salmon, J. A., Ubatuba, F. B., Gryglewski, R. J., and Moncada, S. (1979): Preparation and biochemical properties of PGH₃. *Prostaglandins*, 18:423–438.

88. Spector, A. A., Hoak, J. C., Fry, G. L., Denning, G. M., Stoll, L. L., and Smith, J. B. (1980): Effect of fatty acid modification of prostacyclin production by cultured human endothelial cells. *J. Clin. Invest.*, 65:1003–1012.

89. Sun, F. F., Taylor, B. M., McGuire, J. C., Wong, P. Y.-K., Malik, K. U., and McGiff, J. C. (1979): Metabolic disposition of prostacyclin. In: *Prostacyclin*, edited by J. R. Vane, and S. Bergström, pp. 119–131. Raven Press, New York.

90. ten Hoor, F., de Deckere, E. A. M., Haddeman, E., Hornstra, G., and Quadt, J. F. A. (1980): Dietary manipulation of prostaglandin and thromboxane synthesis in heart, aorta, and blood platelets of the rat. In: *Advances in Prostaglandin and Thromboxane Research*, edited by B. Samuelsson, P. W. Ramwell, and R. Paoletti, pp. 1771–1781. Raven Press, New York.

91. Van de Velde, V., Beetens, J., and Herman, A. G. (1980): Interactions of dipyridamole with prostacyclin biosynthesis. *Acta Therap.*, 6(Suppl.):15.

92. Vermylen, J., Chamone, D. A. F., and Verstraete, M. (1979): Stimulation of prostacyclin release from vessel wall by Bay g 6575, an antithrombotic compound. *Lancet*, 1:518–520.

93. Vermylen, J., Defreyn, G., Carreras, L. O., Machin, S. J., Van Schaeren, J., and Verstraete, M. (1981): Thromboxane synthetase inhibition as antithrombotic strategy. *Lancet*, 1:1073–1075.

94. Villa, S., Cavenaghi, A. E., and de Gaetano, G. (1979): Suloctidil does not inhibit vascular prostacyclin activity in rats. *Thromb. Haemost.*, 42:368(Abstract).

95. Villa, S., Livio, M., and de Gaetano, G. (1979): The inhibitory effect of aspirin on platelet and vascular prostaglandins in rats cannot be completely dissociated. *Br. J. Haematol.*, 42:425–431.

96. Weiss, S. J., Turk, J., and Needleman, P. (1979): A mechanism for the hydroperoxide-mediated inactivation of prostacyclin synthetase. *Blood*, 53:1191–1196.

97. Weksler, B. B., Eldor, A., Falcone, D., Levin, R. I., Jaffe, E. A., and Minick, C. R. (1982): Prostaglandins and vascular endothelium. In: *Cardiovascular Pharmacology of the Prostaglandins*, edited by A. G. Herman, P. Vanhoutte, H. Denolin and A. Goossens, pp. 137–148. Raven Press, New York.

98. Weksler, B. B., Knapp, J., and Tack-Goldman, K. (1979): Prostacyclin (PGI$_2$) is destroyed by superoxide produced by human polymorphonuclear leukocytes. *Clin. Res.*, 27:466A.

99. Weksler, B. B., Ley, C. W., and Jaffe, E. A. (1978): Stimulation of endothelial cell prostacyclin production by thrombin, trypsin and the ionophore A23187. *J. Clin. Invest.*, 62:923–930.

100. Weksler, B. B., Marcus, A. J., and Jaffe, E. A. (1977): Synthesis of prostaglandin I$_2$ (prostacyclin) by cultured human and bovine endothelial cells. *Proc. Natl. Acad. Sci. USA*, 74:3922–3926.

101. Whitaker, M. O., Needleman, P., Wyche, A., Fitzpatrick, F. A., and Sprecher, H. (1980): PGD$_3$ is the mediator of the antiaggregatory effects of the trienoic endoperoxide PGH$_3$. In: *Advances in Prostaglandin and Thromboxane Research*, Vol. 6, edited by B. Samuelsson, P. W. Ramwell, and R. Paoletti, pp. 301–303. Raven Press, New York.

102. Willems, C., and van Aken, W. G. (1979): Production of prostacyclin by vascular endothelial cells. *Haemostasis*, 8:266–273.

103. Willis, A. L., Comai, K., Kuhn, D. C., and Paulsrud, J. (1974): Dihomo-γ-linolenate suppresses platelet aggregation when administered *in vitro* or *in vivo*. *Prostaglandins*, 8:509–519.

5-Hydroxytryptamine in Peripheral Reactions,
edited by Fred De Clerck and Paul M.
Vanhoutte. Raven Press, New York © 1982.

Clinical Syndromes Related to Platelet Activation *In Vivo*

*S. Cortellazzo, *P. Viero, **T. Barbui, and †G. de Gaetano

*Division of Hematology, Ospedale Generale Regionale, Vicenza, Italy; **Division of Hematology, Ospedali Riuniti, Bergamo, Italy; and †Laboratory of Cardiovascular Clinical Pharmacology, Istituto di Ricerche Farmacologiche "Mario Negri," 20157 Milan, Italy*

Normally platelets neither adhere to vascular wall nor aggregate, but they do so if exposed to a number of "inducers" such as thrombin, immune complexes, or damaged vessel wall.

Clinical conditions in which platelet involvement has been documented include glomerulonephritis (15), myeloproliferative disorders (2), and thrombotic microangiopathy (hemolytic uremic syndrome, thrombotic thrombocytopenic purpura, preeclampsia) (9,18).

In all these conditions platelet involvement is reflected by the presence in the circulation of "exhausted" platelets. Patients with disorders progressing to renal failure (for instance, systemic lupus erythematosus) reportedly show lowered intraplatelet 5-hydroxytryptamine, as do patients with chronic myeloid leukemia or hemolytic uremic syndrome. This common laboratory feature may possibly be the consequence of *in vivo* platelet activation triggered, however, by different mechanisms. Indeed, it has been suggested that circulating immune complexes interact with platelets in patients with systemic lupus erythematosus (15) or thrombotic thrombocytopenic purpura (1). It appears that defective intraplatelet mechanisms controlling platelet function might play a pathogenic role in the thrombotic complications of myeloproliferative disorders (5). More recently, a disturbed plasmatic control of vascular prostacyclin production was proposed as being responsible for intravascular platelet activation in some patients with thrombotic microangiopathy (9) or anticoagulant lupus (4). This chapter focuses on the possible mechanisms underlying the reduced intraplatelet levels of 5-hydroxytryptamine in patients with myeloproliferative disorders.

Human platelets contain a high concentration of 5-hydroxytryptamine in storage organelles, called dense granules, together with nucleotides and calcium. 5-Hydroxytryptamine is not synthesized by platelets, but is taken up from the blood. The incorporation process involves three steps: transport through the membrane, accumulation in the cytosol and transport through the storage granule membrane, formation of complexes with adenine nucleotides and divalent cations inside the dense granules (10). Platelet 5-hydroxytryptamine is secreted following stimulation by agents such as thrombin, collagen, or products of prostaglandin biosynthesis (13).

Platelets of patients with myeloproliferative diseases such as polycythemia vera, chronic myelogenous leukemia, idiopathic myelofibrosis, and essential thrombocythemia, have a low 5-hydroxytryptamine content (8,17). This finding has been interpreted as the consequence of a reduction or absence of platelet dense bodies (14,19) or of a release reaction occurring *in vivo* (2). The platelet abnormality in myeloproliferative disease patients has been compared to that occurring in congenital storage pool disease (17). Indeed, besides the very low 5-hydroxytryptamine content, platelets of patients with myeloproliferative disease showed reduced 5-hydroxytryptamine uptake and increased leakage of the amine during prolonged *in vitro* incubation with imipramine (17). Defective active transport of 5-hydroxytryptamine across the platelet plasma membrane has also been reported in myeloproliferative disease patients by Caranobe et al. (3).

In an attempt to clarify if the platelet defect in myeloproliferative disease is due to the presence of an abnormal stem cell line or to exposure of platelets to inducers of the release reaction *in vivo*, we investigated 5-hydroxytryptamine content, uptake, and release in platelets from patients with different myeloproliferative diseases. In some of them 5-hydroxytryptamine content was also measured after 10 days of treatment with aspirin.

PATIENTS AND METHODS

Myeloproliferative disease was diagnosed in 23 patients, 10 males and 13 females (32–74 years old). There were 7 cases of polycythemia vera, 9 cases of chronic myelogenous leukemia, 4 of essential thrombocythemia, and 3 of idiopathic myelofibrosis. Diagnosis was based on pertinent clinical and laboratory data. All patients were newly diagnosed and had not been given drugs known to affect platelet function in the 2 weeks before the study. Routine coagulation tests were within the normal range in all cases. The control group consisted of 23 sex- and age-matched normal subjects, most of them laboratory and hospital personnel.

Platelets were counted by phase contrast microscopy. Blood collection, platelet-rich plasma, and platelet-poor plasma were prepared as previously described (6). Intraplatelet 5-hydroxytryptamine was measured by the formation of a fluorophore with *o*-phthaldialdehyde, in 1 ml volume of platelet-rich plasma according to the spectrofluorometric method of Drummond and Gordon (11). In 6 patients, 5-hydroxytryptamine was also determined after 10 days oral treatment with aspirin (1 g/daily).

Active uptake of 5-hydroxy[G-^{3}H]tryptamine creatinine sulphate (Amersham, specific activity 500 mCi/mmoles) was measured according to Gordon and Olverman (12). Radioactivity was measured by a liquid scintillation counter (Packard Tri Carb Tandem Liquid Scintillation Spectrometer, Model 3385) for 2 min. When the same experiment was conducted at 4°C active transport was abolished and the amount of [^{3}H]5-hydroxytryptamine bound to platelets represented the radioactive amine that remained in the extracellular spaces of the pellet (zero time). Radioactivity values (cpm) obtained at zero time were subtracted from the corresponding values (cpm) obtained at 37°C. Thereafter, cpm were transformed in pmoles/platelets/time calculating the ratio of pmoles to cpm from the standards.

Each concentration of the [^{3}H]5-hydroxytryptamine substrate was plotted against the velocity of uptake expressed in pmoles/platelets/time. Apparent K_m and V_{max} values for [^{3}H]5-hydroxytryptamine were determined by Lineweaver and Burk plot using an appropriate computer program (22). Percentage total (active and passive) [^{3}H]5-hydroxytryptamine taken up by and its leakage from platelets was measured according to Pareti et al. (16).

To inhibit [^{3}H]5-hydroxytryptamine reuptake during prolonged incubation, 20 μM imipramine (Ciba-Geigy, Basel, Switzerland) was added to the platelet-rich plasma (3 ml) preincubated for 15 min at 37°C with [^{3}H]5-hydroxytryptamine. To increase [^{3}H]5-hydroxytryptamine efflux from platelets, (+)fenfluramine HCl (Servier, Paris, France) was added at various concentrations (1,10,50 μM) to the platelet-rich plasma preincubated with [^{3}H]5-hydroxytryptamine as in the experiment with imipramine, and aliquots were removed at fixed times thereafter (30, 60, 120 min). Results are expressed as mean ± SD.

RESULTS

The endogenous platelet 5-hydroxytryptamine concentration values were below the control range in all but 3 patients (Fig. 1). The average 5-hydroxytryptamine content (nmoles/10^8 platelets) was 0.34 ± 0.12 and 0.10 ± 0.11 in controls and patients, respectively ($p < 0.001$, Student's t test). In 6 patients the low concentration of 5-hydroxytryptamine in the platelet did not appear to be modified after treatment with aspirin (Table 1). K_m and V_{max} for [^{3}H]5-hydroxytryptamine platelet active uptake were similar in controls and patients (Table 2).

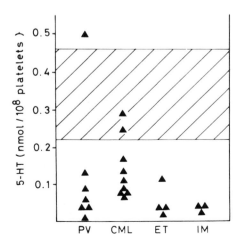

FIG. 1. Platelet 5-hydroxytryptamine (5-HT) concentrations in myeloproliferative disorders: polycythemia vera (PV); chronic myelogenous leukemia (CML); essential thrombocythemia (ET); idiopathic myelofibrosis (IM). The *shaded area* represents the range in normal controls. Note the reduction of platelet-bound 5-hydroxytryptamine in all but 3 patients.

TABLE 1. *Platelet 5-hydroxytryptamine content before and after 10 days administration of aspirin (1 g/daily) to patients with myeloproliferative diseases*

| | | 5-Hydroxytryptamine (nmoles/10^8 platelets) | |
Patients	Diagnosis	Before	After
C.F.	P.V.	0.04	0.04
R.A.	C.M.L.	0.08	0.08
V.M.	C.M.L.	0.07	0.03
R.I.	C.M.L.	0.08	0.06
B.C.	E.T.	0.11	0.13
T.M.	E.T.	0.02	0.13

P.V. = polycythemia vera; C.M.L. = chronic myelogenous leukemia; E.T. = essential thrombocythemia.

TABLE 2. *[^{3}H]5-Hydroxytryptamine (5-HT) uptake by platelets of patients with myeloproliferative diseases*

| | [^{3}H]5-HT uptake | |
Group	K_m (μM)	V_{max} (pmoles/10^8 platelets/10 sec)
Controls ($n=11$)	0.90 ± 0.61	4.9 ± 1.7
Patients ($n=12$)	1.12 ± 0.55	7.6 ± 3.7

TABLE 3. *Percentage of added [^{3}H]5-hydroxytryptamine taken up by platelets of normals and of patients with myeloproliferative diseases*

Incubation time (min)	Controls ($n=13$)	Patients ($n=15$)
5	40.6 ± 6	34.3 ± 14
10	61.5 ± 7	51.0 ± 16
20	78.0 ± 5	64.0 ± 17
30	81.0 ± 4	71.0 ± 13

Prolonging the incubation period, the total (active and passive) amount of [^{3}H]5-hydroxytryptamine taken up by myeloproliferative disease platelets was slightly but not significantly reduced in comparison with controls (Table 3). Following incubation of platelet-rich plasma of controls or patients with [^{3}H]5-hydroxytryptamine, more than 80% of the radioactive amine remained within the platelets for 240 min. The addition of imipramine to platelet-rich plasma 15 min after [^{3}H]5-hydroxytryptamine resulted in an efflux of the amine of about 5% and 12% from control and patient's platelets, respectively (Table 4). When [^{3}H]5-hydroxytryptamine labeled platelets were incubated for 120 min with 50 μM fenfluramine, a monoamine-

TABLE 4. *Percentage of added [³H]5-hydroxytryptamine bound by platelets of normals and of patients with myeloproliferative diseases*

Incubation time (min)	Without imipramine		With imipramine (20 μM f.c.)	
	Controls (n=9)	Patients (n=14)	Controls (n=9)	Patients (n=14)
90	88 ± 3	83 ± 4	78 ± 8	68 ± 10
120	87 ± 2	83 ± 5	78 ± 7	70 ± 8
180	87 ± 2	81 ± 5	79 ± 6	68 ± 9
240	84 ± 4	79 ± 6	79 ± 6	68 ± 9

TABLE 5. *Release of [³H]5-hydroxytryptamine from platelets induced by (+)fenfluramine*

Group	Incubation with (+)fenfluramine (50 μM)		% Release
	Before	After	
Controls (n=6)	86.5 ± 1.37	66.5 ± 5.75	24
Patients (n=6)	85.0 ± 2.0	59.0 ± 10.0	30

releasing drug (22), the efflux of the radioactive amine was similar in platelet-rich plasma of controls and of patients with myeloproliferative disease (24% and 30%, respectively; Table 5).

DISCUSSION

This study confirms that platelets from patients with myeloproliferative diseases have a very low 5-hydroxytryptamine content. This could be due to: (a) a reduction of dense bodies, (b) a defective transport mechanism, or (c) a release reaction following *in vivo* platelet activation. The former hypothesis is supported by other findings of reduction of dense bodies as seen with the electron microscope, or using mepacrine (14,19). Reduced intraplatelet 5-hydroxytryptamine levels in patients with myeloproliferative disease do not seem to be the consequence of defective transport of the amine at the plasma membrane level. Indeed, the kinetic parameters for active uptake of [³H]5-hydroxytryptamine by such platelets were not significantly different from those obtained in control platelets. Passive diffusion of the radioactive amine and its retention within platelets were also similar in patients and controls.

Pharmacological attempts to unmask a possibly deranged storage mechanism were unsuccessful. Inhibition of 5-hydroxytryptamine reuptake by imipramine or induction of moderate release by fenfluramine did not distinguish control from myeloproliferative disease platelets. The possibility that low 5-hydroxytryptamine levels reflect an *in vivo* platelet release reaction is not supported by the failure of aspirin to raise endogenous platelet 5-hydroxytryptamine concentrations. Aspirin was administered daily for 10 days in order to examine a population of platelets fully exposed to this platelet release reaction-inhibiting drug already upon their entry into circulation. The pharmacological efficacy of aspirin was verified by the complete inhibition of platelet arachidonic acid metabolism (7). However, the possibility cannot be ruled out of *in vivo* platelet activation with subsequent degranulation induced by endogenous stimuli such as thrombin or a "platelet deactivating factor" whose effects are not necessarily prevented by aspirin (20,21). The results of the present study do not completely agree with those of previous investigations (3,17), especially as far as 5-hydroxytryptamine platelet uptake and storage is concerned. This discrepancy may be due to some uncontrolled difference in the patients studied or, more likely, to the different experimental procedures utilized. In this respect, it is worth mentioning that the method used in this study to measure [^{3}H]5-hydroxytryptamine uptake (12) differs from the methods used by others in that it rigorously explores the initial *active* transport of the amine and is not influenced by passive diffusion.

ACKNOWLEDGMENT

This work was supported in part by the Italian CNR ("Farmacologia Clinica e Malattie Rare").

REFERENCES

1. Amorosi, E. L., and Karpatkin, S. (1977): Antiplatelet treatment of thrombotic thrombocytopenic purpura. *Ann. Intern. Med.*, 86:102–106.
2. Boughton, B. J., Cobett, W. E. N., and Ginsburg, A. D. (1977): Myeloproliferative disorders: a paradox of *in-vivo* and *in-vitro* platelet function. *J. Clin. Pathol.*, 30:228–234.
3. Caranobe, C., Sie, P., Nouvel, C., Laurent, G., Pris, J., and Boneu, B. (1980): Platelets in myeloproliferative disorders. II. Serotonin uptake and storage: Correlation with mepacrine labelled dense bodies and with platelet density. *Scand. J. Haematol.*, 25:289–295.
4. Carreras, L. O., Defreyn, G., Machin, S. J., Vermylen, J., Deman, R., Spitz, B., and Van Assche, A. (1981): Arterial thrombosis, intrauterine death and "lupus" anticoagulant: Detection of immunoglobulin interfering with prostacyclin formation. *Lancet*, 1:244–246.
5. Cooper, B., and Ahern, D. (1979): Characterization of the platelet prostaglandin D$_2$ receptor. Loss of prostaglandin D$_2$ receptors in platelets of patients with myeloproliferative disorders. *J. Clin. Invest.*, 64:586–590.
6. Cortelazzo, S., Barbui, T., Bassan, R., and Dini, E. (1980): Abnormal aggregation and increased size of platelets in myeloproliferative disorders. *Thromb. Haemost.*, 43:127–130.
7. Cortelazzo, S., Barbui, T., Viero, P., Bassan, R., Dini, E., and Ferro Milone, F. (1979): Platelet malonyldialdehyde and spontaneous aggregation during ischaemic attacks of patients with polycythaemia vera. *Thromb. Haemost.*, 42:1344–1346.
8. Culebras Poza, J. M., Launay, J. M., Briere, J., and Dreux, C. (1977): Blood platelet and "extra-platelet" serotonin in some myeloproliferative disorders. *Biomedicine*, 27:300–303.
9. Donati, M. B., Misiani, R., Marchesi, D., Livio, M., Mecca, G., Remuzzi, G., and de Gaetano, G. (1980): Hemolytic-uremic syndrome, prostaglandins, and plasma factors. In: *Hemostasis, Prostaglandins, and Renal Disease*, edited by G. Remuzzi, G. Mecca, and G. de Gaetano, pp. 283–290. Raven Press, New York.
10. Drummond, A. H. (1976): Interactions of blood platelets with biogenic amines: Uptake, stimulation and receptor binding. In: *Platelets in Biology and Pathology*, edited by J. L. Gordon, pp. 203–239. North-Holland, Amsterdam.

11. Drummond, A. H., and Gordon, J. L. (1974): Rapid sensitive microassay for platelet 5-HT. *Thromb. Diath. Haemorr.*, 31:366–367.
12. Gordon, J. L., and Olverman, H. J. (1978): 5-Hydroxytryptamine and dopamine transport by rat and human blood platelets. *Br. J. Pharmacol.*, 62:219–226.
13. Kinlough-Rathbon, R. L., Packham, M. A., and Mustard, J. F. (1977): Synergism between platelet aggregating agents: The role of the arachidonate pathway. *Thromb. Res.*, 11:567–580.
14. Maldonado, J. E., Pintado, T., and Pierre, R. V. (1974): Dysplastic platelets and circulating megakaryocytes in chronic myeloproliferative diseases. I. The platelets: Ultrastructure and peroxidase reaction. *Blood*, 43:797–809.
15. Parbtani, A., and Cameron, J. S. (1980): Platelet involvement in glomerulonephritis. In: *Hemostasis, Prostaglandins, and Renal Disease*, edited by G. Remuzzi, G. Mecca, and G. de Gaetano, pp. 45–61. Raven Press, New York.
16. Pareti, F. L., Day, H. J., and Mills, D. C. B. (1974): Nucleotide and serotonin metabolism in platelets with defective secondary aggregation. *Blood*, 44:789–800.
17. Pareti, F. I., Mannucci, P. M., Asti, D., Guarini, A., Gugliotta, L., and Tura, S. (1979): Acquired storage pool disease in myeloproliferative disorders. *Thromb. Haemost.*, 42:44.
18. Prentice, C. R. M. (1980): Intravascular coagulation in preeclampsia: Cause or consequence? In: *Hemostasis, Prostaglandins, and Renal Disease,* edited by G. Remuzzi, G. Mecca, and G. de Gaetano, pp. 347–351. Raven Press, New York.
19. Rendu, F., Lebret, M., Nurden, A. T., and Caen, I. P. (1979): Detection of an acquired platelet storage pool disease in three patients with a myeloproliferative disorder. *Thromb. Haemost.*, 42:794–796.
20. Smith, J. B., and Willis, A. L. (1971): Aspirin selectively inhibits prostaglandin production in human platelets. *Nature (New Biol.)*, 231:235–237.
21. Vargaftig, B. B., Chignard, M., Le Couedic, J. P., and Benveniste, J. (1980): One, two or more pathways for platelet aggregation. *Acta Med. Scand. (Suppl.)*, 642:23–29.
22. Wielosz, M., Roncaglioni, M. C., de Gaetano, G., and Garattini, S. (1977): Interference by fenfluramine with the storage of ^{14}C-5-hydroxytryptamine in rat platelets. *Arch. Int. Pharmacodyn. Ther.*, 225:232–239.

5-Hydroxytryptamine in Peripheral Reactions,
edited by Fred De Clerck and Paul M.
Vanhoutte. Raven Press, New York © 1982.

Malignant Hyperthermia: Etiology, Pathophysiology, and Prevention

*L. A. A. Ooms and **A. K. Verheyen

*Department of Veterinary Pharmacology, and **Laboratory of Cell Biology,
Janssen Pharmaceutica, B-2340 Beerse, Belgium*

The predominant clinical features associated with malignant hyperthermia in humans and swine are gross musculature rigidity (not always present in humans), tachycardia, hyperventilation, rapid rise in body temperature resulting in hyperthermia, and blotchy cyanosis. There is a severe metabolic acidosis with a rise in concentration of serum electrolytes, especially of potassium, calcium, inorganic phosphate, and lactate.

In swine, malignant hyperthermia is a manifestation of a generalized susceptibility to stress. In man, malignant hyperthermia develops suddenly either during or shortly after general anesthesia. Malignant hyperthermia in pigs has been studied in most detail and a recent investigation has shown that the pharmacological properties of the muscle are identical during malignant hyperthermia in both human and swine (52).

The malignant hyperthermia is not confined to humans and pigs. Anesthetic-induced malignant hyperthermia has also been described in dogs (60), cats (13), horses (66), birds (30), as well as wild animals during capture (29,30).

GENETICS

In man, the individuals susceptible to malignant hyperthermia have an underlying disease of the muscles. The more common of the two myopathies is predominantly inherited and usually subclinical (14). There may be some muscle wasting, particularly in the lower parts of the thighs. The second myopathy is probably inherited as a recessive characteristic. It occurs in children, usually boys, who also have a number of physical abnormalities including short stature, abnormal facies, webbing of the neck, winging of the scapulae, ptosis, and an undescended testicle (36). Also in patients with Duchenne muscular dystrophy, halothane and/or succinylcholine may cause augmentation of skeletal muscular damage and/or destruction of skeletal muscles (35).

In pigs, it is hypothesized that multiple alleles are involved in the susceptibility to halothane (37). Pietrain pigs and Belgian Landrace pigs have a susceptibility to halothane-induced malignant hyperthermia of up to 100% and 87%, respectively.

Susceptibility of different breeds is indicated in Table 1. Stress-susceptibility increases in the different breeds with breeding patterns designed to produce pigs with rapid growth rates, good feed efficiency, and superior musculature.

TRIGGERING OF MALIGNANT HYPERTHERMIA

Stress

In swine, the whole syndrome of malignant hyperthermia can be triggered by environmental stress such as exercise (34,51), heat stress (16,34,43), anoxia (39), and excitement (51). In bilaterally amygdalectomized animals, the lesions as well as an increase of norepinephrine in plasma were prevented (33). The psychological mechanisms, therefore, are important for the development of the porcine stress syndrome. In humans, triggering by stress has also been described (20). In addition, susceptible families may have an increased incidence of unexplained sudden deaths (67). Susceptible individuals may develop a nonspecific cardiomyopathy (31).

Inhalation Anesthetics

Most inhalation anesthetics (halothane, methoxyflurane, diethyl ether, ethyl chloride, trichloroethylene, cyclopropane) (6,21,56,63) can induce malignant hyperthermia in pigs. In susceptible humans malignant hyperthermia can also be triggered by inhalation anesthetics. Halothane acts beyond the neuromuscular junction (50). It produces a depolarization (5–10 mV) of susceptible skeletal muscle but not of the normal muscle (18), and causes contractures via mechanisms involving surface membrane calcium equilibria (27). The mechanical threshold might be lower than normal in muscle cells from susceptible swine (49).

TABLE 1. *Halothane susceptibility in different breeds of pigs[a]*

Breed	Percent
Pietrain (The Netherlands)	100
Pietrain (USA)	80
Pietrain (France)	20–34
Belgian Landrace (The Netherlands)	85
Belgian Landrace (France)	47
Belgian Landrace (Fed. Rep. Germany)	87
Belgian Landrace (Denmark)	80
German Landrace (Fed. Rep. Germany)	70
Dutch Landrace (The Netherlands)	13–22
Dutch Landrace (Denmark)	18
Irish Landrace (Ireland)	5
Danish Landrace (Denmark)	9
French Landrace (France)	18
Swiss Yorkshire (Switzerland)	13
Norwegian Landrace (Great Britian)	5

[a]From ref. 37, p. 189, with permission.

Depolarizing Substances

Carbachol has effects similar to those of halothane and increases oxygen consumption and lactate production. Drugs that depolarize the myoplasmic membrane, such as succinylcholine (22,42) or decamethonium (13) can induce malignant hyperthermia in pigs. *d*-Tubocurarine has been associated with greater lactate production in susceptible pigs exposed to environmental stress, but is not a triggering agent (26,58). Nondepolarizing relaxants (e.g., *d*-tubocurarine, pancuronium) block the effects of succinylcholine and carbachol in triggering malignant hyperthermia (24).

Sympathetic Nervous System

The sympathetic nervous system appears to be involved with malignant hyperthermia. By fluorescence microscopy it has been shown that some noradrenergic axons may make synaptic contact with both smooth and striated muscle fibers (1). Autonomous innervation of pig and human striated muscle is probably analogous. Pietrain pigs are extremely sensitive to alpha-adrenergic stimulation (phenylephrine) and develop fatal hyperthermia (25). The increase in muscle temperature precedes the increase in lactate, suggesting that the mechanism is due to muscle and cutaneous vasoconstriction, resulting in ischemia and decreased heat loss. Thus, hypoxia or increased temperature may produce the malignant hyperthermia response in susceptible muscles. Unlike alpha-adrenergic-agonists, beta-adrenergic-agonists do not trigger malignant hyperthermia nor cause muscle damage (4,28).

PATHOPHYSIOLOGY

Striated Muscles

Accumulation of calcium is an early reaction of cells and tissues to damage. In muscles this can occur following a variety of insults (e.g., denervation, ischemia, nutritional deficiencies). Calcium accumulates in human dystrophic muscle (19) and it has been postulated that this is the major cause of the muscle necrosis (3). The immediate cause of malignant hyperthermia appears to be a sudden rise in myoplasmic calcium concentration.

Drugs that increase myoplasmic calcium (e.g., lidocaine, cardiac glycosides, and caffeine) worsen the prognosis of malignant hyperthermia (9). On the other hand, drugs that lower myoplasmic calcium (e.g., dantrolene sodium, procaine, and verapamil) improve survival of crises (12,27).

The abnormality that could account for the rapid rise of myoplasmic calcium is not yet known. Among the possibilities are: (a) defective accumulation of calcium in the sarcoplasmic reticulum (8,57); (b) defective accumulation of calcium in the mitochondria (5); and (c) excessively fragile sarcolemma with passive diffusion of calcium into the myoplasm from the extracellular fluid (7,18,45). A freeze-fracture study proposes that in humans the initial change may involve phospholipids (61). In male malignant hyperthermia swine, an elevation in the choline pool and a reduction in phosphatidylcholine and phosphatidylethanolamine was found when compared with normal animals (32). The elevated myoplasmic calcium exerts a number of effects. The activation of inactive phosphorylase increases the catabolism of glycogen to lactic acid, carbon dioxide, and heat. As the muscle temperature rises, the increased temperature eliminates the calcium requirement for myosin-actin interaction (17). The inactivation of the calcium-regulating mechanisms is also potentiated by the decline in adenosine triphosphate (ATP) levels. Some of the excess calcium may be absorbed by the mitochondria. Within the mitochondria, the resulting toxic calcium concentration uncouples oxidative phosphorylation, thereby decreasing ATP production and further accelerating oxygen consumption and output of lactate, carbon dioxide, and heat. ATP levels are well maintained early in the reaction through conversion of creatine phosphate and adenosine diphosphate (ADP) to creatine and ATP (40). In malignant hyperthermia the muscles suffer from a deficiency of adenylate kinase (59). Once ATP depletion occurs, the malignant hyperthermia becomes fatal. Calcium is not taken up again into the sarcoplasmic reticulum and muscles do not relax. The muscle membrane becomes leaky.

Other Organs

Heart function is altered during human and porcine malignant hyperthermia, as is evidenced by the early appearance of tachycardia and arrhythmias, followed by hypotension, declining output, and finally cardiac arrest. The central nervous system appears to be secondarily involved. Pulmonary changes include tachypnea, hyperventilation, and ultimately pulmonary edema. The kidneys and the endocrine system are also involved (see ref. 20).

PREVENTION

Myorelaxants

Prophylaxis of halothane-induced malignant hyperthermia can be performed using dantrolene sodium (27). Dantrolene is known to attenuate calcium release without affecting uptake. It interferes with excitation-contraction coupling between the transverse tubules and the terminal cisternae of the sarcoplasmic reticulum and/or acts directly upon the terminal cysternae (10,38,48).

Nondepolarizing relaxants (e.g., *d*-tubocurarine, pancuronium) can antagonize the effects of succinylcholine or carbachol in triggering malignant hyperthermia but do not inhibit the triggering effects of halothane (24,26).

Neuroleptic Drugs

Droperidol and spiperone protect susceptible pigs from halothane-induced procine malignant hyperthermia (44,46).

Serotonergic 5-Hydroxytryptamine₂ Antagonists

We tried to prevent malignant hyperthermia with ketanserin, a selective serotonergic 5-hydroxytryptamine₂ antagonist, with a high selectivity for blood vessels, blood platelets and bronchial tissue (F. De Clerck et al., *this volume*; refs. 38,64). Ketanserin also has a moderate affinity for the alpha$_1$ and histamine$_1$ receptors (38). In malignant hyperthermia susceptible pigs (20–40 kg) (15), pretreatment with ketanserin (10 mg i.m.) ½ hr before exposure to halothane (for 12 min) prevents halothane-induced malignant hyperthermia (53). Only 2 out of 8 pigs showed muscle stiffness on the backhand and hyperthermia (Fig. 1). The nonpretreated pigs showed the typical symptoms of malignant hyperthermia: muscle stiffness (after 2–7 min), white-red color pattern of the skin, high breathing frequency, and increase in rectal temperature (Fig. 2). These pigs showed the blood values typical of damaged muscle: significantly increased values of potassium, calcium, inorganic phosphate, and cholesterol (Table 2). Postmortem examination of these animals revealed severe muscle damage, focal heart necrosis, and lung edema. Electron microscopy of skeletal muscle tissue of nonpretreated pigs showed severe mitochondrial damage and calcium precipitation (Fig. 3). Ketanserin protects malignant-hyperthermia-susceptible pig muscles from the adverse effects of halothane *in vivo*.

Ketanserin has also been found to inhibit skeletal muscle dystrophy caused by 5-hydroxytryptamine in femoral artery ligated rats (65). In the rat, the combination of a 5-hydroxytryptamine uptake blocker (e.g., chlorpheniramine) plus 5-hydroxytryptamine resulted in muscle necrosis which could be prevented by methysergide (47). The role of 5-hydroxytryptamine in the development of malignant hyperthermia or muscle necrosis is, at present, unknown. It probably increases the cell

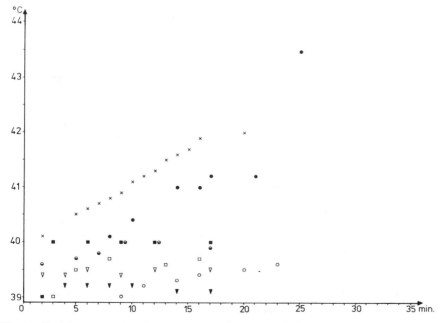

FIG. 1. Rectal temperature of pigs pretreated with ketanserin (0.25–0.5 mg/kg i.m.) during (*t*0–*t*12) and after exposition to halothane. All animals survived.

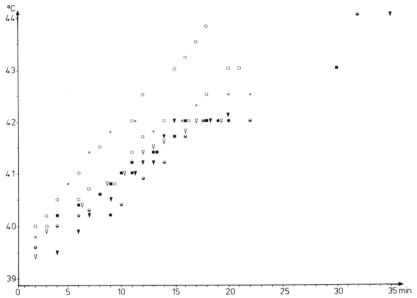

FIG. 2. Rectal temperature of nonpretreated pigs during (*t*0–*t*12) and after exposition to halothane. All animals died.

TABLE 2. *Serum analysis of nonpretreated pigs*

Parameter	Number of animals	Start of anesthesia mean x	SD	Mean (at 19 min)	SD	T-value	Significance
Potassium (mEq/liter)	3	5	0.793	8.8	0	8.29	a
Calcium (mEq/liter)	3	12.066	0.568	13.8	0.458	4.11	b
Inorganic phosphate (mg %)	3	10.7	1.276	17.7	2.007	5.09	a
Lactate (mg %)	5	47.6	40.67	108.8	40.35	2.38	b
LDH (U/liter)	3	928.3	117.6	1,237	249.3	1.93	
Cholesterol (mg %)	3	102.66	2.08	115.6	0.57	10.42	a
Glucose (mg %)	3	163.66	48.26	274.33	63.31	2.40	

[a] $p < 0.01$.
[b] $0.01 > p < 0.05$
SD: standard deviation.

membrane permeability for calcium, in this way increasing the intracellular calcium content, as has been shown in other tissues (2).

In susceptible humans, halothane may increase platelet ATP depletion associated with aggregation, an effect similar to that observed in skeletal muscle (11). In man it was shown that epinephrine stimulates primary platelet aggregation through a specific receptor interaction that results in a selective increase in platelet membrane permeability to calcium (56). Malignant hyperthermia can be induced in susceptible pigs (Pietrain) by i.v. infusion of alpha-adrenergic substances (25). Inhibition of

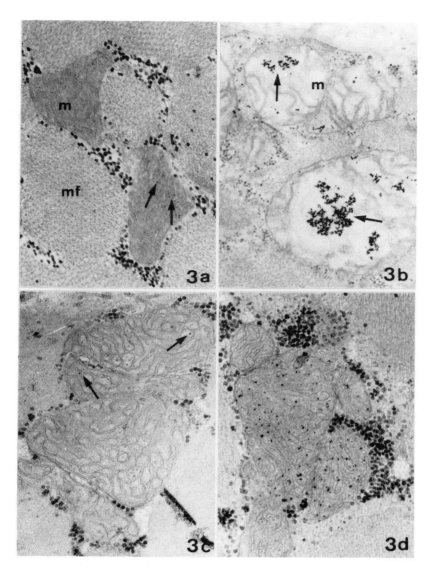

FIG. 3. Ultrastructural localization of calcium in the mitochondria of skeletal muscle tissue observed in four different samples taken from the same pig. **(a):** Pre-anesthesia sample; no pretreatment. The low amount of calcium in the normal mitochondria (m) is visualized by the presence of a few spots of precipitate *(arrows)* in the matrix. Glycogen (g); myofilaments (mf) (×42,500). **(b):** Post-anesthesia sample; no pretreatment. The large conglomerates of precipitate *(arrows)* in the clarified matrix of these swollen mitochondria (m) indicate the presence of large amounts of intramitochondrial calcium (×33,800). The greatly increased amounts of calcium are most probably deleterious to these skeletal muscle mitochondria. **(c):** Preanesthesia sample; pretreatment with ketanserin. A comparably low amount of calcium *(arrows)* is seen in these normal mitochondria as shown in Fig. 3a (×42,500). **(d):** Post-anesthesia sample; pretreatment with ketanserin. The amount of calcium is increased in the otherwise normal looking mitochondria (×42,500). The moderate increase in myoplasmic calcium which may have occurred after halothane anesthesia in this pretreated pig can probably be managed by the mitochondria.

[14]C-epinephrine uptake into isolated chromaffin granules was shown at halothane concentrations of more than 1.3 mM, but there was no effect when the concentration was 0.7 mM or less (62). Complete adrenergic blockade inhibits the contractions of skeletal muscle from Pietrain pigs due to halothane, and the adrenal medulla contributes to this response, as is shown by bilateral adrenalectomy combined with bretylium tosylate administration (41).

The mechanism of action of ketanserin and other serotonergic 5-hydroxytryptamine$_2$ antagonists in the prevention of halothane-induced malignant hyperthermia appears to be due primarily to their effect as 5-hydroxytryptamine$_2$ receptor antagonist. Substances combining several pharmacological properties (dopamine antagonism, alpha$_1$-adrenergic blocking activity and histamine$_1$ blocking activity) are more potent. These experiments suggest the involvement of 5-hydroxytryptamine in the development of malignant hyperthermia. The exact mechanism of action remains a matter of discussion.

ACKNOWLEDGMENT

The authors wish to thank Mr. R. Mostmans for his assistance.

REFERENCES

1. Barker, D., and Saito, M. (1980): Probable innervation of cat striated muscle fibers by autonomic axons. *J. Physiol.*, 307:16P.
2. Berridge, M. J. (1980): Anion and proton transport. In: *The Role of Cyclic Nucleotides and Calcium in the Regulation of Chloride Transport*, edited by W. A. Brodsky. *Ann. NY Acad. Sci.*, 341:156–171.
3. Bonilla, E., Schotland, D. L., Wakayama, Y., and Watts, H. M., Jr. (1978): Duchenne dystrophy: Focal alterations in the distribution of concanavalin A binding sites at the muscle cell surface. *Ann. Neurol.*, 4:117–123.
4. Briskey, E. J. (1964): Etiological status and associated studies of pale, soft, exudative porcine musculature. *Adv. Food Res.*, 13:89–178.
5. Britt, B. A., Endrenyi, L., Cadman, D. L., Ho Man Fan, and Fung, H. Y.-K. (1975): Porcine malignant hyperthermia—effects of halothane on mitochondrial respiration and calcium accumulation. *Anaesthesiology*, 42:292–300.
6. Britt, B. A., Frodis, W., Endrenyi, L., Scott, E., and Kalow, W. (1980): Comparison of effects of several inhalation anaesthetics on caffeine-induced contractures of normal and malignant hyperthermic skeletal muscle. *Can. Anaesth. Soc. J.*, 27:12–15.
7. Britt, B. A., Endrenyi, L., Peters, P. L., Kwong, F. H.-F., and Kadijevic, L. (1976): Screening of malignant hyperthermia susceptible families of CPK measurement and other clinical investigations. *Can. Anaesth. Soc. J.*, 23:263–284.
8. Britt, B. A., Kalow, W., Gordon, A., Humphrey, J. G., and Barry Rewcastle, N. (1973): Malignant hyperthermia—an investigation of five patients. *Can. Anaesth. Soc. J.*, 20:431–467.
9. Britt, B. A., Kwong, F. H.-F., and L. Endrenyi (1977): The clinical and laboratory features of malignant hyperthermia managment. A review. In: *Malignant hyperthermia. Current Concepts*, edited by E. O. Henschel. Appleton-Century Crofts, New York.
10. Brocklehurst, L. (1975): Dantrolene sodium and "skinned" muscle fibers. *Nature*, 254:364.
11. Bronstein, S. L., Ryan, D. E., Solomons, C. C., and Mahowald, M. C. (1979): Dantrolene sodium in the management of patients at risk from malignant hyperthermia. *J. Oral Surg.*, 37:719–724.
12. Csongrady, A., Bake, I., Pfänder, Ch., Farmann, H., Schneider, N., and Buttazzoni, E. (1976): Ein weiterer Fall malignen Hyperpyrexie und seine Behandlung mit Lidocain, Methylprednizolon und Verapamil. *Anaesthesist*, 25:80–81.
13. De Jong, R. H., Heavner, J. E., and Amory, D. W. (1974): Malignant hyperpyrexia in the cat. *Anaesthesiology*, 41:608–609.

14. Denborough, M. A., Ebeling, P., King, J. O., and Zapf, P. (1970): Myopathy and malignant hyperpyrexia. *Lancet*, i:1138–1140.
15. Eikelenboom, G., and Minkema, D. (1974): Prediction of pale, soft, exudative muscle with a non-lethal test for the halothane-induced porcine malignant hyperthermia syndrome. *Tijdschr. Diergeneeskd.*, 99:421–426.
16. Forrest, J. C., Will, J. A., Schmidt, G. R., Judge, M. D., and Briskey, E. J. (1968): Homeostasis in animals *(Sus domesticus)* during exposure to a warm environment. *J. Appl. Physiol.*, 24:33–39.
17. Fuchs, F. (1975): Thermal inactivation of the calcium regulatory mechanism of human skeletal muscle actomyosin: A possible contributing factor in the rigidity of malignant hyperthermia. *Anaesthesiology*, 42:584–589.
18. Gallant, E. G., Godt, R. E., and Gronert, G. A. (1979): Role of plasma membrane defect of skeletal muscle in malignant hyperthermia. *Muscle Nerve*, 2:491–494.
19. Gardner, J., and Frantz, C. (1974): Effects of cations on ouabain binding by intact human erythrocytes. *J. Membr. Biol.*, 16:43–64.
20. Gronert, G. A. (1980): Malignant hyperthermia. *Anaesthesiology*, 53:395–423.
21. Gronert, G. A., Milde, J. H., and Theye, R. A. (1976): Porcine malignant hyperthermia induced by halothane and succinylcholine: Failure of treatment with procaine or procainamide. *Anaesthesiology*, 44:124–132.
22. Gronert, G. A., and Theye, R. A. (1976): Suxamethonium-induced porcine malignant hyperthermia. *Br. J. Anaesthesiol.*, 48:513–517.
23. Gronert, G. A., Thompson, R. L., and Onofrio, B. M. (1980): Human malignant hyperthermia: Awake episodes and correction by dantrolene. *Anesth. Analg.*, 59:377–378.
24. Hall, G. M., Lucke, J. N., and Lister, D. (1976): Porcine malignant hyperthermia. IV. Neuromuscular blockade. *Br. J. Anaesthesiol.*, 48:1135–1141.
25. Hall, G. M., Lucke, J. N., and Lister, D. (1977): Porcine malignant hyperthermia. V. Fatal hyperthermia in the pietrain pig, associated with the infusion of α-adrenergic agents. *Br. J. Anaesthesiol.*, 49:855–863.
26. Harrison, G. G. (1973): The effect or procaine and curare on the initiation of anaesthetic-induced malignant hyperpyrexia. In: *International Symposium on Malignant Hyperthermia*, edited by R. A. Gordon, B. A. Britt, and W. Kalow, pp. 271–286. Charles C Thomas, Springfield, Illinois.
27. Harrison, G. G. (1977): The prophylaxis of malignant hyperthermia by oral dantrolene sodium in swine. *Br. J. Anaesthesiol.*, 49:315–317.
28. Harrison, G. G., Saunders, S. J., Biebuyck, J. F., Hiekman, R., Dent, D. M., Weaver, W., and Terblanche, J. (1969): Anaesthetic-induced malignant hyperpyrexia and a method for its prediction. *Br. J. Anaesthesiol.*, 41:844–855.
29. Hartharn, A. M., Van der Walt, K., and Young, E. (1974): Possible therapy for capture myopathy in captured wild animals. *Nature*, 247:577.
30. Henschel, J. R., and Louw, G. N. (1978): Capture stress, metabolic acidosis and hyperthermia in birds. *S. Afr. J. Sci.*, 74:305–306.
31. Huckell, V. F., Staniloff, H. M., Britt, B. A., Waxman, M. B., and Morck, J. E. (1978): Cardiac manifestations of malignant hyperthermia susceptibility. *Circulation*, 58:916–925.
32. Jardon, D. M., Barak, A. J., Noffsinger, J. K., Chapin, J., and Wingard, D. W. (1980): Phospholipid abnormalities in sarcoplasmic reticulum from malignant hyperthermia swine. *IRCS Med. Sci.*, 8:618–619.
33. Johansson, G., and Jönsson, L. (1979): Porcine stress syndrome. Experimental evidence of psychological mechanisms. *Acta Agricult. Scand. (Suppl.)*, 21:322–329.
34. Judge, M. D., Eikelenboom, G., and Zuidam, L. (1973): Blood acid-base status and oxygen binding during stress-induced hyperthermia in pigs. *J. Anim. Sci.*, 37:776–784.
35. Karpati, G., and Watters, G. V. (1980): Adverse anaesthetic reactions to Duchenne dystrophy. In: *Muscular Dystrophy Research: Advances and New Trends*, edited by C. Angelini, G. A. Danieli, and D. Fontanari, pp. 206–217. *Proceedings of International Symposium on Muscular Dystrophy Research*, Venice, Italy.
36. King, J. O., and Denborough, M. A. (1973): Anesthetic-induced malignant hyperpyrexia in children. *J. Pediatr.*, 83:37–40.
37. Lampo, P. (1980): Stress susceptibility in pigs-inheritance of the halothane-sensitivity. *Vlaams Diergeneeskd. Tijdschr.*, 49:187–194.
38. Leysen, J. E., Awouters, F., Kenis, L., Laduron, P. M., Vandenberk, J., and Janssen, P. A. J. (1981): Receptor binding profile of R 41 468, a novel antagonist at 5-HT$_2$ receptors. *Life Sci.*, 28:1015–1022.

39. Lister, D., Sair, P. A., Will, J. A., Schmidt, G. R., Cassens, R. G., Hoekstra, W. G., and Briskey, E. J. (1970): Metabolism of striated muscle of stress-susceptible pigs breathing oxygen or nitrogen. *Am. J. Physiol.*, 218:102–107.
40. Lohman, K. (1934): Über die enzymatische Aufspaltung der Kreatinphosaure; zugleich ein Beitrag zur Chemismus der Muskelkontraction. *Biochem. Z.*, 271:264–268.
41. Lucke, J. N., Denny, H., Hall, G. M., Lovell, R., and Lister, D. (1978): Porcine malignant hyperthermia. VI. The effects of bilateral adrenalectomy and pretreatment with bretylium on the halothane-induced response. *Br. J. Anaesthesiol.*, 50:241–246.
42. Lucke, J. N., Hall, G. M., and Lister, D. (1976): Porcine malignant hyperthermia. I: Metabolic and physiologic changes. *Br. J. Anaesthesiol.*, 48:297–304.
43. Marple, D. N., Aberle, E. D., Forrest, J. C., Blake, W. H., and Judge, M. D. (1972): Endocrine responses of stress susceptible and stress resistant swine to environmental stresses. *J. Anim. Sci.*, 35:576–579.
44. McGrath, C. J., Rempel, W. E., Jessen, C. R., Addis, P. B., Crimi, A. J., and Ruff, J. (1980): Protection from halothane-induced porcine malignant hyperthermia syndrome by droperidol. *Lab. Anim. Sci.*, 30:992–995.
45. McIntosch, D., and Berman, M. C. (1974): Neutral lipid and phospolipid composition of normal and myopathic skeletal muscle of pigs. *S. Afr. Med. J.*, 48:1221–1226.
46. McLoughlin, J. V., Somers, C. J., Ahern, C. P., and Wilson, P. (1979): Porcine malignant hyperthermia syndrome: Effectiveness of spiperone and dantrolene in prevention and treatment. *Acta Agricult. Scand. (Suppl.)*, 21:343–348.
47. Meltzer, H. Y. (1976): Skeletal muscle necrosis following membrane-active drugs plus serotonin. *J. Neurol. Sci.*, 28:41–56.
48. Morgan, K. G., and Bryant, S. H. (1977): The mechanism of action of dantrolene sodium. *J. Pharmacol. Exp. Ther.*, 201:138–147.
49. Moulds, R. F. W., and Denborough, M. A. (1974): Biochemical basis of malignant hyperpyrexia. *Br. Med. J.*, ii:241–244.
50. Nelson, T. E. (1978): Excitation-contraction coupling: A common etiologic pathway for malignant hyperthermia susceptible muscle. In: *Second International Symposium on Malignant Hyperthermia*, edited by J. A. Aldrete and B. A. Britt, pp. 23–36. Grune & Stratton, New York.
51. Nelson, T. E., Jones, E. W., Hendrickson, R. L., Falk, S. N., and Kerr, D. D. (1974): Porcine malignant hyperthermia: Observations on the occurrence of pale, soft exudative musculature among susceptible pigs. *Am. J. Vet. Res.*, 35:347–350.
52. Okumura, F., Crocker, B. D., and Denborough, M. A. (1979): Identification of susceptibility to malignant hyperpyrexia in swine. *Br. J. Anaesthesiol.*, 51:171–176.
53. Ooms, L., Verheyen, F., and Vandenberghe, J. (1981): The prevention of halothane-induced malignant hyperthermia in susceptible pigs with ketanserin, a serotonin₂ receptor antagonist. *(Unpublished observations.)*
54. O'Steen, W. K. (1967): Serotonin antagonist increases longevity in mice with hereditary muscular dystrophy. *Proc. Soc. Exp. Biol. Med.*, 126:579–583.
55. Owen, N. E., Feinburg, H., and Le Breton, G. C. (1980): Epinephrine induced Ca^{2+}-uptake in human blood platelets. *Am. J. Physiol.*, 239:H483–H488.
56. Relton, J. E. S. (1973): Malignant hyperthermia—anaesthetic techniques and agents. In: *International Symposium on Malignant Hyperthermia*, edited by R. A. Gordon, B. A. Britt, and W. Kalow, pp. 425–429. Charles C Thomas, Springfield, Illinois.
57. Ryan, J. F. (1977): Treatment of malignant hyperthermia. In: *Malignant Hyperthermia—Current Concepts*, edited by E. O. Henschel, pp. 47–56. Appleton-Century-Crofts, New York.
58. Sair, R. A., Lister, D., Moody, W. G., Cassens, R. G., Hoekstra, W. G., and Briskey, E. J. (1970): Action of curare and magnesium on striated muscle of stress-susceptible pigs. *Am. J. Physiol.*, 218:108–114.
59. Schmidt, J., Schmidt, K., and Ritter, H. (1974): Hereditary malignant hyperpyrexia associated with muscle adenylate kinase deficiency. *Humangenetik*, 24:253–257.
60. Short, C. E., and Paddleford, R. R. (1973): Malignant hyperthermia in the dog. *Anaesthesiology*, 39:462–463.
61. Smallbruck, H. (1979): A freeze-fracture study of the plasma membrane of muscle fibers of a patient with chronic creatinine kinase elevation suspected for malignant hyperthermia. *J. Neuropathol. Exp. Neurol.*, 38:407–418.
62. Sumikawa, K., Amakata, Y., Yoshikawa, K., Kashimoto, T., and Izumi, F. (1980): Catecholamine uptake and release in isolated chromaffin granules exposed to halothane. *Anaesthesiology*, 53:385–389.

63. Van den Hende, C., Lister, D., Muylle, E., Ooms, L., and Oyaert, W. (1976): Malignant hyperthermia in Belgian Landrace pigs, rested or exercised before exposure to halothane. *Br. J. Anaesthesiol.*, 48:821–829.
64. Van Nueten, J. M., and Vanhoutte, P. M. (1981): Selectivity of calcium-antagonism and serotonin-antagonism with respect to venous and arterial tissues. *Angiology*, 32:476–484.
65. Verheyen, A., Vlaminckx, E., Remeysen, P., and Borgers, M. (1981): The influence of ketanserin, a new serotonin$_2$ receptor antagonist on experimentally induced skeletal muscle myopathy in the rat. A histological approach. *Virchows Arch. (Pathol. Anat.)*, 393:265–272.
66. Williams, C. H. (1976): Some observations on the etiology of the fulminant hyperthermia—stress syndrome. *Perspect. Biol. Med.*, 20:120–130.
67. Wingard, D. W., and Gatz, E. E. (1978): Some observations on stress-susceptible patients. In: *Second International Symposium on Malignant Hyperthermia*, edited by J. A. Aldrete and B. A. Britt, pp. 363–372. Grune & Stratton, New York.

5-Hydroxytryptamine in Peripheral Reactions,
edited by Fred De Clerck and Paul M.
Vanhoutte. Raven Press, New York © 1982.

The Possible Role of 5-Hydroxytryptamine in Duchenne Muscular Dystrophy

Peter J. Stoward

Department of Anatomy, The University, Dundee DDI 4HN, Scotland

This chapter is concerned with the evidence for and against the hypothesis that 5-hydroxytryptamine, and possibly other vasoactive agents, may initiate Duchenne muscular dystrophy in man. One of the oldest and most actively debated explanations of the pathogenesis of Duchenne muscular dystrophy is the vascular or ischemic theory (5), which suggests that the flow of blood through skeletal muscles is periodically impaired, giving rise to repeated episodes of transient functional ischemia that lead eventually to the degeneration of isolated groups of muscle fibers. As exogenous 5-hydroxytryptamine is known to have marked physiological effects on the vascular system of normal muscle, it is pertinent to enquire whether endogenous 5-hydroxytryptamine might cause similar effects in the early stages of Duchenne muscular dystrophy. The effects might arise if 5-hydroxytryptamine circulating in the blood is temporarily in excess, or if there are more 5-hydroxytryptamine receptor sites than usual in the blood vessels of patients who eventually show the symptoms of the disease.

WHY 5-HYDROXYTRYPTAMINE?

5-Hydroxytryptamine can stimulate the synthesis and release of prostaglandins, which in turn may promote the entry of substantial amounts of calcium ions into skeletal muscle cells, eventually causing them to degenerate and die. Horobin et al. (11) have reviewed this possibility and, therefore, it is not pursued further here. Another reason for regarding 5-hydroxytryptamine as a potential initiator of muscular dystrophy is its well established ability to alter the systemic blood flow and microvasculature of normal skeletal muscle (7). When injected intravenously, 5-hydroxytryptamine usually constricts large blood vessels, but dilates small ones. If small vessels are already neurogenically dilated, 5-hydroxytryptamine does not dilate them any further, but continues to constrict large vessels; the net effect of 5-hydroxytryptamine is, thus, constriction.

EVIDENCE SUGGESTING THE INVOLVEMENT OF 5-HYDROXYTRYPTAMINE IN DUCHENNE MUSCULAR DYSTROPHY

The evidence in support of a role of 5-hydroxytryptamine in the pathogenesis of Duchenne muscular dystrophy is mostly indirect.

Platelets

Until 1979 the most incriminating evidence suggesting a role for 5-hydroxytryptamine was that the platelets of patients with Duchenne muscular dystrophy took up and stored significantly less 5-hydroxytryptamine than those of age-matched controls (23). Since the average level of 5-hydroxytryptamine in the plasma of patients with Duchenne muscular dystrophy is normal (23), it was argued that the 5-hydroxytryptamine not taken up by platelets must be stored or inactivated by other receptor cells, the most obvious candidates being the endothelium and smooth muscle cells of the vasculature.

However, using a more sensitive technique, Andornato et al. (1) have recently found that the average amounts of 5-hydroxytryptamine in platelets of normal subjects and patients with Duchenne muscular dystrophy are the same. On the other hand, they also discovered that platelets of patients with Duchenne muscular dystrophy contained significantly fewer dense bodies, which are stores for 5-hydroxytryptamine, implying that platelets of patients with Duchenne muscular dystrophy release 5-hydroxytryptamine faster or more readily than normal platelets. Thus, in Duchenne muscular dystrophy there may be temporary local excesses of free 5-hydroxytryptamine in the blood.

Dilatation of Capillaries

Capillaries in dystrophic muscle are significantly dilated compared to those in normal muscle (13). This would be expected if the "excess" 5-hydroxytryptamine just referred to acts in the same way that exogenously administered 5-hydroxytryptamine does on the vasculature of normal muscle (7).

Carcinoid Tumors

A myopathy develops, albeit slowly, in humans with carcinoid tumors, which are known to produce large amounts of circulating 5-hydroxytryptamine (27).

Induction of Myopathies with 5-Hydroxytryptamine

When 5-hydroxytryptamine is given repeatedly in low doses to rats or mice over a period of several weeks, the lower limb muscles acquire histopathological lesions consistent with a myopathy (22,25). The induction of the lesions is accelerated if either the aorta or the femoral artery is ligated beforehand (20,30).

Serotonergic Antagonists

Drugs antagonistic to 5-hydroxytryptamine prevent the induction of the experimental myopathy described above (6,30), thus implying that 5-hydroxytryptamine is responsible for initiating the myopathy rather than the ligation procedure. This is supported by the absence of myopathic lesions in animals whose femoral artery has been ligated but to whom no 5-hydroxytryptamine has been administered (10).

Serotonergic antagonists also improve the muscle performance of chickens with an inherited myopathy (2), prolong the life of genetically dystrophic mice (24), and lower the high levels of plasma creatine kinase in dystrophic chickens and hamsters (2).

EVIDENCE AGAINST THE INVOLVEMENT OF 5-HYDROXYTRYPTAMINE IN DUCHENNE MUSCULAR DYSTROPHY

Several observations, open to conflicting interpretations, argue against a primary role for 5-hydroxytryptamine in the etiology of Duchenne muscular dystrophy.

Ligation Experiments

Myopathic lesions can be produced in rats by ligating their aorta alone; giving 5-hydroxytryptamine in addition makes little further difference (15).

Histology

The histological patterns of the myopathies induced by 5-hydroxytryptamine in rats and the myopathic muscle of patients with carcinoid tumors (see previous sections), do not resemble the histological picture characteristic of the early and midphases of Duchenne muscular dystrophy (22). For example, in 5-hydroxytryptamine-associated myopathies, there are no enlarged "hyalinized" fibers, no increase in the endomysial and perimyseal connective tissue, and no progressive loss of muscle fibers—all diagnostic features of Duchenne muscular dystrophy. Moreover, the preferential damage of the high oxidative fibers (type I) in 5-hydroxytryptamine-associated myopathies does not occur in Duchenne muscular dystrophy (22). Instead, the histological pattern most resembles that seen in polymyositis and atherosclerotic occlusive vascular disease.

Blood Flow Rates

Total blood flow rates and capillary diffusion rates through human dystrophic muscles do not differ significantly from those in normal muscles (3,16). However, it is highly improbable that measurements of total blood flow (such as those based on ^{133}Xe-clearance rates) will ever reveal the small periodic fluctuations in blood flow in limited regions of the microvasculature of putative dystrophic muscle predicted by the vascular theory. The falls in some capillaries, and the increases in others (particularly in the larger blood vessels and the precapillary arterioles), require measurements to be carried out on local blood flows, for example, using the hydrogen electrode (21) or by measuring the Doppler shift of laser light scattered by erythrocytes flowing through a capillary exposed at biopsy (28). The first-named technique has so far revealed substantial differences in local muscle blood flow of different muscles, particularly in their response to epinephrine. Preliminary data obtained with the light scattering technique (28) suggest that in patients with muscle disorders such as polymyositis, the microvascular hemodynamics differ considerably from those in control subjects and in patients with neuropathic diseases.

Heterogeneity of the Microvasculature

Many of the arguments arraigned against the vascular theory of Duchenne muscular dystrophy, and by implication against a role for 5-hydroxytryptamine, ignore the complexity of the vascular tree in skeletal muscle (14) and its extraordinary capacity to compensate for regions that are destroyed or compromised. This has recently been demonstrated in rabbits and rats by ligating the femoral artery and observing the development of an anastomizing collateral circulation with a radioopaque dye (12). As well as being structurally complex, the vascular tree also displays very marked biochemical, and presumably functional, variations as it ramifies through a particular muscle. Thus, for example, some capillaries contain alkaline phosphatase (26), aminopeptidase A (18), and dipeptidylpeptidase IV (8,17), whereas other capillaries in the same muscle appear, histochemically, to be completely devoid of these enzymes *(unpublished observations)*. Since these enzymes may modulate the action of vasoactive agents such as angiotensin II acting on the various cells of the vascular wall, it is necessary to investigate the effects of these agents on each part of the vascular bed separately. This is now possible with the quantitative histochemical and histological techniques which have become available recently.

ROLE OF OTHER VASOACTIVE AGENTS

Other agents that have been considered for explaining the etiology of Duchenne muscular dystrophy include angiotensin II, alpha- and beta-adrenergic agents, cholinergic substances, and various metabolites such as the adenine nucleotides (4,19,29,31). However, it is difficult to obtain proof of their possible involvement for the same reasons as those given for 5-hydroxytryptamine.

CAPILLARIES AND METABOLISM

It is possible, but not proven, that capillaries affect the metabolism of muscle fibers. The metabolism and the efficient functioning of a muscle cell is generally assumed to depend on the rapid diffusion of oxygen and essential metabolic precursors (carbohydrates, amino acids) across the capillary walls into it. Consequently, if a capillary becomes altered in any way, the supply of nutrients to the muscle cell it serves will also change. Thus a muscle fiber will presumably become dystrophic (in the literal sense of the word) if either the number or surface area of the capillaries supplying it decreases, or if the oxygen concentration drops. The evidence to justify this presumption is neither clear-cut nor encouraging. For example, it is not known how many capillaries (and, hence, how much endothelial surface area) are required to ensure the diffusion of sufficient oxygen into a muscle fiber, bearing in mind the varied needs of fibers of different types. Thus type I "aerobic" fibers ought to have a greater capillary density than type II "anaerobic" fibers. This seems to be true since "slow-red" fibers have up to nearly twice as many capillaries as "fast-white" ones, but when estimates of the oxygen utilized by different fiber types are taken into account, "anaerobic" (type II; fast-white) fibers appear to have an excessive capillary supply, whereas "aerobic" (type I; slow-red) fibers are considerably undersupplied for their oxygen requirements (9). Therefore, muscles composed largely of aerobic fibres, such as the soleus, should, if the vascular hypothesis is correct, be more susceptible to shortcomings in their blood supply and prone to dystrophy than anaerobic, fast muscles. In fact, aerobic muscles are the most affected in Duchenne muscular dystrophy.

The heterogeneity in the distribution and function of capillaries (see also the section on heterogeneity of the microvasculature) suggests that it is invalid to draw conclusions about the functioning of whole muscles from morphological measurements on capillaries selected at random without reference to the metabolism of the muscle fibers adjacent to them. Therefore, it does not necessarily follow that the microcirculation in Duchenne muscular dystrophy is not abnormal, as Jerusalem et al. (13) have argued, simply because the muscle fiber area served per capillary in muscles from Duchenne muscular dystrophy patients and controls are virtually the same.

CONCLUSIONS AND PERSPECTIVES

5-Hydroxytryptamine undoubtedly induces a myopathy and ischemia in rats. However, this does not signify that 5-hydroxytryptamine is involved in Duchenne-type muscular dystrophies in man. The histological patterns of 5-hydroxytryptamine-induced myopathies and Duchenne muscular dystrophy are too dissimilar (22). Further, the argument that serotonergic antagonists reverse 5-hydroxytryptamine-induced myopathies in animals is a circular one, and may have little bearing on the pathogenesis of Duchenne muscular dystrophy. These negative conclusions do not mean that 5-hydroxytryptamine plays no part in the etiology of Duchenne muscular dystrophy. It may do, although unambiguous positive evidence is lacking at present. Before obtaining such evidence, it should be proved first, one way or the other, that some regions of the microvasculature of patients with Duchenne muscular dystrophy are relatively more ischemic than in normal subjects. When this proof is forthcoming, it might be worthwhile investigating if the ischemia is instigated by 5-hydroxytryptamine or some other vasoactive agent, using experimental strategies other than those deployed previously. One approach might be to find out if the administration of very low doses of a vasoactive substance over a long period of time to an *appropriate* animal model: (a) eventually induces the histological lesions characteristic of a human myopathy; (b) reduces local blood flow in capillaries supplying the region of muscle that eventually becomes dystrophic; and (c) leads to a gradual reduction in the activity of cytochrome *c* oxidase (as an indicator of the diffusion and utilization of oxygen) in those muscle fibers whose surrounding capillaries show ultrastructural and histochemical signs of being compromised (e.g., the thickening of the basal lamina). The cytochrome *c* oxidase activity can be determined in individual muscle fibers with a validated quantitative histochemical technique.

The major problem the researcher is confronted with is to find a suitable animal model of Duchenne muscular dystrophy. What is needed is an animal in which the cellular distribution and metabolism of 5-hydroxytryptamine is similar to that in man. This rules out most of the experimental animals used previously. The favorite example, the rat, is unsuitable because circulating 5-hydroxytryptamine is largely concentrated in mast cells and not platelets (32).

REFERENCES

1. Adornato, B. T., Corash, L., Costa, J., Shafer, B., Stark, H., Murphy, D., and Engel, W. K. (1979): Abnormality of platelet dense bodies in Duchenne dystrophy. *Neurology*, 29:567.
2. Barnard, E. A., and Barnard, P. J. (1979): Use of genetically dystrophic animals in chemotherapy trials and applications of serotonin antagonists as antidystrophic drugs. *Ann. NY Acad. Sci.*, 37:374–397.
3. Bradley, W. G., O'Brien, M. D., Walder, D. N., Murchison, D., Johnson, M., and Newall, D. J. (1975): Failure to confirm a vascular cause of muscular dystrophy. *Arch. Neurol.*, 32:466–474.
4. Devynck, M.-A., Pernollet, M.-G., Meyer, P., Fermandjian, S., and Fromageot, P. (1973): Angiotension receptors in smooth muscle membranes. *Nature (New Biol.)*, 245:55–57.
5. Engel, W. K. (1976): Workshop on the aetiology of Duchenne muscular dystrophy. The vascular hypothesis. In: *Recent Advances in Myology*, edited by W. G. Bradley, D. Gardner-Medwin, and J. N. Walton, pp. 166–177. American Elsevier, New York.
6. Engel, W. K., and Derrer, E. C. (1976): Drugs blocking the muscle-damaging effects of 5HT and noradrenaline in aorta-ligated rats. *Nature*, 254:151–152.
7. Garattini, S., and Valzelli, L. (1965): *Serotonin*. Elsevier, Amsterdam.
8. Gossrau, R. (1979): Peptidasen II. Zur Lokalisation der Dipeptidylpeptidase IV (DPPIV). Histochemische und biochemische Untersuchung. *Histochemistry*, 60:231–248.
9. Gray, S. D., and Renkin, E. M. (1978): Microvascular supply in relation to fiber metabolic type in mixed skeletal muscles of rabbits. *Microvasc. Res.*, 16:406–425.
10. Hathaway, P. W., Engel, W. K., and Zellweger, H. (1970): Experimental myopathy after microarterial embolization. Comparison with childhood X-linked pseudohypertrophic muscular dystrophy. *Arch. Neurol.*, 22:365–378.
11. Horobin, D. F., Morgan, R., Karmali, R. A., Manku, M. S., Karmazyn, M. K., Ally, A., and Mtabaji, J. P. (1977): The roles of prostaglandins and calcium accumulation in muscular dystrophy. *Med. Hypotheses*, 1:150–153.
12. Jaya, Y. (1980): Effect of ligation of various vessels ischaemia and collateral circulation in rabbits and rats. *Acta Anat.*, 106:10–14.
13. Jerusalem, F., Engel, A. G., and Gomez, M. R. (1974): Duchenne dystrophy. I. Morphometric study of the muscle microvasculature. *Brain*, 97:115–122.
14. Johnson, P. C. (1977): Landis Award Lecture. The myogenic response and the microcirculation. *Microvasc. Res.*, 13:1–18.
15. Kelts, K. A., and Kaiser, K. K. (1979): Experimental ischaemic myopathy. Effects of aortic ligation and serotonin. *J. Neurol. Sci.*, 40:23–27.
16. Leinonen, H., Juntunen, J., Somer, H., and Rapola, J. (1979): Capillary circulation and morphology in Duchenne muscular dystrophy. *Eur. Neurol.*, 18:249–255.
17. Lojda, Z. (1979): Studies on dipeptidyl(amino)peptidase IV (glycylproline naphthylamidase). II. Blood vessels. *Histochemistry*, 59:153–166.
18. Lojda, Z., and Gossrau, R. (1980): Study on aminopeptidase A. *Histochemistry*, 67:267–290.
19. McGiff, J. C., Malik, K. U., and Terragno, N. A. (1976): Prostaglandins as determinants of vascular reactivity. *Fed. Proc.*, 35:2382–2387.
20. Mendell, J. R., Engel, W. K., and Derrer, E. C. (1971): Duchenne muscular dystrophy: Functional ischaemia reproduces its characteristic lesions. *Science*, 172:1143–1145.
21. Mishra, S. K., and Haining, J. L. (1980): Measurement of local skeletal muscle blood flow in animals by the hydrogen electrode technique. *Muscle Nerve*, 3:285–288.

22. Munsat, T. L., Hudgson, P., and Johnson, M. A. (1977): Experimental serotonin myopathy. *Neurology*, 27:772–782.
23. Murphy, D. L., Mendell, J. R., and Engel, W. K. (1973): Serotonin and platelet function in Duchenne muscular dystrophy. *Arch. Neurol.*, 28:239–242.
24. O'Steen, W. K. (1967): Serotonin antagonist increases longevitiy in mice with hereditary muscular dystrophy. *Proc. Soc. Exp. Biol. Med.*, 126:579–583.
25. O'Steen, W. K., Barnard, J. L., and Yates, R. D. (1967): Serotonin induced changes in skeletal muscle of mice as revealed with the light and electron microscopes. *Anat. Rec.*, 154:380.
26. Romanul, F. C. A., and Bannister, R. G. (1962): Localized areas of high alkaline phosphatase activity in the terminal arterial tree. *J. Cell Biol.*, 15:73–84.
27. Swash, M., Fox, K. P., and Davidson, A. R. (1975): Carcinoid myopathy: Serotonin-induced muscle weakness in man. *Arch. Neurol.*, 32:572–574.
28. Tahmoush, A. J., Bowen, P. D., Bonner, R. F., and Engel, W. K. (1981): Open-biopsy muscle blood flow in patients with neuromuscular diseases and controls. A new technique. *Neurology*, 31:116.
29. Vanhoutte, P. M., Verbeuren, T. J., and Webb, R. C. (1981): Local modulation of adrenergic neuroeffector interaction in the blood vessel wall. *Physiol. Rev.*, 61:151–247.
30. Verheyen, A., Vlaminckx, E., Remeysen, P., and Borgers, M. (1981): The influence of ketanserin, a new S_2 receptor antagonist on experimentally induced skeletal muscle myopathy in the rat. *Virchows Arch. (Pathol. Anat.)*, 393:242–265.
31. Whelan, R. F. (1967): *Control of the Peripheral Circulation in Man.* Charles C Thomas, Springfield, Illinois.
32. Benditt, E. P., Holcenberg, J., and Lagunoff, D. (1963): The role of serotonin (5-hydroxytryptamine) in mast cells. *Ann. NY Acad. Sci.*, 103:179–184.

5-Hydroxytryptamine in Peripheral Reactions,
edited by Fred De Clerck and Paul M.
Vanhoutte. Raven Press, New York © 1982.

Does 5-Hydroxytryptamine Play a Role in Shock and Trauma?

*David H. Lewis and **Claes Post

*Clinical Research Center and **Department of Clinical Pharmacology,
University Hospital, S-581 85, Linköping, Sweden

The purpose of this brief chapter is to review our own studies on the effect of shock and trauma on the microcirculation in skeletal muscle and on the metabolism of the lung, indicating, for each, where 5-hydroxytryptamine may play a role and where further studies are indicated.

EFFECT OF TRAUMA ON SKELETAL MUSCLE BLOOD FLOW

Blunt trauma to the soft tissues, i.e., skeletal muscle, of the hind leg of an anesthetized animal causes an immediate, marked, and transient vasodilatation of the blood vessels in the skeletal muscle. Angiograms taken before and after the injury reveal that the entire vascular bed of the affected leg is dilated. All visible vessels are dilated even those proximal to the injured area (ascending vasodilatation) and the rate of transport of the bolus of contrast material through the tissues is increased (11). Measurement of blood flow in the femoral artery reveals an immediate increase to near maximal values which, within 5 to 10 min, goes over to a moderate to slight flow increase lasting 60 to 90 min (15).

Flow through the leg has been divided into "nutritional" and "nonnutritional," based on the first pass uptake by the muscle of tracer amounts of radioactive rubidium (^{86}Rb) ion (5). It has been shown that the flow increase due to trauma is almost exclusively due to an increase in nonnutritional flow (8). This is, however, not due to the opening up of arteriovenous shunts, as some have suggested, but rather to an increased velocity of flow through the capillary bed (9). It is, therefore, physiological and not anatomical shunting.

Using missile trauma it has been possible to quantitate the amount of energy delivered to the tissues. Results of this type of study indicate that the degree of vasodilatation is proportional to the degree of trauma produced (14). Furthermore, there is a vasodilator agent (or agents) released into the venous effluent from the traumatized area, the amount of which is proportional to the degree of trauma (16).

Studies were then carried out to block the vasodilatation caused by trauma. It was found that administration of the broad spectrum proteinase inhibitor, aprotinin (Trasylol®), before trauma decreased or abolished the initial rapid vasodilator response without altering the second more moderate and longer-lasting vasodilator phase (10). Since the vasodilatation was also potentiated by using British antilewisite, it seemed likely that kinin release was playing an important role in the vasodilatation caused by trauma. However, in a number of instances, the broad spectrum anti-amine, B 400 (Sandoz) also inhibited the vasodilatation, suggesting that one or more amines, possibly 5-hydroxytryptamine, might also play an important role. This point certainly needs further investigation, especially with the advent of more powerful and more specific amine blockers.

EFFECT OF SHOCK ON CAPILLARY BLOOD FLOW AND CAPILLARY TRANSPORT CAPACITY

The transport of substances, especially water soluble molecules, across the capillary wall depends in part on the level of capillary blood flow but also on the permeability-surface area product of the capillary wall (13). With acute hemorrhage there is a marked increase in permeability-surface area product but transport is reduced because of the very low capillary blood flow. In a prolonged shock situation capillary blood flow may return towards normal levels but the situation is not normal, because permeability-surface area product is low, out of proportion to the flow level. Thus, even if flow becomes normal, transport does not (1). Even in the prolonged low flow state transport can be returned to normal by the administration of colloid-containing fluids (2).

In an attempt to understand what role various endogenously-produced vasoactive substances could play in the alteration in transport seen in the prolonged low flow state, a series of studies was carried out examining the effect of a number of blocking agents. Hypovolemic shock was produced using a model of intestinal stasis produced by temporary exteriorization of the intestines (7). With no therapy there was a progressive decline in capillary blood flow and transport, and the transport decrease was, at all levels, low out of proportion to the change in flow. Complete blockade of alpha-adrenergic receptors was able to restore flow, but not transport. Aprotinin increased, temporarily, transport to its theoretical maximum but did not affect flow. Beta-adrenergic blockade, high doses of corticosteroids, acetylsalicylic acid, and a detergent, Pluronic F-68, had no effect either on flow or on transport (7). Here again, highly specific and effective amine blockers, as well as other specific blockers, need to be investigated.

Recent studies from our laboratory (6) have indicated that ischemia interferes with the ability of the capillary endothelial cell to regulate its volume properly. This swelling of the endothelial cell can encroach upon the capillary lumen and can be a factor impairing both flow and transport. The role of various endogenously produced vasoactive factors is under study.

THE METABOLISM OF THE LUNG

In addition to its respiratory function the lung has an important metabolic function, among other things detoxifying and activating a variety of substances (3). Our interest has been directed towards seeing if changes in the metabolic function of the lung play a role in the development of acute respiratory insufficiency seen after trauma. In the initial studies, anesthetized pigs were used and the first pass uptake of the local anesthetic agent, lidocaine, was studied (4). The handling of this agent could be defined as an initial extraction from the blood into the lung and extraction of lidocaine when 95% of the bolus of an accompanying inert substance (e.g., indocyanine green) had passed the lung. Studies up to 1 hr after severe hind leg trauma indicate no change in lidocaine uptake by the lung (12), but recently it has been shown that at longer times after trauma (e.g., 5–10 hr) lidocaine uptake by the lung is depressed *(unpublished observations)*. In patients with respiratory insufficiency both initial extraction of lidocaine and the so-called 95% uptake are reduced in comparison to values obtained in patients with normal respiratory function.

Recent studies from this laboratory indicate that the degree of trauma which interferes with lidocaine uptake by the lung does not appear to alter the first pass uptake of 5-hydroxytryptamine. Further studies here are in progress and the effect of a specific 5-hydroxytryptamine blocker both in the normal and in the pathological state should be interesting to determine.

CONCLUSIONS

Trauma, the prolonged low flow state, and ischemia cause major alterations in the microcirculation and metabolic function in many organs. We have described a few of the reactions seen in skeletal muscle and in lung. Even if many changes have been described operationally, detailed mechanisms in the cellular level are poorly understood. Specific pharmacological agents, such as the recently described specific $5-HT_2$ receptor-blocking drug ketanserin may help us to understand these mechanisms and, it is hoped, lead to improved therapy. Such studies are awaited with great interest. Until then, the question raised in the title of this chapter will remain unanswered.

ACKNOWLEDGMENTS

The original results reported in this communication were supported in part by grants-in-aid from the Swedish Medical Research Council (02042-15C), from the Swedish National Defence Research Institute (H-564), from Linköpings University, and from the County Council of Östergötland.

REFERENCES

1. Appelgren, L., and Lewis, D. H. (1972): Capillary flow and capillary transport in dog skeletal muscle in hemorrhagic shock. *Eur. Surg. Res.*, 4:29–45.
2. Appelgren, L., and Lewis, D. H. (1970): Capillary flow and capillary transport in dog skeletal muscle after induced intravascular RBC aggregation and dis-aggregation. *Eur. Surg. Res.*, 2:161–170.
3. Bakhle, Y. S., and Vane, J. R. (1974): Pharmacokinetic function of the pulmonary circulation. *Physiol. Rev.*, 54:1007–1045.

4. Bertler, Å., Lewis, D. H., Löfström, J. B., and Post, C. (1978): *In vivo* lung uptake of lidocaine in pigs. *Acta Anaesthesiol. Scand.*, 22:530–536.
5. Friedman, J. J. (1965): Microvascular flow distribution and rubidium extraction. *Fed. Proc.*, 24:1099–1103.
6. Gidlöf, A., Hammersen, F., Larsson, L., Lewis, D. H., and Liljedahl, S.-O. (1982): Is capillary endothelium in human skeletal muscle an ischemic shock tissue? In: *Induced Skeletal Muscle Ischemia in Man*, edited by D. H. Lewis, pp. 63–79. Karger, Basel.
7. Lewis, D. H. (1972): Effect of various pharmacological treatment schedules on the capillary blood flow and capillary transport function in dog skeletal muscle in surgical shock. In: *New Aspects of Trasysol Therapy. Protease Inhibition in Shock Therapy*, edited by W. Brendel, and G. L. Haberland, pp. 183–192. Schattauer Verlag, Stuttgart.
8. Lewis, D. H., and Lim, R. C., Jr. (1970): Studies on the circulatory pathophysiology of trauma. I. Effect of acute soft tissue injury on nutritional and non-nutritional shunt flow through the hindleg of the dog. *Acta Orthop. Scand.*, 41:17–36.
9. Lewis, D. H., and Lim, R. C., Jr. (1970): Studies on the circulatory pathophysiology of trauma. II. Effect of acute soft tissue injury on the passage of macroaggregated albumin (^{131}I) particles through the hindleg of the dog. *Acta Orthop. Scand.*, 41:37–43.
10. Lewis, D. H., Rybeck, B., Sandegård, J., Seeman, T., and Zachrisson, B. (1975): Activation of the kinin system in trauma. *Life Sci.*, 16:828–829.
11. Lewis, D. H., Sandegård, J., Seeman, T., and Zachrisson, B. E. (1975): Angiography of the dilator response in extremity trauma. *Acta Radiol. (Diagn.)*, 16:679–688.
12. Post, C., and Lewis, D. H. (1979): Effect of bullet wounding in thigh on the uptake of lidocaine by the lung. *Acta Chir. Scand. (Suppl.)*, 489:205–209.
13. Renkin, E. M. (1959): Transport of potassium-42 from blood to tissue in isolated mammalian skeletal muscles. *Am. J. Physiol.*, 197:1205–1210.
14. Rybeck, B., Lewis, D. H., Sandegård, J., and Seeman, T. (1975): The immediate circulatory response to high-velocity missiles. *J. Trauma*, 15:328–335.
15. Rybeck, B., Lewis, D. H., Sandegård, J., and Seeman, T. (1975): Early changes in capillary flow and transport following missile wounds. *Microvasc. Res.*, 10:267–275.
16. Rybeck, B., Lewis, D. H., Sandegård, J., and Seeman, T. (1975): Cardiovascular effects of venous blood from missile wounds. *Eur. Surg. Res.*, 7:193–204.

5-Hydroxytryptamine in Peripheral Reactions,
edited by Fred De Clerck and Paul M.
Vanhoutte. Raven Press, New York © 1982.

Endotoxemic Shock: An Implied Role for 5-Hydroxytryptamine

*G. L. Makabali, **A. K. Mandal, and †J. A. Morris
(with J. Brown, J. Chang, J. Bankhead, and B. A. Reeves)

*Division of Reproductive Sciences, Department of Obstetrics and Gynecology,
**Department of Surgery, The Charles R. Drew Postgraduate Medical School,
Los Angeles, California 90059; and †Department of Pharmacology, Obstetrics and
Gynecology, Medical University of South Carolina, Charleston, South Carolina 29425

The pathophysiology of endotoxin (septic) shock is uncertain and complex, notwithstanding the well documented hemodynamic, metabolic, and hematologic changes observed in different animal species and in man (2,3,7,15). Many vasoactive substances have been incriminated including kinins (17), 5-hydroxytryptamine (5,11, 18,19), histamine (5,9,19) and prostaglandins (1,8,25,26), along with sympathoadrenal hyperactivity, mechanical obstruction of the microcirculation, volume insufficiency due to vascular leaks, pooling in the peripheral and portal circulation, and other mechanisms (22). The humoral stimuli which cause pulmonary hypertension and systemic hypotension but result in a significant increase in both pulmonary and systemic vascular resistance are not well characterized. 5-Hydroxytryptamine causes platelet aggregation and pulmonary hypertension; it is a potent vasoconstricting agent and amplifies vasoconstriction induced by other vasoactive substances, particularly catecholamines, and by anoxia (6). Serotonergic receptors, based on *in vitro* binding studies, have recently been classified as 5-HT_1 and 5-HT_2 (13,20). Binding to the 5-HT_2 receptor correlates with *in vitro* and *in vivo* pharmacologic effects of 5-hydroxytryptamine. The possible participation of 5-hydroxytryptamine in the hemodynamic responses to endotoxin was evaluated using a selective 5-HT_2 receptor antagonist ketanserin (Janssen Pharmaceutica, Belgium). This antagonist reportedly has a high selectivity for 5-HT_2 receptors in blood vessels, blood platelets, and bronchial tissue.

MATERIAL AND METHODS

A pool of 45 Beagle dogs (Marshall Beagles for Research, North Rose, New York) was prepared in two stages, as previously described (16), prior to the administration of either the endotoxin or the modifying drug. Briefly, a precalibrated electromagnetic flowmeter transducer (Micron Industries, Los Angeles, California) of appropriate size (12–14 mm i.d.) was implanted under general anesthesia on the pulmonary artery. The implantation of a precalibrated pressure sensor into the left atrium, previously reported (16), was discontinued because of chronic malfunction and zero baseline instability. The chest wound was closed, the connecting cables buried under the skin, and the animal allowed to recover over a 6-week period after which an interval splenectomy was accomplished. Six to 9 weeks later each dog was premedicated with i.m. morphine sulfate (1 mg/kg), restrained in the lateral recumbency; the femoral artery was exposed and cannulated under local anesthesia so as to measure systemic arterial blood pressure and to collect arterial blood samples for various assays.

The jugular vein was exposed and a 7Fr triple lumen Swan-Ganz balloon catheter advanced into the pulmonary artery so as to measure pulmonary arterial pressure. This catheter has a port 20 cm distal from the tip which lies in the right atrium to allow measurement of right atrial pressure. Intermittent inflation of the balloon and advancement of the catheter tip into the "wedge" position measured pulmonary artery wedge pressure, the hemodynamic equivalent of left arterial pressure. The buried chest leads were exposed and connected, along with the other inserts to appropriate devices, to a physiologic recorder (Electronics for Medicine VR-6, White Plains, New York) for continuous and concomitant signal display.

Each animal was allowed to ventilate spontaneously. Supplemental i.v. injections of morphine (0.25–0.50 mg/kg) were used if the animal became restless. All catheters were filled and flushed with a heparinized normal saline solution, 1,000 U.S.P. units/liter.

Arterial blood samples were collected and pH, pO_2, pCO_2, HCO_3^-, hematocrit and colloidal osmotic pressure were measured (Model IL-213 Digital pH blood gas analyzer and Model IL-186 Weil Oncometer System, Lexington, Massachusetts). Lactic acid and pyruvic acid were measured using Sigma kits (Sigma Chemical Co., St. Louis, Missouri). "Excess" lactate (Xl), a measure of oxygen debt, was calculated after Huckabee (10). Base excess was calculated from the Siggard-Anderson nomogram.

After preparation the animals were studied over a 30 to 40 min control period during which all hemodynamic parameters were recorded continuously. From this common pool of 45 dogs, 19 were assigned to 2 populations. Population I ($n = 10$), the control, untreated animals, received purified *E. coli* lipopolysaccharide endotoxin (Difco 026:B6, lot 613872, Westphal) in the dose of 1 mg/kg, i.v. That dosage is sublethal in our experience with the model. The lyophilized moiety was reconstituted in normal saline 2 hr prior to injection and kept at 37°C; the injection volume (5 ml) was administered as a bolus over 15 sec.

A second group of dogs, Population II ($n = 9$), were pretreated with the 5-HT$_2$ receptor antagonist, ketanserin, 0.2 mg/kg. This drug was available in 2 ml ampoules, at 5 mg/ml; the proper dosage was diluted to 5 ml in normal saline and given as an i.v. bolus over 15 sec. Thirty min later, the endotoxin was administered as above.

Selected hemodynamic parameters were measured at periodic intervals prior to and after the use of ketanserin and in response to the endotoxin. These measures included cardiac output (as $\dot{Q}_{PA}$ = pulmonary flow in ml/kg/min), Δ systemic arterial blood pressure (= systemic arterial blood pressure − right atrial pressure in mm Hg), Δ pulmonary arterial pressure (= pulmonary arterial pressure − left atrial pressure in mm Hg), systemic vascular resistance where systemic vascular resistance = Δ systemic arterial pressure × $10/\dot{Q}_{PA}$ and pulmonary vascular resistance (PVR = ΔPAP × $10/\dot{Q}_{PA}$); both systemic arterial pressure and peripheral vascular resistance are expressed in resistance units.

Arterial blood samples were obtained prior to the endotoxin administration and again 1 hr and 2 hr later.

Differences between treatment groups were analyzed using a repeated measures analysis of variance and covariance. A p value < 0.05 was considered statistically significant. The data are presented as the mean ± 1 SEM.

RESULTS

Figure 1 evaluates the pretreatment effects of ketanserin so as to answer the question: Has the drug significantly modified the animals hemodynamic status even before the endotoxin was administered? No cardiac output studies were available in 4 animals in this group. These results indicate that the two populations were not

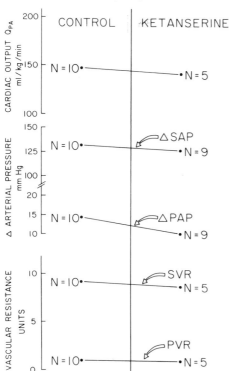

FIG. 1. Effect of treatment with ketanserin, a 5-HT$_2$ receptor antagonist, on cardiac output ($\dot{Q}_{PA}$ = pulmonary flow), Δ systemic arterial pressure (ΔSAP) = systemic arterial pressure − right atrial pressure, Δ pulmonary arterial pressure (ΔPAP) = pulmonary arterial pressure − left atrial pressure, systemic vascular resistance (SVR) = ΔSAP/$\dot{Q}_{PA}$ × 10 and peripheral vascular resistance (PVR) = Δ Pulmonary arterial pressure/$\dot{Q}$ × 10 prior to induction of endotoxin shock. The changes are not significant from control (p < 0.05).

significantly different notwithstanding the apparent decline in pulmonary arterial pressure; peripheral vascular resistance was not altered. Preliminary trials in mongrel dogs *(unpublished data)* with higher dosages of ketanserin (1 mg/kg) significantly reduced *preshock* systemic arterial blood pressure whereas the selected dosage used in this report (0.2 mg/kg) did not.

Figures 2 to 6 illustrate the changes in the hemodynamic parameters of interest in both animal populations in response to the i.v. endotoxin. While the fall in pulmonary flow (Fig. 2) was equally abrupt in the first 5 min, recovery was significantly better in the control dogs. Δ Systemic arterial blood pressure fell to the same extent (Fig. 3) in both populations and there was no recovery of systemic pressure back to control values thereafter. Systemic vascular resistance rose abruptly, as depicted in Fig. 4, then gradually declined, falling below preshock values 1 hr after endotoxin administration. Thus, there was little apparent effect of pretreatment with the 5-HT$_2$ receptor antagonist on these indices of flow, systemic pressure, and systemic vascular resistance, although the fall in cardiac output was more pronounced in the pretreated dogs.

The pulmonary vascular bed response contrasted sharply with the systemic circulation as depicted in Figs. 5 and 6. The transient pulmonary hypertension, typically observed and reported (15) in the untreated dog, was significantly reduced by pretreatment with ketanserin. The transient and minimal elevation in pulmonary arterial pressure noted in this group of dogs was not significantly different from the pretreatment values. Concomitantly, the significant attenuation in peripheral vascular resistance (see Fig. 6) in Population II as compared to Population I, was striking. Nevertheless, a significant but attenuated increase in peripheral vascular resistance persisted after pretreatment with ketanserin indicating that additional humoral factors other than 5-hydroxytryptamine may participate in the pulmonary hypertension.

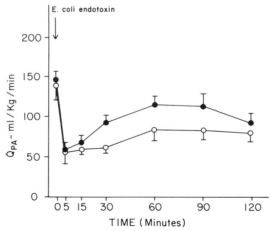

FIG. 2. Changes in pulmonary flow ($\dot{Q}_{PA}$) in response to *E. coli* endotoxin. The *solid dots* represent the control population (*n* = 10), and the *open dots* the dogs (*n* = 5) pretreated with the 5-HT$_2$ receptor antagonist ketanserin. Each datum is the mean value ± SEM.

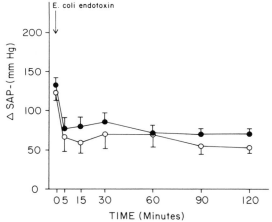

FIG. 3. Changes in the net systemic arterial pressure (ΔSAP) where Δ systemic arterial pressure (ΔSAP) = systemic arterial pressure − right atrial pressure in response to *E. coli* endotoxin. The *solid dots* are the control animals, the *open dots* are the animals pretreated with the 5-HT$_2$ receptor antagonist ketanserin. Mean values ± SEM are plotted.

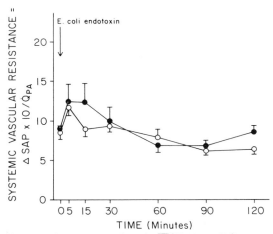

FIG. 4. Changes in systemic vascular resistance (SVR) where SVR = Δ systemic arterial pressure (ΔSAP) × 10/Q$_{PA}$, expressed as units, in response to *E. coli* endotoxin. Control animals are the *solid dots*, the animals pretreated with the 5-HT$_2$ receptor antagonist ketanserin are the *open dots*. Each data point is the mean ± 1 SEM.

Table 1 depicts the changes in the metabolic parameters in hematocrit and in plasma colloidal osmotic pressure. The metabolic changes were not significantly different in the two groups; both developed a metabolic acidosis, an oxygen debt, and hemoconcentration. As a group, the dogs in Population II, pretreated with ketanserin, appeared more acidotic and with higher hematocrits than the control animals (Population I). No apparent problems with gas diffusion were noted but the extent to which the seemingly good arterial po$_2$ reflects pulmonary arteriovenous

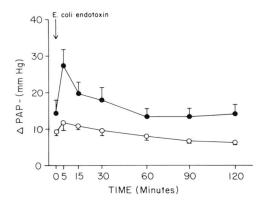

FIG. 5. Changes in net pulmonary arterial pressure where Δpulmonary arterial pressure (ΔPAP) = pulmonary arterial pressure − left atrial pressure or pulmonary arterial wedge pressure, in response to *E. coli* endotoxin in two populations of dogs. The *solid dots* are the control animals, the *open circles* are the animals pretreated with the 5-HT$_2$ receptor antagonist ketanserin. Mean values, ± 1 SEM, are plotted.

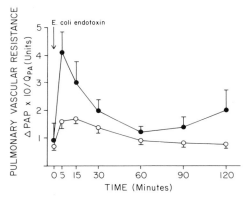

FIG. 6. Changes in pulmonary vascular resistance (PVR) where Δ pulmonary arterial pressure (ΔPAP) × 10/$\dot{Q}_{PA}$ in response to *E. coli* endotoxin. Control animals are the *solid dots*, the animals pretreated with the 5-HT$_2$ receptor antagonist ketanserin, are the *open dots*. Each data point is the mean ± 1 SEM.

shunting was not evaluated. Plasma colloidal osmotic pressure measures were available only in Population II and reflect a significant reduction.

DISCUSSION

The genesis of the pulmonary hypertension and the increased pulmonary vascular resistance in endotoxemia is unclear. 5-Hydroxytryptamine is a well known potent pulmonary vasoconstrictor in many animal species (4). Pulmonary hypertension has been avoided with other serotonergic antagonists, notably methysergide and cyproheptadine (14,18,21). Increased plasma 5-hydroxytryptamine levels have been measured in the pulmonary veins in the intact animal after induction of endotoxin shock (5,12). The reduction in endotoxin-induced pulmonary vasoconstriction in our dogs by pretreatment with ketanserin provides further support for the participatory role of 5-hydroxytryptamine. Little participation of serotonergic responses in the systemic circulation was evident, however.

So far, no particular physiologic role for 5-hydroxytryptamine has been defined and its physiopathological significance is unclear other than that of being both able to cause vasoconstriction and vasodilation. 5-Hydroxytryptamine, like the prosta-

TABLE 1. Changes in arterial blood pH, blood gases (O$_2$, CO$_2$), bicarbonate (HCO$_3^-$), hematocrit (HCT), calculated base excess (BE), and excess lactate (XI), both pre- and postadministration of E. coli endotoxin in two populations[a] of beagle dogs

	pH (units)	pO$_2$ (mm Hg)	pCO$_2$ (mm Hg)	BE (mEq/liter)	HCO$_3^-$ (mEq/liter)	XI (mg %)	HCT (vol %)	COP[b] (mm Hg)
Preshock								
Control (n=10)	7.29 ± 0.01	80.8 ± 3.0	50.4 ± 2.2	−2.9 ± 0.7	23.6 ± 1.1		39.4 ± 0.6	NA
Ketanserin (n=9)	7.25 ± 0.01	91.2 ± 2.2	52.1 ± 1.1	−5.3 ± 0.4	22.2 ± 0.2		44.5 ± 0.8	15 ± 0.6
Shock (60 min)								
Control	7.27 ± 0.00	85.8 ± 3.4	40.4 ± 0.9	−7.2 ± 0.5	19.2 ± 0.5	5.3 ± 1.0	43.2 ± 1.1	NA
Ketanserin	7.21 ± 0.01	94.6 ± 5.8	40.2 ± 0.8	−11.5 ± 0.8	15.8 ± 0.4	7.0 ± 1.3	50.6 ± 1.5	11.5 ± 0.4
Shock (120 min)								
Control	7.30 ± 0.00	96.8 ± 4.6	36.8 ± 1.2	−7.4 ± 0.4	18.2 ± 0.5	6.6 ± 2.3	42.2 ± 0.8	NA
Ketanserin	7.20 ± 0.02	101.1 ± 4.3	39.5 ± 1.3	−12.4 ± 1.3	15.1 ± 0.6	7.4 ± 1.4	49.4 ± 1.7	10.9 ± 0.3

[a]Population I = the control group and Population II = animals pretreated with the 5-HT$_2$ receptor antagonist, ketanserin. Plasma colloidal osmotic pressure (COP) was measured only in Population II dogs. Each data point is a mean value ± 1 SEM.
[b]Lab standard: 16.7 ± 0.2 (±1 SEM).
NA: not available.

glandins, is produced in response to some abnormal stimulus, i.e., endotoxin. Conceptually, it may act as an "amplifier" of other vasoconstricting or platelet-aggregating agents such as the catecholamines. More recently, Shepro and associates (23) reported that 5-hydroxytryptamine released from platelets somehow maintains microvascular integrity. If so, then the inhibition of 5-hydroxytryptamine activity with ketanserin, however beneficial to cardiopulmonary hemodynamics, may have contributed to the substantive loss of plasma volume noted in our experiments, as evidenced by the rise in hematocrit and the fall in plasma colloidal osmotic pressure.

If, indeed, ketanserin is a potent antagonist of the vasoconstrictor but not the vasodilator effects of 5-hydroxytryptamine, as reported by Van Nueten et al. (24), then the similar changes in cardiac output and in the systemic circulation noted in our two dog populations are understandable. Presumably the reduction in cardiac output is the result of pooling and stagnation of the circulating volume, compounded by the leakage of plasma from the vascular bed; none of these effects were prevented by pretreatment with ketanserin. The peripheral effects of serotonergic antagonists on venomotor tone and venous compliance are speculative.

It is noteworthy that a small residual of pulmonary hypertension and increased peripheral vascular resistance still developed after pretreatment with ketanserin. Perhaps the dose used was insufficient to antagonize all serotonergic receptors involved; alternatively, some other vasoactive substance may be responsible. Current experimental findings *(unpublished)* with larger doses of ketanserin alone, or in combination with prostaglandin cyclooxygenase inhibitors, suggest this may be so. Nevertheless, in our experience with this and similar dog preparations, ketanserin is unique in significantly attenuating the pulmonary hypertension and vascular resistance which acutely follows the administration of i.v. bolus of *E. coli* endotoxin. Published and unpublished trials wherein dogs were *pretreated* with a variety of autonomic system blocking drugs (dibenzyline, trimethaphan), with vasodilators (hydralazine, isoproterenol), with corticosteroids (dexamethasone), with prostaglandin cyclooxygenase inhibitors (indomethacin), with thromboxane synthetase inhibitors (imidazole), and even with full heparinization, have not yielded comparable results.

While it is hazardous to transpose animal data to human disease, a possible role for this $5-HT_2$ receptor antagonist seems likely in a number of other conditions characterized by pulmonary hypertension and increased pulmonary vascular resistance. Pulmonary embolism, both infant and adult respiratory disease, congestive heart failure, and decompression sickness are but a few that come to mind. Future animal experimentation to test these premises is indicated.

ACKNOWLEDGMENTS

The authors are grateful to Dr. C. B. Loadholt, Professor, Biometry Department, Medical University of South Carolina for his assistance with the statistical analyses, and to Dr. Perry Halushka, Associate Professor, Department of Pharmacology, Medical University of South Carolina for his review and critique of this manuscript.

This study was supported by grant No. 5 S06 RR01840 from the National Heart, Lung and Blood Institute.

REFERENCES

1. Anderson, F. I., Jubiz, W., Tsagaris, T. J., and Kuida, H. (1975): Endotoxin-induced prostaglandin E and F release in dogs. *Am. J. Physiol.*, 228(2):410–414.
2. Blaisdell, F. W., and Lewis, F. R. (1977): *Respiratory Distress Syndrome of Shock and Trauma.* Saunders, Philadelphia.
3. Cavanaugh, D., Rao, R. S., and Comas, M. R. (1977): *Septic Shock in Obstetrics and Gynecology.* Saunders, Philadelphia.
4. Chand, N. (1981): 5-Hydroxytryptamine induces relaxation of goat pulmonary vein evidence for M and D-tryptamine receptors. *Br. J. Pharmacol.*, 72:233–237.
5. Davis, R. B., Bailey, W. I., and Hanson, N. P. (1963): Modification of serotonin and histamine release after *E. coli* administration. *Am. J. Physiol.*, 205(3):560–566.
6. Douglas, W. W. (1975): Histamine and antihistamines; 5-hydroxytryptamine and antagonists. In: *The Pharmacologic Basis of Therapeutics*, edited by L. S. Goodman and A. Gilman, pp. 590–629. Macmillan, New York.
7. Duff, P. (1980): Pathophysiology and management of septic shock. *J. Reprod. Med.*, 24:109–117.
8. Fletcher, J. R., Ramwell, P. W., and Herman, C. M. (1976): Prostaglandins and the hemodynamic course of endotoxin shock. *J. Surg. Res.*, 20:589–594.
9. Hinshaw, L. B., Jordan, M. M., and Vick, J. A. (1961): Mechanisms of histamine release in endotoxin shock. *Am. J. Physiol.*, 200:987–989.
10. Huckabee, W. E. (1958): Relationship of pyruvate and lactate during anaerobic metabolism. II. Exercise and formation of O_2 debt. *J. Clin. Invest.*, 37:255–263.
11. Koehler, J. A., Tsagaris, T. J., Kuida, H., and Hecht, H. H. (1963): Inhibition of endotoxin-induced pulmonary vasoconstriction in dogs by alpha-methyldopa. *Am. J. Physiol.*, 204:987–990.
12. Kobold, E. E., Lovell, R., Katz, W., and Thal, A. P. (1964): Chemical mediators released by endotoxin. *Surg. Gynecol. Obstet.*, 118:807–813.
13. Leysen, J. E., Niemegeers, C. J. E., Tollenaere, J. P., and Laduron, P. M. (1978): Serotonergic components of neuroleptic receptors. *Nature*, 272:168–171.
14. Malligan, I. J., Oleksyn, T. W., and Schwartz, S. I. (1972): Effects of sergide on pulmonary capillary perfusion in experimental pulmonary embolism. *Surg. Forum*, 23:212–213.
15. Morris, J. A. (1967): Bacteremic shock in obstetrics. In: *Advances in Obstetrics and Gynecology*, edited by S. L. Marcus and C. C. Marcus, pp. 150. Williams & Wilkins, New York.
16. Morris, J. A., O'Grady, J. P., and Toapanta, P. (1979): Endotoxin shock in the beagle dog. *Am. J. Obstet. Gynecol.*, 134:120–126.
17. Nies, A. S., Forsyth, R. P., Williams, H. E., and Melmon, K. L. (1964): Contribution of kinins to endotoxin shock in unanesthetized Rhesus monkey. *Circ. Res.*, 22:155–164.
18. Ozdemir, I. A., Kusajima, K., Wax, S. D., and Webb, W. R. (1972): The effects of serotonin on pulmonary vascular resistance and microcirculation. *Circulation*, (Suppl. II), 45–46, 2:46.
19. Parratt, J. R., and Sturgess, R. M. (1977): The possible roles of histamine, 5-hydroxytryptamine and prostaglandin $F_{2\alpha}$ as mediators of the acute pulmonary effects of endotoxin. *Br. J. Pharmacol.*, 60:209–219.
20. Peroutka, S. J., and Snyder, S. H. (1979): Multiple serotonin receptors: Differential binding of [³H]5-hydroxytryptamine, [³H]lysergic acid diethylamide and [³H]spiroperidol. *Mol. Pharmacol.*, 16:687–699.
21. Pitzele, S., Sze, S., and Sobell, A. R. C. (1973): The inhibition of serotonin-induced blood cell aggregation in the dog. *Surgery*, 73:416–422.
22. Rao, P. S., Dahn, C. H., and Cavanagh, D. (1977): Pathophysiology. In: *Septic Shock in Obstetrics and Gynecology*, edited by D. Cavanagh, P. S. Rao, and M. R. Comas, pp. 5–76. Saunders, Philadelphia.
23. Shepro, D., and Hechtman, H. (1981): Loss of microvascular integrity with fluoxetine, a serotonin antagonist. *Fed. Proc.*, 40(3):774.
24. Van Nueten, J. M., Janssen, P. A. J., Van Beek, J., Xhonneux, R., Verbeuren, T. J., and Vanhoutte, P. M. (1981): Vascular effects of ketanserin (R 41 468), a novel antagonist of $5\text{-}HT_2$ serotonergic receptors. *J. Pharmacol. Exp. Ther.*, 218:217–230.

25. Wise, W. C., Cook, J. A., Eller, T., and Halushka, P. V. (1980): Ibuprofen improves survival from endotoxic shock in the rat. *J. Pharmacol. Exp. Ther.*, 215:160–164.
26. Wise, W. C., Cook, J. A., Halushka, P. V., and Knapp, D. R. (1980): Protective effects of thromboxane synthetase inhibitors in rats in endotoxic shock. *Circ. Res.*, 46:854–859.

5-Hydroxytryptamine in Peripheral Reactions,
edited by Fred De Clerck and Paul M.
Vanhoutte. Raven Press, New York © 1982.

5-Hydroxytryptamine, Vasospasm, and Hypertension

Paul M. Vanhoutte

*Department of Physiology and Biophysics, Mayo Clinic and Foundation,
Rochester, Minnesota 55905*

To allow normal cellular life there must be a continuous stream of nutrients from the outside world to the extracellular space and a continuous stream of waste products from the cells to the outside world. This is achieved by the cardiovascular system, whereby its different components (blood, blood vessels, heart) have a particular contribution to the functioning of the whole. Whenever the cardiovascular system fails to meet the demands of an individual tissue, cellular intoxication and impaired tissue function follow. To avoid this, the blood flow through each organ has to match the metabolic demands of the tissue cells. This is achieved by altering the local arteriolar diameter in function of the cellular requirements, while maintaining the perfusion pressure (arterial blood pressure) relatively constant. The latter implies coordinated adjustments of cardiac function and peripheral vascular tone. Active changes in wall tension or in diameter of the blood vessels are caused by the contraction or the relaxation of the vascular smooth muscle cells. In the large conduit arteries, changes in wall stiffness contribute to the adjustment of the impedance encountered by the left ventricle; together with the systemic peripheral resistance this determines the afterload of the cardiac pump. Active variations in arteriolar diameter help ensure an appropriate blood supply to the tissues and determine the pressure within the capillaries, the venules, and the veins, thus controlling both fluid exchanges at the capillary level and the amount of blood held passively in the postcapillary vessels; the degree of opening of the systemic arterioles also is the major determinant of the peripheral vascular resistance, and together with the cardiac output determines the arterial blood pressure. Constriction of the venules and veins, by altering the pre- and postcapillary resistance ratio, affect the capillary hydrostatic pressure and, thus, the capillary fluid exchanges. The contraction and relaxation of venous smooth muscle cells also permit active alteration of the vascular capacity and so adjust the filling pressure of the right heart, and through the Frank-Starling mechanism, the stroke volume (see refs. 21,23). The coordination of the degree of activity of the muscle cells in the wall of the heart and the blood vessels to maintain the appropriate perfusion pressure to all tissues rests with the central nervous system. It integrates information from various sensors within the cardiovascular system and

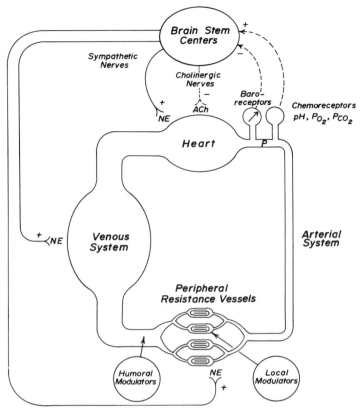

FIG. 1. Nervous, humoral, and local regulation of the cardiovascular system. Peripheral receptors sense either changes in blood pressure (mechanoreceptors) or variations in the chemical composition of the blood (chemoreceptors). The degree of activity of these receptors is conveyed by afferent nerves to centers in the brainstem which control the function of the heart and blood vessels by altering the activity of the sympathetic and cholinergic nerves. When the activity of the former is increased, the neurotransmitter norepinephrine (NE) is released, which stimulates the heart and constricts the blood vessels (+). When the cholinergic nerves are activated, the released acetylcholine (ACh) depresses the heart (−). The activity of both heart and blood vessels is also modulated by substances released into the circulation from endocrine glands (e.g., epinephrine from the adrenal medulla). In the tissues products of metabolism (e.g., adenosine) regulate the local blood flow in accordance with their needs. The degree of opening of the arterioles determines the resistance to flow, and the individual perfusion rate in each tissue; the systemic resistance to flow, together with the cardiac output, determines the arterial blood pressure. The largest part of the blood volume is contained in the systemic veins. These form a dynamic reservoir which continuously adjusts the capacity of the cardiovascular system in order to maintain an appropriate filling pressure of the heart, and thus an appropriate stroke volume. P = pressure. (From ref. 23, by permission.)

modulates the function of its components via the peripheral autonomic nerves and certain endocrine cells (Fig. 1). In addition, other blood-borne substances, the products of cellular metabolism, and autocoids produced in the vicinity of vascular smooth muscle cells, can cause their contraction or relaxation (see refs. 21–23,26,28).

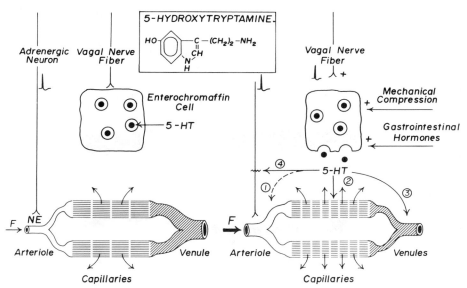

FIG. 2. Mechanisms of release and vascular effect of 5-hydroxytryptamine (5-HT) in the gastrointestinal wall. Mechanical compression by the contraction of the gastrointestinal muscle, or release evoked by vagal nerve activity or gastrointestinal hormones (e.g., gastrin), cause the enterochromaffin cells to discharge 5-hydroxytryptamine. The released 5-hydroxytryptamine: (1) dilates arterioles; (2) increases vascular permeability; (3) constricts venules; and (4) inhibits adrenergic neurotransmission. These effects combine to increase the blood flow (F) and the exudation of fluid to meet the metabolic requirements of the gastrointestinal wall and sustain the secretion of the gastrointestinal juices. NE = norepinephrine. (From ref. 23, by permission.)

This overview briefly discusses the vascular effects of one of the autocoids, 5-hydroxytryptamine, in relationship to the potential role it may play in certain pathological situations. With few exceptions, the references cited in the first two sections will be monographs or review articles to which the reader is referred for more detailed descriptions and references.

VASCULAR EFFECTS OF 5-HYDROXYTRYPTAMINE

Depending upon the type of blood vessel studied, the concentration of 5-hydroxytryptamine used and the experimental condition applied, the monoamine can cause either relaxation or contraction of vascular smooth muscle (Fig. 2).

Vasoconstrictor Effects

5-Hydroxytryptamine causes contraction of most isolated vascular preparations (see refs. 21,24). There are, however, important differences in sensitivity to the monoamine among various blood vessels (see refs. 26,29; J. M. Van Nueten, *this volume*). At the microcirculatory level the direct constrictor effect of the monoamine predominates on the venules (see refs. 1,26). The contraction of vascular smooth muscle cells in presence of 5-hydroxytryptamine can be due to: (a) direct-activation

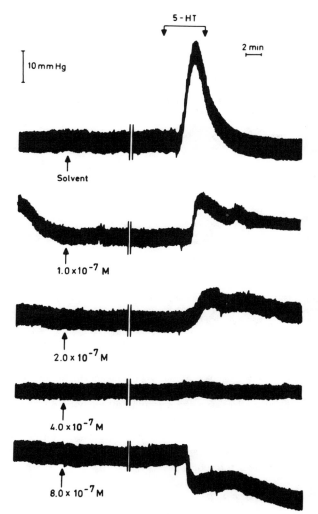

FIG. 3. Demonstration, in the isolated perfused guinea pig stomach that increasing concentrations of the 5-HT$_2$-serotonergic antagonist ketanserin (R41468) inhibit the vasoconstrictor response to 5-hydroxytryptamine and eventually reverse it to a vasodilator reaction. (From ref. 30, by permission.)

of serotonergic receptors on the cell membrane of the vascular smooth muscle cells. The available evidence suggests that the receptors involved belong to the serotonergic 5-HT$_2$-subtype, and that their activation triggers the contractile process mainly by increasing the entry of extracellular Ca^{2+} into the vascular smooth muscle cells (see refs. 29–32); (b) amplification of the response to other vasoconstrictor agonists. The available evidence suggests that this effect is also mediated by 5-HT$_2$-receptors (see ref. 29, J. M. Van Nueten, *this volume*); (c) activation of alpha-adrenoceptors

PULMONARY
CAPILLARY LUMEN

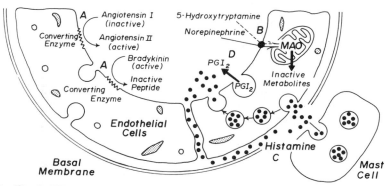

FIG. 4. The handling of bioactive substances by the pulmonary capillaries. **A:** Substances such as angiotensin I and bradykinin are transformed "on" the endothelium by converting enzymes, with resulting formation of active and inactive components, respectively. **B:** Substances such as norepinephrine and 5-hydroxytryptamine are actively taken up *(solid circles)* and degraded enzymatically by monoamine oxidase (MAO). Other substances metabolically degraded by the lung capillaries include certain prostaglandins. **C:** During allergic and anaphylactic reactions, substances such as histamine can overflow into the capillary lumen. **D:** It is likely that the lung capillaries can produce certain prostaglandin-like substances such as prostacyclin (PGI$_2$) and release them into the bloodstream. (From ref. 23, by permission.)

on the vascular smooth muscle cells. This effect is particularly obvious in cutaneous vessels and presumably involves mainly the alpha$_1$-subtype of the alpha-adrenoceptor population (3,7,30; see refs. 26,29); and (d) displacement of endogenous norepinephrine from adrenergic nerve endings and subsequent activation of alpha-adrenoceptors on the vascular smooth muscle cells (see refs. 26,28).

Vasodilator Effects

The vasodilator effect of 5-hydroxytryptamine has been observed mainly in the intact organism, in particular at the level of the small arteries, although certain isolated vascular preparations tissues may relax when exposed to it (see refs. 24,26). The dilatation caused by 5-hydroxytryptamine could be due to: (a) inhibition of norepinephrine release, through activation of prejunctional receptors for 5-hydroxytryptamine which are not blocked by the available serotonergic antagonists (10,16,30; see refs. 17,18,28); (b) activation of nonadrenergic noncholinergic inhibitory nerves present in certain blood vessels (20; see ref. 26); (c) activation of beta-adrenergic receptors (9; see ref. 28); and (d) activation of inhibitory receptors, with yet unknown pharmacological characteristics, on the vascular smooth muscle cells (see ref. 28). It is likely that in certain vascular beds the inhibitory effects of the monoamine are overcome by the potent vasoconstriction it causes; thus 5-HT$_2$-serotonergic antagonists, which inhibit the latter, may unmask the vasodilator properties of 5-hydroxytryptamine (Fig. 3; ref. 30).

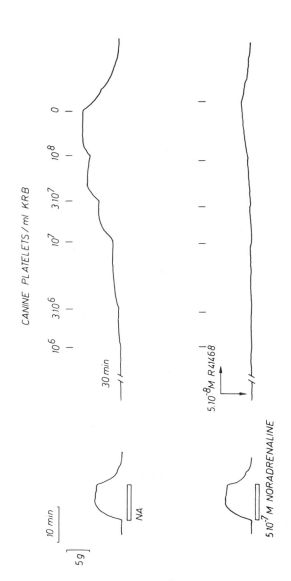

FIG. 5. Isometric recording in a canine femoral artery demonstrating that canine platelets, added in increasing numbers suspended in Krebs-Ringer bicarbonate solution (KRB), cause progressive contraction of the vascular smooth muscle cells (*upper*). This contraction is due in part to the release of 5-hydroxytryptamine since it is inhibited by the 5-HT$_2$-serotonergic antagonist ketanserin (R 41 468) (*lower*). The *left* part of the illustration shows the response to the ED$_{50}$ of norepinephrine (NE). (J. De Mey and P. M. Vanhoutte, *unpublished observations*.)

5-HYDROXYTRYPTAMINE AND VASOSPASM

Exaggerated contraction of the smooth muscle cells of the blood vessel wall may cause an abnormal reduction in vascular diameter and thus endanger tissue perfusion (see refs. 14,27,31,32). Although the etiology of such vasospasm is not known, and may vary among individuals, one possibility is that 5-hydroxytryptamine released from aggregating platelets may activate the contractile process. This may be the case during extravascular clotting and during arterial occlusion; it would primarily occur at sites with endothelial lesions, since the endothelium not only generates prostacyclin which inhibits platelet aggregation, but also destroys the monoamine enzymatically (Fig. 4; see refs. 23,26,31). Preliminary experiments indicate that when platelets aggregate on the blood vessel wall, they release 5-hydroxytryptamine in sufficient amounts to cause contraction of the vascular smooth muscle cells (Fig. 5; J. De Mey and P. M. Vanhoutte, *unpublished observations*).

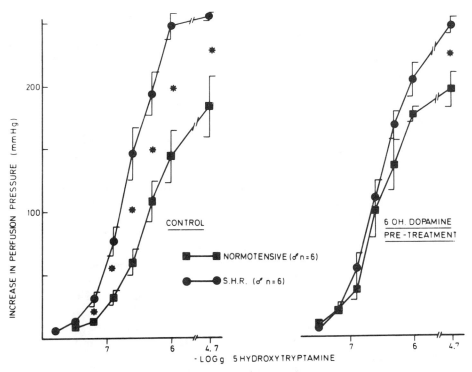

FIG. 6. Left: Log dose-response curves to 5-hydroxytryptamine in kidneys from 6 to 7-week-old spontaneously hypertensive and control rats, before treatment with 6-hydroxydopamine. **Right:** After treatment. Mean increases in perfusion pressure of kidneys from spontaneously hypertensive *(circles)* and control rats *(squares)*. Significant differences between kidneys from spontaneously hypertensive and control rats are indicated by *asterisks*. These experiments demonstrate that the indirect sympathanimetic effect of the monoamine is more pronounced in the young spontaneously hypertensive rat than in the control animals. (From ref. 4, by permission of the American Heart Association.)

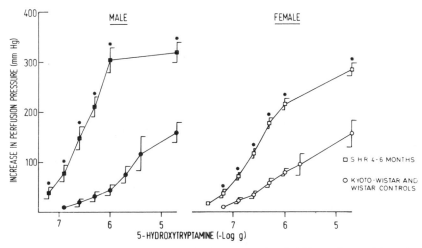

FIG. 7. Log dose-response curves to 5-hydroxytryptamine in kidneys from adult male and female spontaneously hypertensive and control rats. Mean increases in perfusion pressure of kidneys from female control rats *(open circle)*; female spontaneously hypertensive rats *(open square)* **(right panel)**; male control rats *(solid circle)*; male spontaneously hypertensive rats *(solid square)* **(left panel)**. Significant differences between kidneys from spontaneously hypertensive and control rats are indicated by *asterisks*. (From ref. 5, by permission of the American Heart Association.)

5-HYDROXYTRYPTAMINE AND HYPERTENSION

In the isolated, Tyrode-perfused kidney of the young, spontaneously hypertensive rat, the indirect sympathomimetic effect of 5-hydroxytryptamine is more pronounced than in kidneys from normotensive controls (Fig. 6; ref. 4). Isolated blood vessels of renal and desoxycorticosterone acetate hypertensive animals are hyperreactive to 5-hydroxytryptamine (Fig. 7); the same is true for the mesenteric and renal vascular beds of the adult spontaneously hypertensive rats (5,6,8,11–13,25). In the kidney of the latter strain, the exaggeration of the constrictor response to the monoamine is more pronounced than that to catecholamines (5). In rats, including spontaneously hypertensive animals, systolic arterial blood pressure is correlated to the maximal vasoconstrictor response of the renal vasculature to 5-hydroxytryptamine (Fig. 8). The kidneys from the adult spontaneously hypertensive rat develop tachyphylaxis to the vasoconstrictor effect of 5-hydroxytryptamine more slowly than those from control animals (Fig. 9; refs. 5,6,8). The delayed tachyphylaxis to 5-hydroxytryptamine in the kidney of the spontaneously hypertensive rat is less pronounced in older animals; it is due to a specific alteration of the vascular smooth muscle cells exposed to chronic high pressure (6,8). Although these findings all suggest that the increased vascular reactivity to 5-hydroxytryptamine is a marker of the hypertensive process, they do not allow to conclude to a causal relationship between the hyperreactivity to the monoamine and the occurrence of the high blood pressure. However, other observations point in that direction. In the genetically hypertensive New Zealand rat, inhibition of 5-hydroxytryptamine synthesis lowers

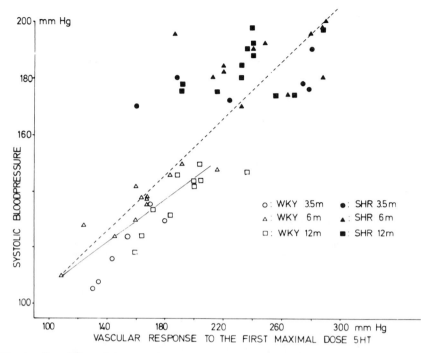

FIG. 8. Correlation of the vascular response (increase in perfusion pressure, mm Hg) to a high dose of 5-hydroxytryptamine (2×10^{-5} g) in the isolated perfused kidney of spontaneously hypertensive and normotensive rats, with the indirectly measured systolic blood pressure (mm Hg). (From ref. 8, by permission of the American Heart Association.)

arterial blood pressure (15); in the same strain the serotonergic antagonist methysergide has an hypotensive effect, albeit presumably due to a central nervous action (2). In the Japanese spontaneously hypertensive rat, methysergide does not lower arterial blood pressure (13); however, methysergide has agonistic properties in vascular smooth muscle (29), which, in view of the hyperreactivity of the vascular smooth muscle cells to serotonergic activation, could mask its peripheral antihypertensive properties. This interpretation is supported by the observations that ketanserin, in doses which are devoid of agonistic properties and do not affect adrenergic responsiveness in the spontaneously hypertensive rat, decreases its arterial blood pressure more than in normotensive controls (Fig. 10; ref. 30). With the demonstration of increased vasoconstrictor responses and delayed tachyphylaxis to the monoamine, and in particular with the positive correlation between systolic blood pressure and vascular responsiveness to 5-hydroxytryptamine, these observations favor the hypothesis that in the intact spontaneously hypertensive rat, increased or normal levels of 5-hydroxytryptamine in the vicinity of the vascular smooth muscle cells may contribute to the etiology of the hypertensive process (8,30). The 5-hydroxytryptamine could act directly on the hyperresponsive vascular smooth mus-

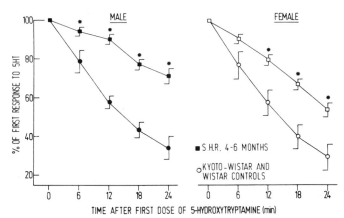

FIG. 9. The rate of development of tachyphylaxis to 5-hydroxytryptamine in kidneys from male and female spontaneously hypertensive and sex-matched control rats. Mean percentage decrease in response amplitude to repeated doses (2 × 10⁻⁵ g) of 5-hydroxytryptamine in kidneys from female control rats *(open circle)*; female spontaneously hypertensive rats *(open square)* **(right panel)**; male control rats *(solid circle)*; male spontaneously hypertensive rats *(solid square)* **(left panel)**. Significant differences between kidneys from spontaneously hypertensive and control rats are indicated by *asterisks*. (From ref. 5, by permission of the American Heart Association.)

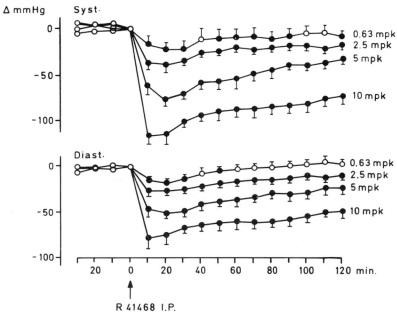

FIG. 10. Effect of increasing doses of ketanserin (R 41 468) on systolic (syst.) and diastolic (diast.) blood pressure in spontaneously hypertensive rats. Ketanserin was given intraperitoneally (I.P.). Full symbols indicate that the values obtained in the presence of ketanserin are significantly different from control. mpk = mg/kg. (From ref. 30, by permission.)

cle cells and/or amplify their response to the existing adrenergic tone. Compounds such as ketanserin would be effective in lowering arterial blood pressure because they inhibit the vasoconstrictor effects of 5-hydroxytryptamine and, at the same time, allow the full expression of the pre- and postjunctional vasodilator properties of the monoamine (30). The observations that ketanserin is effective in lowering arterial blood pressure in hypertensive patients (J. DeCrée et al., *this volume*) suggests that also in the human, 5-hydroxytryptamine may play a role in the etiology of the disease.

REFERENCES

1. Altura, B. M. (1981): Pharmacology of venules: Some current concepts and clinical potential. *J. Cardiovasc. Pharmacol.*, 3:1413–1428.
2. Antonaccio, M. J., and Coté, D. (1976): Centrally mediated antihypertensive and bradycardic effects of methysergide in spontaneously hypertensive rats. *Eur. J. Pharmacol.*, 36:451–454.
3. Apperley, E., Humphrey, P. P. A., and Levy, G. P. (1976): Receptors for 5-hydroxytryptamine and noradrenaline in rabbit isolated ear artery and aorta. *Br. J. Pharmacol.*, 58:211–221.
4. Collis, M. G., De Mey, Ch., and Vanhoutte, P. M. (1979): Renal vascular reactivity in the young spontaneously hypertensive rat. *Hypertension*, 2:45–52.
5. Collis, M. G., and Vanhoutte, P. M. (1977): Vascular reactivity of isolated perfused kidneys from male and female spontaneously hypertensive rats. *Circ. Res.*, 41:759–767.
6. Collis, M. G., and Vanhoutte, P. M. (1981): Tachyphylaxis to 5-hydroxytryptamine in perfused kidneys from spontaneously hypertensive and normotensive rats. *J. Cardiovasc. Pharmacol.*, 3:229–235.
7. Curro, F. A., Greenberg, S., Verbeuren, T. J., and Vanhoutte, P. M. (1978): Interaction between alpha-adrenergic and serotonergic activation of canine saphenous veins. *J. Pharmacol. Exp. Ther.*, 207:936–949.
8. De Mey, Ch., and Vanhoutte, P. M. (1981): Effect of age and spontaneous hypertension on the tachyphylaxis to 5-hydroxytryptamine and angiotensin II in the isolated rat kidney. *Hypertension*, 3:718–724.
9. Edvinsson, L., Hardebo, J. E., and Owman, C. (1978): Pharmacological analysis of 5-hydroxytryptamine receptors in isolated intracranial and extracranial vessels of cat and man. *Circ. Res.*, 42:143–151.
10. Feniuk, W., Humphrey, P. P. A., and Watts, A. D. (1979): Presynaptic inhibitory action of 5-hydroxytryptamine in dog isolated saphenous vein. *Br. J. Pharmacol.*, 67:247–254.
11. Field, F. P., Janis, R. A., and Triggle, D. J. (1973): Relationship between aortic reactivity and blood pressure of renal hypertensive, hyperthyroid and hypothyroid rats. *Can. J. Physiol. Pharmacol.*, 51:344–353.
12. Finch, L. (1974): Vascular reactivity in hypertensive rats after treatment with antihypertensive agents. *Life Sci.*, 15:1827–1863.
13. Haeusler, G., and Finch, L. (1972): Vascular reactivity to 5-hydroxytryptamine and hypertension in the rat. *Naunyn Schmiedebergs Arch. Pharmacol.*, 272:101–110.
14. Hillis, L. D., and Braunwald, E. (1978): Coronary-artery spasm. *N. Engl. J. Med.*, 299:695–702.
15. Jarrott, B., McQueen, A., Graf, L., and Louis, W. J. (1975): Serotonin levels in vascular tissue and the effects of a serotonin synthesis inhibition on blood pressure in hypertensive rats. *Clin. Exp. Pharmacol. Physiol.*, (Suppl.) 2:201–205.
16. McGrath, M. A. (1977): 5-Hydroxytryptamine and neurotransmitter release in canine blood vessels. Inhibition by low and augmentation by high concentrations. *Circ. Res.*, 41:428–435.
17. McGrath, M. A., and Shepherd, J. T. (1978): Histamine and 5-hydroxytryptamine-inhibition of transmitter release mediated by H_2- and 5-hydroxytryptamine receptors. *Fed. Proc.*, 37:195–198.
18. McGrath, M. A., and Vanhoutte, P. M. (1978): Vasodilatation caused by peripheral inhibition of adrenergic neurotransmission. In: *Mechanisms of Vasodilatation*, edited by P. M. Vanhoutte and I. Leusen, pp. 248–257. Karger, Basel.
19. Moncada, S., and Vane, J. R. (1978): Prostacyclin (PGI_2), the vascular wall and vasodilatation. In: *Mechanisms of Vasodilatation*, edited by P. M. Vanhoutte and I. Leusen, pp. 107–121. Karger, Basel.

20. Myers, H. A., Schenk, E. A., and Honig, C. R. (1975): Ganglion cells in arterioles of skeletal muscle: Role in sympathetic vasodilation. *Am. J. Physiol.*, 229:126–138.
21. Shepherd, J. T., and Vanhoutte, P. M. (1975a): *Veins and Their Control.* Saunders, Philadelphia.
22. Shepherd, J. T., and Vanhoutte, P. M. (1975b): Skeletal muscle blood flow-neurogenic determinants. In: *Peripheral Circulations*, edited by R. Zelis, pp. 3–55. Grune & Stratton, New York.
23. Shepherd, J. T., and Vanhoutte, P. M. (1979): *The Human Cardiovascular System.* Raven Press, New York.
24. Somlyo, A. P., and Somlyo, A. V. (1970): Vascular smooth muscle. II. Pharmacology of normal and hypertensive vessels. *Pharmacol. Rev.*, 22:249–353.
25. Vacek, L. (1970): Susceptibility of rabbit aorta strips to serotonin in endocrine hypertension. *Arch. Int. Pharmacodyn. Ther.*, 124:461–465.
26. Vanhoutte, P. M. (1978): Heterogeneity of vascular smooth muscle. In: *Microcirculation*, Vol. II, edited by G. Kaley and B. M. Altura, pp. 181–309. University Park Press, Baltimore.
27. Vanhoutte, P. M. (1981): Calcium entry blockers and cardiovascular failure. *Fed. Proc.*, 40:2882–2887.
28. Vanhoutte, P. M., Verbeuren, T. J., and Webb, R. C. (1981): Local modulation of the adrenergic neuroeffector interaction in the blood vessel wall. *Physiol. Rev.*, 61:151–247.
29. Van Nueten, J. M., Janssen, P. A. J., and Vanhoutte, P. M. (1982): Pharmacological properties of serotonergic responses in vascular, bronchial and gastrointestinal smooth muscle. In: *Vascular Neuroeffectors and Other Smooth Muscle*, edited by J. A. Bevan et al. Raven Press, New York *(in press)*.
30. Van Nueten, J. M., Van Beek, J., and Vanhoutte, P. M. (1980): Inhibitory effect of lidoflazine on contractions of isolated canine coronary arteries caused by norepinephrine, 5-hydroxytryptamine, high potassium, anoxia and ergonovine maleate. *J. Pharmacol. Exp. Ther.*, 213:179–187.
31. Van Nueten, J. M., and Vanhoutte, P. M. (1981a): Calcium entry blockers and vasospasm. In: *Vasodilatation*, edited by P. M. Vanhoutte and I. Leusen, pp. 459–468. Raven Press, New York.
32. Van Nueten, J. M., and Vanhoutte, P. M. (1981): Calcium entry blockers and vascular smooth muscle heterogeneity. *Fed. Proc.*, 40:2862–2865.

5-Hydroxytryptamine in Peripheral Reactions,
edited by Fred De Clerck and Paul M.
Vanhoutte. Raven Press, New York © 1982.

Hypertension Following Extracorporeal Circulation

*P. J. A. Van der Starre, *J. Bach Kolling, *H. Scheijgrond, and
**R. S. Reneman

*Department of Cardiovascular Anaesthesia, Medisch Centrum De Klokkenberg,
4800 RA Breda; and **Department of Physiology, University of Limburg,
6200 MD Maastricht, The Netherlands*

Hypertension is a common complication following heart valve replacement and coronary artery bypass surgery, using extracorporeal circulation. The incidence of this complication is reported in 30 to 60% of the patients during the first 4 to 6 hr of recovery in Intensive Care Units (2,5,6,9,12). The incidence of hypertension during the first 4 to 6 hr after extracorporeal circulation for coronary artery bypass surgery performed by our unit is 46%, notwithstanding the conventional precautions. Hypertension following extracorporeal circulation constitutes a major problem for several reasons. Firstly, following extracorporeal circulation heart rate is higher than before surgery, often reaching values of 90 to 110 beats/min. In combination with an elevated arterial blood pressure, this may jeopardize the myocardium.

Secondly, the tension generated during the hypertensive crisis may be deleterious to the suture sites of the coronary anastomoses or valvular rings. Thirdly, hypertension may induce general complications like cerebral vascular accidents or pulmonary edema.

Several factors may contribute to the development of hypertension in patients subjected to extracorporeal circulation (Table 1). They include consequences of anesthesia and surgery like arousal, nasopharyngeal and tracheal stimulation, and pain. Considering nonpulsatile flow in extracorporeal circulation as a state of "con-

TABLE 1. *Factors possibly contributing to the development of postoperative hypertension following extracorporeal circulation*

1. Increased levels of angiotensin-renin
2. Increased levels of catecholamines
3. Neurogenic reflexes of the large vessels
4. Hypothermia
5. Pain
6. Arousal from anesthesia
7. Nasopharyngeal and tracheal stimulation
8. Release of 5-hydroxytryptamine, mainly from blood platelets

trolled shock," an increase in circulating catecholamines represents a normal defense mechanism of the body. High dose fentanyl anesthesia techniques or pulsatile flow during bypass were in some respects not unsuccessful in controlling this mechanism (8,13,15,16).

During extracorporeal circulation the number of circulating blood platelets drops drastically beyond the level which can be accounted for by the hemodilution. Such a thrombycytopenia may be explained by an activation of platelets and subsequent formation of aggregates. This activation can be caused by the suction during blood removal from the operation field. Alternatively, platelets might be activated by the stress imposed by the nonpulsatile flow generated by the roller pump and sequestered temporarily in the spleen from which they are gradually released during the postoperative period (16).

In addition, heparinization of the patients before the start of extracorporeal circulation may activate the platelets or sensitize them for other stimuli, including contact with foreign surfaces and catecholamines (4). In suitable conditions activated platelets may release their granular content and/or synthesize prostaglandins. Of the products released or formed by such processes, 5-hydroxytryptamine and thromboxane A_2 are known to be vasoconstrictors and amplifiers of the vasoconstrictive effect of catecholamines. Therefore, these substances may increase systemic vascular resistance and, hence, induce hypertension.

In view of the nature of the contributing factors involved, the logical treatment of such hypertensive patients mainly aims at lowering the systemic vascular resistance. For that purpose vasodilators such as sodium nitroprusside, nitroglycerin, or hydralazine have been used. This type of treatment, however, produces reflex tachycardia (1,10,11,14) which can be considered as a major disadvantage. Moreover, some patients are resistant to the therapy, at least when nontoxic doses of the drugs are used. Newly developed compounds acting as angiotensin II antagonists or converting enzyme inhibitors seem to be devoid of reflex tachycardia, but their efficacy needs further evaluation (3). Assuming that 5-hydroxytryptamine (serotonin), among others, released from activated platelets plays a role in the development of postoperative hypertension, the effect of ketanserin (R 41 468, Janssen Pharmaceutica), a selective 5-HT$_2$ receptor antagonist, was studied in patients with hypertension following coronary artery bypass surgery.

METHODS

Patients

Thirteen out of 27 patients (48%) developed hypertension during early recovery after selective coronary artery bypass surgery and entered the study. In all of them coronary artery disease had been recognized from weeks to years before operation and was confirmed, in all instances, by coronary arteriography.

The age and weight distribution, the duration of anesthesia and surgery, and the number of bypass grafts for this group of patients are described in Table 2. Extra-

TABLE 2. *Patients and procedure description*

Parameter	Parameter values and number of patients					
Age (years)	41–50	51–68	61–70			
	2	7	4			
Weight (kg)	61–70	71–80	81–90	91–100		
	8	2	2	1		
Anesthesia (min)	151–180	181–210	211–240	241–270	271–300	301–330
	1	3	4	3	1	1
Surgery (min)	154–180	181–210	211–240	241–270	271–300	301–330
	4	5	3	0	1	0
Number of (bypass)	1	2	3	4	5	
	2	0	3	2	6	

corporeal bypass time varied from 31 to 111 (median: 80) min. No serious complications occurred during the operation with any of the patients.

Coronary arterial lesions were bypassed by saphenous vein grafts; surgery involved 1 to 5 coronary arteries. Maintenance therapy, usually consisting of beta-adrenergic blockers, long-acting nitrates and, incidentally, Ca^{2+} entry blockers, was continued during hospitalization until the night before surgery.

Patients did not receive anticoagulants before or after surgery. Recognizing the large number of patient variables and intraoperative and postoperative variations we tried to standardize anesthesia and the postoperative care period.

Anesthesia

At arrival in the operating theatre, ECG leads (II and V5) were connected, as well as an intravenous catheter (16 gauge) and a radial arterial cannula (18 gauge) inserted before induction of anesthesia. After induction, a catheter (16 gauge) was introduced through the internal jugular vein for monitoring of the central venous pressure.

Peripheral circulation was monitored by plethysmography of the ear lobe. A nasopharyngeal and a forehead skin temperature probe were placed in position. At the end of the extracorporeal circulation period, a catheter was placed in the left atrium at its junction with the superior pulmonary vein for registration of left atrial pressure. All catheters were left in place for at least 48 hr postoperatively.

Premedication with scopolamine (0.005 mg/kg) and morphine (0.125 mg/kg) i.m. was given 45 min before induction. Anesthesia was induced with etomidate (0.3 mg/kg), fentanyl (0.5 mg), and pancuronium bromide (0.15 mg/kg) and the patient was mechanically ventilated with a mixture of 50% nitrous oxide and 50% oxygen. Ventilation was guided by capnographically monitored CO_2 and blood gases measured in arterial blood samples. Before median sternotomy, during cardiopulmonary bypass, and before closure of the sternum incremental doses of 250 to 500 μg fentanyl and of 0.1 mg/kg pancuronium bromide were given. Unconsciousness, analgesia, and muscle relaxation were adjusted to blood pressure, heart rate, peripheral circulation, and the EEG. Accidental hypertension was treated with nitroglycerin intravenously. Before extracorporeal circulation heparin (3 mg/kg) was administered i.v. The priming solution of the heart-lung machine consisted of dextrose 5% Ringer's lactate, 20 mg/kg body weight, with 50 mEq sodium bicarbonate and 50 mg heparin/liter of the priming solution. The calculated flow was 50 ml/kg body weight. Extracorporeal circulation was performed by a roller-pump (Harvey), using a bubble-oxygenator. Mean arterial pressure during extracorporeal circulation was regulated by vasodilating drugs like trimetaphan and nitroglycerin. The patients were cooled down to 28°C nasopharyngeal temperature with a heat exchanger. The heart was stopped by ventricular fibrillation or by a hyperkalemic cardioplegic solution, with 30 mM KCl, 15 mM $MgCl_2$, 5 mM $NaHCO_3$ and 2 mM $CaCl_2$ in a 5% glucose solution with 0.45% NaCl. Topical cooling of the heart was added. After the distal anastomosis was installed the patient was rewarmed to normothermia (1°C per 3 min). Heparin was antagonized by protamin chloride (1.2 mg/kg) after extracorporeal circulation was stopped. The mean hematocrit at the end of extracorporeal circulation was aimed at 28%. The mean blood loss during surgery was 400 ml. The residual priming solution was transfused to the patient through a transfusion system.

Postoperative Care

During transfer to the intensive care unit, and as long as the patient remained asleep, artificial ventilation was continued aiming at a Pco_2 of 33 to 45 mm Hg and a Po_2 of 100 to 150 mm Hg.

At arrival in the intensive care unit the nasopharyngeal temperature probe was replaced by a rectal probe. Arterial blood pressure, heart rate, ECG, central venous pressure, left atrial pressure, and rectal temperature were monitored for at least 48 hr.

The infusion regimen consisted of 1 ml/kg/hr dextrose 5% Ringer's lactate and the aimed urine production was 0.8 ml/kg/hr. Care was taken that all patients had adequate sedation and analgesia and were free of respiratory difficulties. Blood losses were calculated and were replaced as indicated by the patient's general condition as well as by changes in arterial blood pressure, central venous pressure, and left atrial pressure.

Hypertension

A hypertensive episode was defined as a period of sustained raised systolic blood pressure (>150 mm Hg) provided that this rise was not reversed by simple sedation or analgesia and that there was no evidence of hypoxia, hypercapria, shivering, fighting the ventilator, or intolerance of the endotracheal tube. Besides, right and left filling pressures of the heart had to be sufficient (central venous pressure: 5–10 mm Hg; left atrial pressure: 5–12 mm Hg).

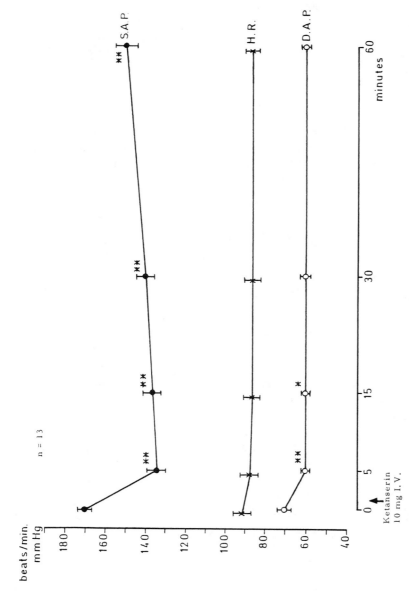

FIG. 1. Effect of 10 mg ketanserin on arterial blood pressure (SAP and DAP) and heart rate (HR) in 13 patients with hypertension following coronary artery bypass surgery. The mean values and standard errors are presented. *p ≤ 0.01, **p ≤ 0.001 Student's *t*-test.

Treatment

Patients with hypertension were treated with a single intravenous dose of 10 mg/kg ketanserin injected over a period of 5 min. Systolic and diastolic blood pressure, heart rate, central venous pressure, left atrial pressure, rectal body temperature, and urine production were registered at 5, 15, 30, and 60 min after the start of treatment.

Statistics

Changes induced by the injection of ketanserin were evaluated for statistical significance by comparing the values of the various variables after injection with those before administration of the compound, using the Student's t-test.

Results

Between 110 and 180 (median: 125) min after the end of anesthesia, 13 patients rapidly developed hypertension. The recorded systolic arterial blood pressure values at the start of treatment varied from 154 to 200 (median: 170) mm Hg. Diastolic arterial pressure varied from 50 to 92 (median: 70) mm Hg and heart rate from 58 to 115 (median: 91) beats/min.

The effect on arterial blood pressure and heart rate of a single, slowly given, intravenous dose of 10 mg ketanserin is illustrated in Fig. 1. The decrease of systolic arterial blood pressure was significant ($p < 0.001$) at 5, 15, 30, and 60 min after the start of treatment. Systolic pressure gradually increased over this period, reaching hypertensive levels again after 60 min. Diastolic arterial blood pressure was significantly decreased at 5 ($p < 0.001$) and 15 ($p < 0.01$) min after the administration of the compound. Heart rate did not change significantly. During 1 hr after treatment central venous pressure and left atrial pressure remained unaffected by the therapy (Table 3). Three other patients did not respond to ketanserin treatment but lowered their arterial blood pressure significantly when a low dose of nitroglycerine (0.4 γ/kg/min) was given.

Urine production remained stable and normal during and after the treatment with ketanserin. Rectal body temperature remained unchanged: None of the patients developed hyperthermia during the first 4 postoperative hours. No untoward effects were noticed.

TABLE 3. *Central venous pressure and left atrial pressure values before and after ketanserin treatment (mean ± SE)*

Pressure	Before	+5 min	+15 min	+30 min	+60 min
Central nervous pressure	6.31 ± 0.38	6.08 ± 0.42	6.08 ± 0.4	5.85 ± 0.36	6.08 ± 0.38
Left atrial pressure	6.64 ± 0.41	6.45 ± 0.53	6.64 ± 0.53	6.55 ± 0.62	6.55 ± 0.62

DISCUSSION

Hypertension following cardiac surgery, especially coronary artery bypass surgery, is a common problem in intensive care units. The percentage of patients suffering from hypertension in the first hours postoperatively varies from 30 to 60% according to several reports.

The multiple hypertensive factors that have been proposed can be divided into two groups, i.e., those related and those not related to anesthesia. Factors not related to anesthesia such as hemodilution, increased antidiuretic hormone and catecholamine levels, variations in angiotensin levels following nonpulsatile extracorporeal circulation, as well as pressor reflexes from the heart and great vessels might be responsible for the frequently reported postoperative hypertension. In the latter mechanism 5-hydroxytryptamine has been considered to play an important role (7). This substance can also be released from platelets activated during the extracorporeal circulation, and gradually released from, for example, the spleen in the postoperative period (16).

In the present study, a 5-hydroxytryptamine receptor-blocking agent (ketanserin) was given as a bolus injection when the systolic arterial blood pressure exceeded 150 mm Hg. The results demonstrate a significant drop in both systolic and diastolic arterial blood pressure, causing a normalization of the pulse pressure. Heart rate, central venous pressure, and left atrial pressure did not change significantly. Systolic blood pressure gradually increased, starting 15 min after the injection of ketanserin and reaching hypertensive levels again after 60 min. This increase in systolic arterial blood pressure can likely be avoided by starting a continuous infusion of ketanserin, immediately following the bolus injection *(preliminary findings)*.

The findings in the present study indicate that 5-hydroxytryptamine might play a role in the hypertension seen after coronary artery bypass surgery.

REFERENCES

1. Armstrong, P. W., Walker, M. D., and Burton, J. R. (1975): Vasodilator therapy in acute myocardial infarction. A comparison of sodium nitroprusside and nitroglycerin. *Circulation*, 52:118–129.
2. Balasaraswathi, K., Glisson, S. N., El-Etr, A. A., and Pifarre, R. (1978): Serum epinephrine and norepinephrine during valve replacement and aorta-coronary bypass. *Can. Anaesth. Soc. J.*, 25:198–203.
3. Editorial (1980): Inhibitors of angiotensin I converting enzyme for treating hypertension. *Br. Med. J.*, 281:630–631.
4. Eiha, C. (1972): On the mechanism of platelet aggregation induced by heparin, protamin and polybrene. *Scand. J. Haematol.*, 9:248–259.
5. Estafanous, F. G., and Tarazi, R. C. (1980): Systemic arterial hypertension associated with cardiac surgery. *Am. J. Cardiol.*, 46:685–694.
6. Estafanous, F. G., Tarazi, R. C., Viljoen, J. F., and El Tawil, M. Y. (1973): Systemic hypertension following myocardial vascularization. *Am. Heart J.*, 85:732–738.
7. James, T. N., Isobe, J. H., and Urthaler, F. (1975): Analysis of components in a cardiogenic hypertensive chemoreflex. *Circulation*, 52:840–845.
8. Lin, W. S., Bidwai, A. V., Lunn, J. K., and Stanley, T. H. (1977): Urine catecholamine excretion after large doses of fentanyl, fentanyl and diazepam and fentanyl, diazepam and pancuronium. *Can. Anaesth. Soc. J.*, 24:371–379.

9. McQueen, M. J., Watson, M. E., and Bain, W. H. (1971): Transient systolic hypertension after aortic valve replacement. *Br. Heart J.*, 34:227–231.
10. Mehta, J., Pepine, C. J., and Conti, R. C. (1978): Haemodynamic effects of hydralazine and of hydralazine plus glyceryl trinitrate paste in heart failure. *Br. Heart J.*, 40:845–856.
11. Moffitt, E. A. (1978): Anaesthetic management for coronary artery bypass surgery. *Can. Anaesth. Soc. J.*, 25:462–467.
12. Roberts, A. J., Niarchos, A. P., Subramanian, V. A., Abel, R. M., Herman, S. D., Sealey, J. E., Case, D. B., White, R. P., Johnson, G. A., Laragh, J. H., and Gay, W. A. (1977): Systemic hypertension associated with coronary artery bypass surgery. *J. Thorac. Cardiovasc. Surg.*, 74:846–859.
13. Salerno, T. A., Henderson, M., Keith, F. M., and Charrette, E. J. (1981): Hypertension after coronary operation. Can it be prevented by pulsatile perfusion? *J. Thorac. Cardiovasc. Surg.* 81:396–399.
14. Stetson, J. B. (1978): Intravenous nitroglycerin, a review. In: *International Anesthesiology Clinics*, edited by W. D. Owens, pp. 261–298. Little Brown, Boston.
15. Taylor, K. M., Morton, I. J., Brown, J. J., Bain, W. H., and Caves, Ph. K. (1977): Hypertension and renin-angiotensin system following open-heart surgery. *J. Thorac. Cardiovasc. Surg.*, 74:840–845.
16. Wenzel, E., Volkmer, I., Laux, E., Limbach, H. G., Mierendorf, M., and Muller, M. (1979): Blood trauma and hypercoaguability produced by extracorporeal circulation. In: *Basic Aspects of Blood Trauma*, edited by H. Schmidt-Schönbein and P. Teitel, pp. 159–183. Martinus Nijhoff Publishers, London.

5-Hydroxytryptamine in Peripheral Reactions,
edited by Fred De Clerck and Paul M.
Vanhoutte. Raven Press, New York © 1982.

Are Serotonergic Mechanisms Involved in High Blood Pressure?

J. De Crée, J. Leempoels, H. Geukens,
W. De Cock, and H. Verhaegen

*Clinical Research Unit St. Bartholomeus, Jan Palfijnziekenhuis,
B-2060 Merksem, Belgium*

In the search for the substance in serum which might be responsible for the increased tone of blood vessels, serotonin was isolated in 1948 by Rapport et al. (11). Because of its possible interest in the study of high blood pressure, clinical studies were undertaken with a few so-called serotonergic antagonists (17,18). These experiments had to be interrupted in a very early stage because of the obvious central side effects of the compounds (17,18). Recently two pharmacologically different subtypes of serotonergic receptors have been identified (5-HT$_1$ and 5-HT$_2$). Whereas 5-HT$_1$ binding sites cannot be associated with any known physiological and pharmacological effects of 5-hydroxytryptamine, binding to 5-HT$_2$ receptors correlates will with *in vivo* and *in vitro* action of 5-hydroxytryptamine (7,10). The availability of ketanserin (R 41 468), a pure and potent 5-HT$_2$ receptor blocking agent, without intrinsic agonistic activity, devoid of central effects, and with a high selectivity for blood vessels and blood platelets (16; F. DeClerck et al., *this volume*) provides a tool to reinvestigate the potential role of 5-hydroxytryptamine in the etiology of hypertension.

The present study was aimed at investigating the effects of ketanserin in patients with high blood pressure.

MATERIALS AND METHODS

Table 1 outlines the general characteristics of the four separate studies performed.

Subjects

A total of 67 subjects were studied. The elderly hypertensive patients were hospitalized (Study I) or attended a home for the elderly (Study III). They all suffered from benign hypertension with superimposed atherosclerosis. There was no evidence of renal functional impairment, endocrine disturbances, or electrolyte imbalances. Fundoscopic examination revealed hypertensive lesions between grade 1 and 3 of Keith-Wagener. The patients of Study II were hospitalized and suffered

TABLE 1. *General outline of four studies to assess the antihypertensive effects of ketanserin*

	Studies			
	I	II	III	IV
Subjects				
Number	23	20	14	10
Ratio males/females	8/15	10/10	0/14	4/6
Median age	71	57	80	54
Age range	62–90	34–80	67–87	34–71
Elderly hypertensive patients	X		X	
Essential hypertension		X		X
Chronic emphysema		X		
Medication				
Ketanserin 10 mg i.v.	X	X		
Ketanserin 20 mg t.i.d. orally				X
Ketanserin 40 mg t.i.d. orally			X	
Duration of treatment				
Single dose	X	X		
Weeks (number)			1/3/30	4
Type of study				
Open	X	X		
Double-blind cross-over				X
Double-blind cross-over/open			X	
Assessment and techniques				
Systolic and diastolic blood pressure	X	X	X	X
Systolic time intervals	X			X
Heart rate	X			X
Deformability of RBCs		X		
Venous blood gases		X		
Hematocrit		X		
Plasma fibrinogen		X		

from essential hypertension or chronic emphysema with acute respiratory distress. The patients of Study IV were outpatients who had been suffering from essential hypertension for a period of 1 to 18 (median: 6.75) years, and without a history of myocardial infarction or cerebrovascular disease.

Techniques

Systolic and diastolic blood pressure was measured with a sphygmomanometer and a stethoscope. Heart rate was evaluated using a peripheral electrocardiographic (ECG) lead from a 4-channel Elema recorder (Siemens). Systolic time intervals were measured from simultaneous recordings of a peripheral lead of the ECG, phonocardiogram (TNO, Leiden), and carotid pulse wave (TNO, Leiden). The tracings were obtained on a modified 4-channel mingograph recorder, at a paper speed of 100 mm/sec (Elema-Siemens). At least five consecutive cardiac cycles were analyzed and averaged for the following parameters: QS_2, total electromechanical systole; LVET, left ventricular ejection time; PEP, preejection period; and the ratio PEP/LVET.

The red blood cell (RBC) deformability was measured by a filtration technique. A 45% RBC suspension in autologous plasma, devoid of leukocytes and platelets, was filtered through a 13 mm circular Unipore polycarbonate filter with a mean pore diameter of 5 μm. All experiments were performed with filters of the same batch. The filters were held in a Millipore plastic filter holder connected to a 1 ml B-D tuberculine syringe. Filtration was performed at room temperature at a negative driving pressure of 20 cm H_2O. After the filter holder and the syringe had filled with the RBC suspension and steady flow through the filter itself began, a volume of 0.5 ml was pressed and the time necessary for this was measured. All measurements were done in duplicate. Results were expressed as flow rate (ml/min).

Venous blood gases were determined with a 40 μl whole blood sample, using an automatic blood gas and Acid/Base microanalyzer (automatic gas check AVC 940). The following parameters were measured: pH, P_{CO_2}, and P_{O_2}. From these data HCO_3 was calculated.

Medication, Treatment, and Procedure

In Study I the acute effects of an intravenous injection of ketanserin were investigated on blood pressure and heart function. The patients were examined in a quiet room after resting in a supine position for at least 15 min. During the subsequent half-hour heart rate and blood pressure were evaluated four times and systolic time intervals twice. The mean values were taken as baseline values. Ten mg of ketanserin (2 ml), diluted in 4 ml saline, were injected intravenously in an antecubital vein over a period of 3 min. Blood pressure and heart rate were measured every minute up to 8 min after the start of the injection, and thereafter every 5 min up to 33 min. Systolic time intervals were measured at 3 and 5 min and at 5 min intervals up to 33 min. Concomitant antihypertensive medication in 16 out of 23 patients were kept unchanged during the experiment.

In Study II an intravenous injection of 10 mg ketanserin was given over a period of 3 min. Before and 5 min after the end of this injection, blood was withdrawn from an antecubital vein for the determination of blood gases, RBC deformability, plasma fibrinogen, and hematocrit. Systolic and diastolic blood pressure was measured before and every minute up to 8 min after the start of the injection, on the same arm, by the same observer. Only the lowest value after the administration was recorded and compared to the pretreatment value. Associated medication was kept unchanged during the experiment.

Study III was a double-blind placebo-controlled cross-over study. Each patient received 40 mg ketanserin or placebo t.i.d. in random sequence for 8 days with an interval of 1 week between both agents. Ketanserin and placebo were supplied in coded boxes containing capsules identical in appearance. Blood pressure was measured on days 1, 4, and 8, three times daily, at fixed hours in the morning, at noon, and in the late afternoon. Measurements were always performed by the same observer on the right arm in the sitting position, after a rest of 5 min. The mean value was computed of three consecutive readings. A total of 126 blood pressure values was thus recorded both during the ketanserin and placebo periods. Ten patients were further treated with 40 mg ketanserin t.i.d. for 3 weeks and blood pressure was measured at the end of treatment. Nine patients were further followed for 7 months during maintenance therapy with 40 mg ketanserin t.i.d. After discontinuation, blood pressure was evaluated until initial high blood pressure values were recorded. Associated antihypertensive medications were clonidine in 5, diuretics in 7, and no medication in 2 patients. This medication was kept unchanged throughout the whole period of study.

Study IV was also a double-blind placebo-controlled cross-over study. Before entering the study antihypertensive medication of the patients was tapered off during a period of at least 2 weeks. Hypertension was ascertained on two successive occasions at a 1 week interval (systolic blood pressure $\geqslant 160$ mm Hg and/or diastolic blood pressure $\geqslant 95$ mm Hg). Patients were allocated in random sequence to either oral treatment with 20 mg ketanserin or placebo t.i.d. at meal time. Ketanserin and placebo were supplied in coded boxes containing tablets identical in appearance. After 4 weeks the alternative medication was given for another 4 weeks. During the double-blind phase lasting for 8 weeks, blood pressure was measured every other week on the same day of the week and at the same time. ECG and systolic time intervals were investigated before entering the double-blind phase, and thereafter every other week.

Statistical Analysis

Statistical methods used were the Student's t-test (4) (Study I) and the Wilcoxon matched-pairs signed-ranks test, two-tailed probability (14) (Studies II, III, and IV).

RESULTS

Study I

An intravenous injection of 10 mg ketanserin significantly reduced both systolic and diastolic blood pressure in elderly hypertensive patients. The onset of action was immediate and the effect lasted for the whole observation period (Fig. 1). Ketanserin had virtually no effect on heart rate and systolic time intervals.

Study II

The effects of an intravenous injection of 10 mg ketanserin on blood pressure, RBC deformability, and venous blood gases of patients suffering from essential hypertension or chronic emphysema are shown in Fig. 2. Ketanserin normalized systolic and diastolic blood pressure ($p < 0.01$). RBC deformability improved after treatment with ketanserin ($p < 0.01$). A significant increase in Po_2 ($p < 0.01$), a decrease in Pco_2 ($p < 0.05$), and an increase in the pH ($p < 0.01$) of the venous blood could be observed. The hematocrit and the fibrinogen content were not affected by ketanserin.

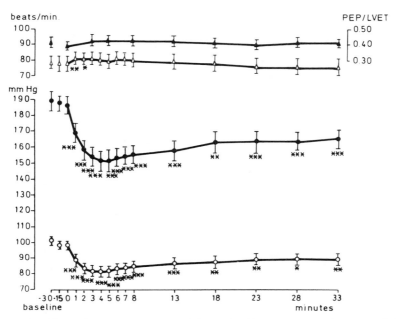

FIG. 1. The effects of acute intravenous administration of 10 mg ketanserin on systolic blood pressure *(solid circle)*, diastolic blood pressure *(open circle)*, heart rate *(open triangle)* and systolic time intervals (PEP/LVET, *solid triangle*) in 23 elderly hypertensive patients. Mean values ± SE. *p*-value: * ≤ 0.01; ** ≤ 0.001; *** ≤ 0.0001.

Study III

In 14 hypertensive elderly patients, treated orally with either placebo or ketanserin (40 mg t.i.d.) for 1 week each, the mean systolic and diastolic blood pressure values were significantly lower during ketanserin treatment than during the corresponding placebo treatment (Fig. 3). Maintenance therapy for 3 weeks with 40 mg ketanserin t.i.d. in 10 patients showed a further decrease of blood pressure necessitating a reduction of the daily dose in 4 patients (Fig. 4). Finally, discontinuation of treatment with ketanserin in 9 patients after 7 months of maintenance therapy showed a progressive return to initial high blood pressure values within 3 months.

No orthostatic hypotension was observed in any of the 14 patients during the treatment with ketanserin. Dizziness and nausea were temporarily seen in the 2 patients with transient hypotension during the first day of the ketanserin period. These symptoms regressed completely without discontinuation of the ketanserin treatment. Four patients necessitated reduction of the dose of ketanserin after 3 weeks of maintenance therapy due to complaints of dizziness and tiredness, which also subsided after reduction of the daily dose.

Study IV

Systolic and diastolic blood pressure did not markedly increase during the weaning phase in 7 out of 10 patients with essential hypertension. At the start of the double-

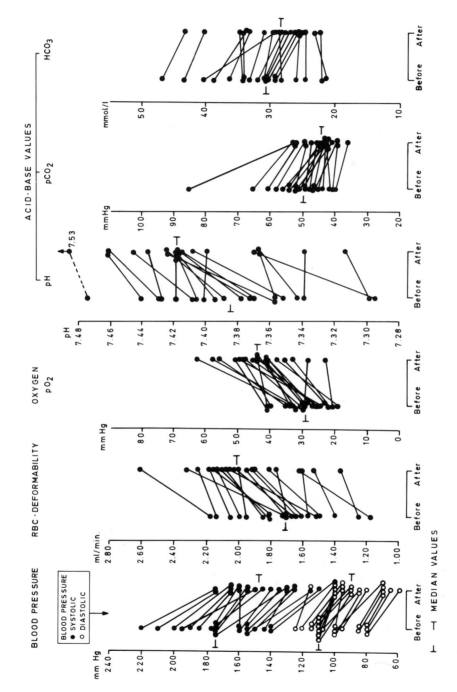

FIG. 2. Systolic and diastolic blood pressure, RBC deformability and venous blood gas values of 20 patients suffering from essential hypertension or chronic emphysema before and after an acute intravenous injection of 10 mg ketanserin.

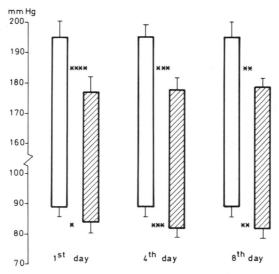

FIG. 3. Systolic and diastolic blood pressure (mean daily values ± SE) in 14 elderly patients during a double-blind cross-over study with oral ketanserin 40 mg t.i.d. *(striped bar)* or placebo *(open bar).* *p*-value: * ≤ 0.05; ** ≤ 0.01; *** ≤ 0.001; **** ≤ 0.0001.

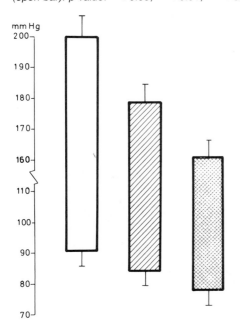

FIG. 4. Systolic and diastolic blood pressure (mean ± SE) in 10 elderly hypertensive patients during a double-blind crossover study with oral ketanserin 40 mg t.i.d. *(striped bar)* and placebo *(open bar)* for 1 week each and during a subsequent 3-week maintenance therapy with ketanserin 40 mg t.i.d. *(cross-hatched bar).*

blind study the mean systolic blood pressure of the ten patients was 173.5 (range: 155–200) mm Hg and the mean diastolic blood pressure was 105.5 (range: 90–120) mm Hg. Ketanserin 20 mg t.i.d. significantly reduced systolic and diastolic blood pressure as compared with control values, whereas no significant changes occurred during the placebo period (Fig. 5). Blood pressure values after 4 weeks of ketanserin treatment were significantly lower than after 2 weeks. No significant changes in heart rate were observed during the whole double-blind study. Systolic time intervals remained unchanged during the ketanserin period, whereas the pre-ejection period (PEP) significantly ($p < 0.05$) increased, the left ventricular ejection time (LVET) significantly ($p < 0.01$) decreased, and the ratio PEP/LVET signif-

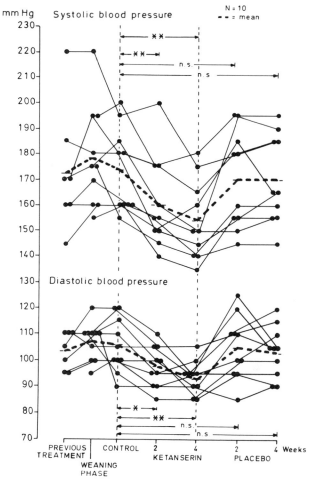

FIG. 5. Systolic and diastolic blood pressure in 10 patients with essential hypertension during a double-blind cross-over study with oral ketanserin 20 mg t.i.d. and placebo for 1 month each. p-value: n.s., not significant; * ≤ 0.05; ** ≤ 0.01.

icantly ($p < 0.01$) increased during the 4-week placebo period, as compared with control values.

DISCUSSION

The obtained results demonstrate that ketanserin is a potent antihypertensive drug, acting both on systolic and diastolic blood pressure; it is active both after intravenous administration and during oral therapy. The effect is immediate after intravenous administration, but rather slow during oral treatment in patients with essential hypertension. In elderly patients the oral effects are more rapid and more pronounced. A rebound hypertension has not been observed so far after discontinuation of the treatment, but there is a long-lasting after-effect. The effects are tolerated uneventfully, in the absence of changes in heart rate and cardiac output. No orthostatic hypotension was reported in any of these patients during treatment with ketanserin.

Our data, thus, suggest that ketanserin should be considered for treating hypertensive crises, as well as for the oral maintenance treatment of essential hypertension and hypertension of the elderly.

The underlying mechanisms in hypertension are still a matter of discussion. The pathophysiology of the disease is mainly determined by a disproportion between the cardiac output and the peripheral vascular resistance, elevation of blood pressure often being explained by an increased vascular resistance subsequent to arteriolar narrowing (13). On the other hand, venous function may also be impaired, as demonstrated both in experimental and human essential hypertension (6,15). According to others, blood viscosity may be another component contributing to the increased peripheral vascular resistance and, hence, high blood pressure (9,12).

It is still a matter of speculation whether the rigidity of RBC is causally related to high blood pressure. Yet, the marked improvement of RBC deformability after ketanserin certainly accounts for an additional decrease in peripheral vascular resistance and, in turn, for a lowering of blood pressure (12).

Substantial evidence supports the contention that 5-hydroxytryptamine is involved in the development of hypertension. Indeed increased vasoconstrictive responses and delayed tachyphylaxis to the monoamine, the positive correlation between systolic blood pressure and vascular responsiveness to 5-hydroxytryptamine, as observed in spontaneously hypertensive rats, favor the hypothesis of such a serotonergic involvement (1,2,3,5). Such 5-hydroxytryptamine may be derived from activated blood platelets as suggested by the increased beta-thromboglobulin levels in hypertensive patients, indicative for the release reaction (8). 5-Hydroxytryptamine then could act directly on the hyperresponsive vascular smooth muscle cell and/or amplify their reaction to the preexisting adrenergic tone (16; P. M. Vanhoutte, *this volume*). Ketanserin antagonizes the direct and the amplification effects of 5-hydroxytryptamine on blood vessels and platelets (16; F. de Clerck et al., *this volume*) and improves the red blood cell deformability. Our present observations that this selective 5-hydroxytryptamine receptor antagonist lowers systolic and diastolic blood pressure in hypertensive patients, therefore, suggests that, in man also, 5-hydroxytryptamine may contribute to the development of this disease.

REFERENCES

1. Collis, M. G., De Mey, C., and Vanhoutte, P. M. (1979): Renal vascular reactivity in the young spontaneously hypertensive rat. *Hypertension*, 2:45–52.
2. Collis, M. G., and Vanhoutte, P. M. (1977): Vascular reactivity of isolated perfused kidneys from male and female spontaneously hypertensive rats. *Circ. Res.*, 41:759–767.
3. Collis, M. G., and Vanhoutte, P. M. (1981): Tachyphylaxis to 5-hydroxytryptamine in perfused kidneys from spontaneously hypertensive and normotensive rats. *J. Cardiovasc. Pharmacol.*, 3:229–235.
4. Davies, O. L. (1947): Student *t*-test. In: *Statistical Methods in Research and Production*, pp. 57–58. Oliver and Boyd, London.
5. De Mey, C., and Vanhoutte, P. M. (1981): Effect of age and spontaneous hypertension on the tachyphylaxis to 5-hydroxytryptamine and angiotensin II in the isolated rat kidney. *Hypertension*, 3:718–724.
6. Greenberg, S. (1980): Venous function in hypertension. *Trends in Pharmacological Sciences*, 1:121–125.
7. Leysen, J. E., Awouters, F., Kennis, L., Laduron, P. M., Vandenberk, J., and Janssen, P. A. J. (1981): Receptor binding profile of R 41 468, a novel antagonist at 5-HT_2 receptors. *Life Sci.*, 28:1015–1022.
8. Mehta, J., and Mehta, P. (1981): Platelet function in hypertension and effect of therapy. *Am. J. Cardiol.*, 47:331–334.
9. Page, J. H. (1966): Die Mosaiktheorie der Hypertonie. In: *Essentielle Hypertonie*, edited by K. D. Bock and R. Cottier. Springer Verlag, Berlin.
10. Peroutka, S. J., and Snyder, S. H. (1979): Multiple serotonin receptors: differential binding of [^{3}H]-5-hydroxytryptamine, [^{3}H]-lysergic acid diethylamide and [^{3}H]-spiroperidol. *Mol. Pharmacol.*, 16:687–699.
11. Rapport, M. M., Green, A. A., and Page, I. H. (1948): Crystalline serotonin. *Science*, 108:329–330.
12. Scholz, P. M., Karis, J. H., Gump, F. E., and Chien, S. (1975): Correlation of blood rheology with vascular resistance in critically ill patients. *J. Appl. Physiol.*, 39:1008.
13. Short, D. (1967): The nature of the increased vascular resistance in chronic hypertension. *Am. Heart J.*, 73:840.
14. Siegel, S. (1956): Wilcoxon matched-pairs signed-ranks test. In: *Nonparametric Statistics for the Behavioral Sciences*, pp. 75–83. McGraw-Hill, New York.
15. Ulrych, M. (1979): Pathogenesis of essential hypertension. Role of the postcapillary segment of the circulation. *Angiology*, 30:104–116.
16. Van Nueten, J. M., Janssen, P. A. J., Van Beek, J., Xhonneux, R., Verbeuren, T. J., and Vanhoutte, P. M. (1981): Vascular effects of R 41 468, a novel antagonist of 5-HT_2 serotonergic receptors. *J. Pharmacol. Exp. Ther.*, 218:217–230.
17. Woolley, D. W., and Shaw, E. N. (1953): An antiserotonin which is active when fed. *Pharmacology*, 108:87–93.
18. Woolley, D. W., and Shaw, E. N. (1956): Antiserotonins in hypertension and the antimetabolite approach to chemotherapy. *Science*, 124:34.

5-Hydroxytryptamine in Peripheral Reactions,
edited by Fred De Clerck and Paul M.
Vanhoutte. Raven Press, New York © 1982.

General Pharmacological Profile of Ketanserin (R 41 468), a Selective 5-HT$_2$ Receptor Antagonist

F. Awouters, J. E. Leysen, F. De Clerck, and J. M. Van Nueten

Department of Pharmacology, Janssen Pharmaceutica, B-2340 Beerse, Belgium

Ketanserin (R 41 468) or 3-{2-[4-(4-fluorobenzoyl)-1-piperidinyl]ethyl}-2,4(1*H*, 3*H*)-quinazolinedione is a quinazolinedione derivative, the tartrate salt of which is soluble in water (Fig. 1). As evidenced by pharmacological work in several species including rat, cat, dog, pig, and man, the compound is a potent and selective antagonist of the peripheral effects of 5-hydroxytryptamine (J. Symoens, *this volume*). The present chapter reviews some of the evidence supporting this concept.

EARLY PHARMACOLOGICAL WORK

The first pharmacological observations made with ketanserin were obtained when using compound 48/80 in rat screening tests. To study histamine H$_1$-antagonists, in 1977, we started to use a lethal shock test in which rats were injected intravenously with a dose of 0.5 mg/kg of compound 48/80. Control rats died from cardiovascular collapse in about 30 min. Treatment with specific histaminergic H$_1$-antagonists prevented the lethal shock (3), but within 4 hr extensive hemorrhagic ulceration developed in the stomach, accompanied by thickening of the stomach wall, regurgitation of intestinal contents, and a large rise in serum pepsinogen.

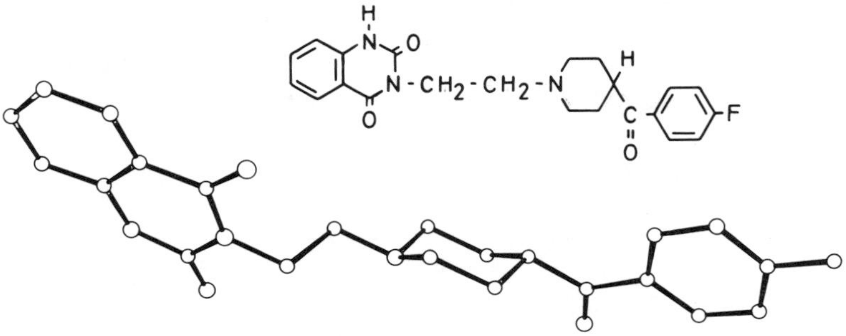

FIG. 1. Chemical and tridimensional crystal structure (from crystallography performed by C. De Ranter) of ketanserin (R 41 468) corresponding to 3-{2-[4-(4-fluorobenzoyl)-1-piperidinyl]ethyl}-2,4(1*H*,3*H*)-quinazolinedione.

193

Attempts were made to prevent this gastric pathology by additional oral treatment of rats, protected from the lethal shock by a high dose of a specific H_1-antagonist. Table 1 is a partial list of compounds tested in this way. It illustrates that high doses of specific antagonists of histaminergic H_1-receptors, such as pyrilamine, could not prevent the occurrence of the ulcers. This was expected, but the same result applied to high doses of specific H_2-antagonists, dopaminergic antagonists, alpha-adrenergic blocking agents, opiate agonists, and inhibitors of prostaglandin biosynthesis. Full protection from the ulcer development was obtained with relatively high doses of compounds which have a common denominator to possess serotonergic antagonistic properties, such as phenoxybenzamine, azatadine, mianserin, cyproheptadine, pipamperone, and spiperone. The more specific 5-hydroxytryptamine antagonists, cinanserin (at high doses) and the ergoline derivatives, methysergide and metergoline (at low doses), were also active. The detailed pharmacological analysis of these results suggests that the ability of compounds to prevent ulcers in this rat model is a measure of 5-hydroxytryptamine antagonism *in vivo*. This conclusion is in agreement with the known releasing effect of compound 48/80 on mast cells of the rat, which contain both histamine and 5-hydroxytryptamine. When tested in this model, ketanserin was very potent, with an ED_{50} of 0.15 mg/kg.

PURITY AND SELECTIVITY

Generally speaking, the serotonergic antagonists, except methysergide, are very active in counteracting tryptamine-induced bilateral convulsions and tremors in the rat. The comparison of the effect, of oral treatment 2 hr before challenge with either tryptamine or compound 48/80, indicated a similar potency in both tests for most compounds (Table 2). However, methysergide and ketanserin antagonized tryptamine-induced tremors only at doses 70 and 96 times higher, respectively, than those effective in preventing gastric ulcers in the test with compound 48/80. Methysergide is known to produce relatively weak lysergic acid diethylamine-(LSD)-like effect in man. In animals trained to discriminate LSD from saline (1) methysergide produced full generalization with LSD, the ED_{50} being 6.1 mg/kg. Ketanserin was inactive even at 40 mg/kg. Thus, in the rat, ketanserin is a potent antagonist of

TABLE 1. *Oral ED_{50}-values (mg/kg) of various drugs in the gastric ulcer test in the rat*

Pyrilamine (H_1)	>80	Cinanserin	43
Cimetidine (H_2)	≥160	Mianserin	16
Haloperidol (DA)	>10	Cyproheptadine	5.4
Prazosin (α_1)	>10	Pipamperone	2.0
Morphine (OP)	>40	Spiperone	0.34
Indomethacin (PG-I)	>10	Methysergide	0.22
Phenoxybenzamine	65	Metergoline	0.19
Azatadine	25	Ketanserin	0.15

TABLE 2. *Comparison between central tryptamine antagonism and mast cell-derived 5-hydroxytryptamine antagonism*

Compound	Oral ED_{50}-values (mg/kg)		Ratio A/B
	A Tryptamine tremors	B Gastric ulcers	
Mianserin	4.7	16	0.3
Cyproheptadine	5.4	5.4	1.0
Metergoline	0.26	0.19	1.3
Cinanserin	65	43	1.5
Spiperone	0.51	0.34	1.5
Pipamperone	4.7	2.0	2.5
Methysergide	16	0.22	70
Ketanserin	14	0.15	96

TABLE 3. *5-Hydroxytryptamine antagonism on isolated tissues[a]*

Compound	Rat caudal artery	Human blood platelets	Guinea pig trachea	Guinea pig ileum	Rat fundus
Methysergide	0.0012	0.016	0.00020	>10.0	0.033
Cyproheptadine	0.00080	0.0041	0.0035	0.032	0.12
Morphine	>10.0	>10.0	⩾10.0	0.079	>10.0
Ketanserin	0.00067	0.0070	0.00097	⩾10.0	>10.0

[a]Inhibition of 5-hydroxytryptamine-induced contractions *in vitro* for rat caudal artery, guinea pig trachea and ileum, rat fundus, and of 5-hydroxytryptamine-induced human platelet aggregation. (From refs. 5,6; F. De Clerck et al., *this volume*.)
ED_{50} values in µg/ml.

vascular congestion induced by endogenous 5-hydroxytryptamine, is a very weak antagonist of central reactions to tryptamine, and lacks central LSD-like effects.

In vitro (Table 3), ketanserin is a potent and reversible antagonist of 5-hydroxytryptamine-induced contractions of isolated rat caudal arteries as well as canine basilar, carotid, coronary, and gastrosplenic arteries, and canine gastrosplenic and saphenous veins (5,6). The ED_{50} of ketanserin in the rat arteries is 0.67 ng/ml, a value suggesting that it is at least as potent as methysergide and cyproheptadine. In contrast to the latter compounds, ketanserin does not induce 5-hydroxytryptamine-like vascular contractions but prevents the agonistic effects of methysergide (5,6). Similar to cyproheptadine and methysergide, low concentrations of ketanserin also inhibit the 5-hydroxytryptamine-induced aggregation of human and cat platelets and the contraction of the guinea pig trachea (5; F. De Clerck et al., *this volume*). Concentrations of ketanserin which fully block the 5-hydroxytryptamine-induced platelet aggregation do not affect the active uptake of the monoamine by human platelets (F. De Clerck et al., *this volume*).

Experiments performed on platelets and isolated vessel preparations demonstrate that ketanserin, in concentrations which do not affect the reaction of the target tissues to other agonists, abolishes the amplifying effect of low concentrations of 5-hydroxytryptamine on various other mediators (5; F. De Clerck et al., *this volume*). Unlike methysergide and cyproheptadine, ketanserin is devoid of serotonergic antagonism in the rat fundus and the guinea pig ileum preparations (6).

Thus, ketanserin appears to be a *pure* serotonergic antagonist, devoid of mixed agonist-antagonist properties. Furthermore, this compound is a *selective* serotonergic antagonist since it blocks only part of the known peripheral actions of the monoamine.

Comparative Receptor Binding Profile

As proposed by Peroutka and Snyder (4) receptors for 5-hydroxytryptamine have been recently reclassified into 5-HT$_1$ binding sites, labeled with [^{3}H]5-hydroxytryptamine in rat hippocampus preparations, and 5-HT$_2$, labeled with [^{3}H]spiperone in the frontal cortex; these receptors are different from the pharmacologically defined D- and M-types since morphine is inactive in both 5-HT$_1$ and 5-HT$_2$-receptor binding models and phenoxybenzamine is only weakly active (2). A variety of drugs with known 5-hydroxytryptamine antagonistic properties including ketanserin were tested in a series of receptor binding assays (2). As indicated in Table 4, LSD binds with similar affinity to both 5-HT$_1$ and 5-HT$_2$ receptors. Methysergide and metergoline have also rather high affinity for the 5-HT$_1$ binding sites and most other compounds show significant binding. The K_i-value for ketanserin, however, is higher than 10 mM, in contrast to its high potency in the 5-HT$_2$ assay, where its K_i is 2.1 nM. When the binding of ketanserin to other receptor sites was measured, rather high binding affinities were found for histamine H$_1$ and alpha$_1$-adrenergic receptor preparations (2). This implies that high doses of ketanserin may antagonize certain effects of histamine and catecholamines. Indeed, in the rat the orally effective dose of the compound for H$_1$-antagonism (histamine skin reaction test) is 10.8 mg/kg

TABLE 4. *Binding to 5-hydroxytryptamine (5-HT) receptors (K$_i$, nM)^a*

Compound	5-HT$_1$	5-HT$_2$	Ratio 5-HT$_1$/5-HT$_2$
LSD	20	8.2	2.4
Methysergide	99	12	8.3
Metergoline	20	0.9	22
Mianserin	1,100	13	85
Cyproheptadine	700	6.5	108
Spiperone	160	1.2	133
Ketanserin	>10,000	2.1	>4,700

^{a}Displacement by compounds of specific binding of ^{3}H-ligands from receptor sites. 5-HT$_1$ receptors labelled with [^{3}H]5-hydroxytryptamine in rat hippocampal membranes; 5-HT$_2$ labeled with [^{3}H]spiperone in rat frontal cortex preparations.

K_i-values represent equilibrium dissociation constants of the compound (inhibitor)-receptor complex versus the ^{3}H-ligand. Specific binding of ketanserin to 5-HT$_2$ receptor sites. (From ref. 2.)

TABLE 5. Receptor binding profiles (K_i, nM) for various serotonergic antagonists[a]

Compound	5-HT$_2$	5-HT$_1$	H$_1$	α_1	α_2	DA	AcCh-M
Metergoline	0.9	20	1100	38	380	23	Inactive
Ketanserin	2.1	Inactive	10	10	Inactive	220	Inactive
LSD	8.2	20	Inactive	160	58	20	Inactive
Methysergide	12	99	Inactive	2,300	2,600	200	Inactive
Cyproheptadine	6.5	700	2.7	100	760	31	19
Mianserin	13	1100	2.9	82	60	620	Inactive
Metitepine	1.9	62	4.9	0.47	48	4.0	Inactive
Spiperone	1.2	160	Inactive	10	Inactive	0.16	Inactive

[a]Equilibrium dissociation constants (K_i-values) for various compounds versus specific [3H]-ligands: 5-HT$_2$ (5-hydroxytryptamine) = [3H]spiperone in rat frontal cortex; 5-HT$_1$ = [3H]5-hydroxytryptamine in rat hippocampus; H$_1$ (histamine = [3H]pyrilamine in guinea pig cerebellum; α_1 (alpha-adrenergic receptor) = [3H]WB 4101 in rat forebrain; α_2 = [3H]clonidine in rat cortex: DA (dopaminergic receptor) = [3H]haloperidol in rat striatum; Ac Ch-M (acetylcholine muscarinic receptor) = [3H]dexetimide in rat striatum.
High selectivity of ketanserin for 5-HT$_2$ receptor sites. (From ref. 2.)

and for alpha-adrenergic antagonism (norepinephrine-induced lethality test) is 12.4 mg/kg. The receptor binding profile of other compounds shows a different specificity: Cyproheptadine, mianserin and pizotifen are primarily active on histamine H$_1$-receptors, metitepine and phenoxybenzamine primarily on alpha$_1$-adrenergic receptors, and spiperone and haloperidol primarily on dopaminergic receptors.

ACKNOWLEDGMENT

Part of this work was supported by a grant from the I.W.O.N.L. (Instituut tot Aanmoediging van het Wetenschappelijk Onderzoek in Nijverheid en Landbouw, Brussel).

REFERENCES

1. Colpaert, F. C., Niemegeers, C. J. E., and Janssen, P. A. J. (1982): A drug discrimination analysis of lysergic acid diethylamide (LSD) (1982): *In vivo* agonist and antagonist effects of purported 5-hydroxytryptamine antagonists and of pirenperone, a LSD-antagonist. *J. Pharmacol. Exp. Ther.*, 221:206–214.

2. Leysen, J. E., Awouters, F., Kennis, L., Laduron, P. M., Vandenberk, J., and Janssen, P. A. J. (1981): Receptor binding profile of R 41 468 a novel antagonist at 5-HT$_2$ receptors. *Life Sci.*, 28(2):1115–1122.

3. Niemegeers, C. J. E., Awouters, F., Van Nueten, J. M., De Nollin, S., and Janssen, P. A. J. (1978): Protection of rats from compound 48/80-induced lethality. A simple test for inhibitors of mast cell-mediated shock. *Arch. Int. Pharmacodyn. Ther.*, 234:164–176.

4. Peroutka, S. J., and Snyder, S. H. (1979): Multiple serotonin receptors: Differential binding of [3H]-5-hydroxytryptamine, [3H]-lysergic acid diethylamide and [3H]-spiroperidol. *Mol. Pharmacol.*, 16:687–699.

5. Van Nueten, J. M., Janssen, P. A. J., Van Beek, J., Xhonneux, R., Verbeuren, T. J., and Vanhoutte, P. M. (1981): Vascular effects of ketanserin (R 41 468), a novel antagonist of 5-HT$_2$ serotonergic receptors. *J. Pharmacol. Exp. Ther.*, 218:217–230.

6. Van Nueten, J. M., and Vanhoutte, P. M. (1981): Selectivity of calcium antagonism and serotonin antagonism with respect to venous and arterial tissues. *Angiology*, 32:476–484.

5-Hydroxytryptamine in Peripheral Reactions,
edited by Fred De Clerck and Paul M.
Vanhoutte. Raven Press, New York © 1982.

Are the Therapeutic Effects of Ketanserin Compatible with a Serotonergic Mechanism?

J. Symoens

Department of Clinical Research, Janssen Pharmaceutica, B-2340 Beerse, Belgium

5-Hydroxytryptamine is a potent vasoactive substance that constricts or dilates blood vessels and causes platelet aggregation (40). It amplifies vasoconstriction and platelet aggregation induced by other substances such as epinephrine, angiotensin II, prostaglandins, etc. (49,50; F. De Clerck et al., *this volume*). In the animal, 5-hydroxytryptamine can induce systemic and pulmonary hypertension (29,36), oliguria (3), muscular dystrophy (1), gastric lesions (52) and paw edema (35). Its role in human pathology is ill defined; it may contribute to diseases such as migraine, carcinoid syndrome, and dumping syndrome (20). The evaluation of the role of 5-hydroxytryptamine in disease is made difficult by the fact that most available 5-hydroxytryptamine antagonists both block and mimic the effects of the monoamine (7), or are relatively unspecific; in particular, they can cause neuroleptic or other side effects not related with interference with 5-hydroxytryptamine receptors (20,28).

Ketanserin is a highly selective antagonist of 5-hydroxytryptamine at 5-HT$_2$ receptors (28). It antagonizes vasoconstriction, bronchoconstriction, and platelet aggregation which is induced by 5-hydroxytryptamine either directly or indirectly through an amplification mechanism (9,49). It does not possess agonistic properties on serotonergic receptors (49). At doses that block 5-HT$_2$ receptors, it does not block the effects of other amines, calcium, cholinergic agents, or prostaglandins (49). Its effects are essentially peripheral and not central (F. Awouters et al., *this volume*). Blood levels of therapeutic doses of ketanserin in man (10 mg i.v. or 40 mg orally) exceed 10 ng/ml for 8 hr, which is more than the concentrations needed for 5-hydroxytryptamine blockade *in vitro* (0.5–10 ng/ml) (23). Ketanserin, thus, may be a valuable tool to study 5-hydroxytryptamine-induced pathology. Its effects may reflect an involvement of 5-hydroxytryptamine. Unlike with other 5-hydroxytryptamine antagonists, central nervous system side effects are not expected to occur at therapeutic doses. Clinical research with ketanserin started in February 1979. After an initial period of trial and error, ketanserin proved to be of potential benefit in a large range of diseases which are characterized by systemically or locally increased vascular resistance. Ketanserin has profound effects on arterial blood pressure, on systemic, pulmonary, and peripheral circulation, on blood gases, and on platelet aggregation. The present chapter will summarize the information available on the therapeutic effects of ketanserin. It is based to a large extent on unpublished data.

CLINICAL PROFILE OF KETANSERIN

Hemodynamic Effects

Arterial Blood Pressure

Ketanserin has no overt effect on blood pressure of normotensive individuals (24). It reduces systolic and diastolic blood pressure to normal in patients with an acute hypertensive episode, e.g., during a cerebrovascular accident (25), after surgery (25; P. A. J. Van der Starre et al., *this volume*), and during preeclampsia (26). The effect is maximal within minutes after the intravenous injection and lasts 1 to 8 hr. It can be maintained by continuous intravenous infusion (P. A. J. Van der Starre, *this volume*) (Fig. 1). The rapid decrease in arterial blood pressure is well tolerated.

A similar rapid normalization of systolic and diastolic blood pressure is observed after the intravenous injection of ketanserin in patients with essential hypertension (11,12). The first preliminary hemodynamic data (37,51) indicate that the reduction in blood pressure is accompanied by a reduction of peripheral vascular resistance (Table 1), while heart rate, cardiac output, glomerular filtration rate, and renal plasma flow remain unchanged.

During chronic oral treatment with ketanserin in the absence of any other antihypertensive medication, systolic and diastolic blood pressure are progressively reduced in most patients with essential hypertension (Fig. 2). After discontinuation of treatment, there is a gradual return to pretreatment blood pressure values without rebound hypertension. There is no evidence of orthostatic hypotension (38); alpha$_1$-adrenergic blockade does not seem to contribute to the reduction of blood pressure (M. Schalekamp and H. Kulbertus, *personal communications*).

Heart rate remains virtually unchanged after oral or parenteral treatment with ketanserin (11,12,37,51). It is reduced to normal when it is abnormally elevated, e.g., after a cerebrovascular accident or postoperatively (25).

Systemic and Pulmonary Circulation

The hemodynamic effects of ketanserin were studied in patients with hemodynamic disorders such as hypertension (51), refractory heart failure (15), and pulmonary edema (47). Ketanserin reduces elevated systemic and pulmonary vascular resistances and blood pressure in such patients. It reduces pre- and afterload (Fig. 3). Cardiac index and stroke work index improve when they are low but they do not increase above normal level. Heart rate remains virtually unchanged. Diuresis is restored in patients with septic or cardiogenic shock (14,17,47) (Fig. 4).

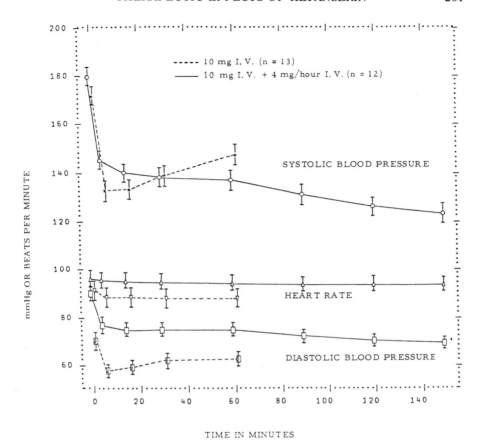

FIG. 1. Effect of intravenous administration of ketanserin on blood pressure and heart rate in 25 patients with hypertension after coronary bypass grafting. (P. A. J. Van der Starre, *this volume.*)

Peripheral Circulation

The effects of ketanserin on the peripheral circulation were studied in healthy volunteers, in patients with peripheral vascular disease such as Raynaud's disease, pregangrene, and thrombosis, and in patients with peripheral vasoconstriction after an operation or during shock.

In healthy volunteers, oral or intravenous treatment with ketanserin prevents the constriction caused by injecting 5-hydroxytryptamine into a finger vein (24). The digital rest flow increases after ketanserin treatment and the cold-induced vasoconstriction is prevented (19).

In patients with septic or traumatic shock and in patients with postoperative vasoconstriction, the peripheral circulation improves within minutes after the intravenous injection of ketanserin (32). Skin temperature rises and the skin color improves (Fig. 4).

TABLE 1. *The effects of a single intravenous dose of 10 mg ketanserin in 8 patients with essential hypertension*

Hemodynamic effects	t_0	$t_{5\,min}$
Systolic blood pressure (mm Hg)	175 ± 15	158 ± 12[a]
Diastolic blood pressure (mm Hg)	87 ± 9	79 ± 6[a]
Mean blood pressure (mm Hg)	116 ± 11	105 ± 8[a]
Heart rate (b/min)	71 ± 16	78 ± 16
Cardiac index (1/min/m²)	4.04 ± 1.48	4.17 ± 1.38
Stroke index (ml/m²)	56 ± 9	53 ± 8
Total peripheral resistance index (dynes sec cm^{-5}/m²)	$2,569 \pm 960$	$2,189 \pm 652$[b]

[a] $p < 0.01$
[b] $p < 0.05$
Mean $\pm$ SD (ref. 37).

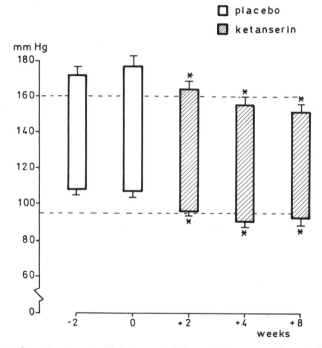

FIG. 2. Effect of oral treatment with ketanserin (40 mg t.i.d.) on systolic and diastolic blood pressure in 10 patients with essential hypertension. *Significant $p < 0.05$ (Wilcoxon MPSR). (G. Sieben, *personal communication.*)

In patients with Raynaud's disease, cold-induced vasoconstriction is prevented after the injection of ketanserin (Fig. 5) (19). The vascular response to cold challenge is markedly reduced after prolonged oral treatment (19).

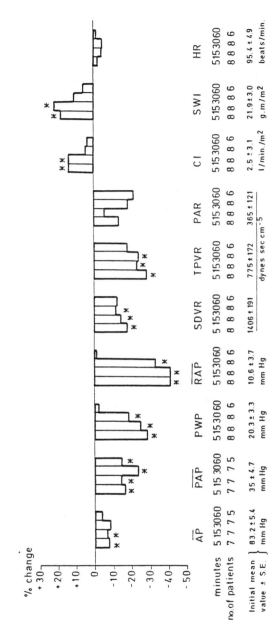

FIG. 3. Hemodynamic effects of a single intravenous injection of 10 mg ketanserin in patients with acute heart failure . AP = mean systemic arterial pressure; PAP = mean pulmonary arterial pressure; PWP = pulmonary wedge pressure; RAP = mean right atrium pressure; SDVR = systematic dynamic vascular resistance; TPVR = total pulmonary vascular resistance; PAR = pulmonary arterial resistance; CI = cardiac index; SWI = stroke work index; HR = heart rate. (From ref. 15.)
*: p ≤ 0.05 (Wilcoxon matched pairs signed ranks test, one tailed).

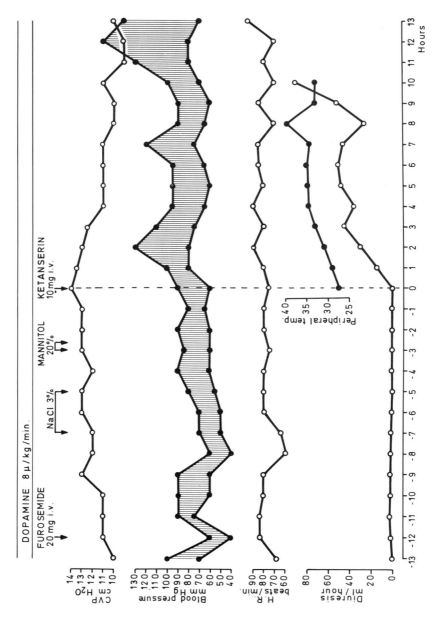

FIG. 4. Effects of a single intravenous injection of 10 mg ketanserin in a patient with septic shock. CVP = central venous pressure; HR = heart rate. (From ref. 14.)

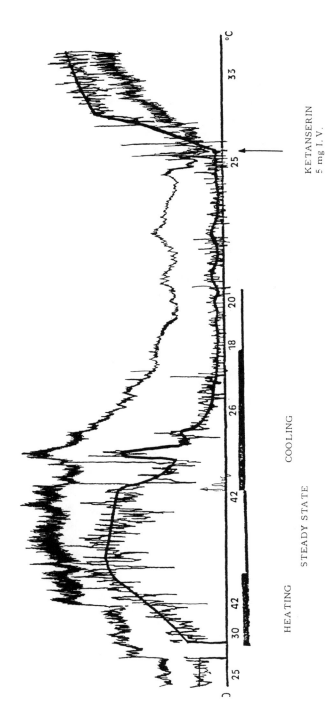

FIG. 5. Effect of a single intravenous injection of 5 mg ketanserin on digital arterial blood flow *(full line)* in a patient with Raynaud's disease. (A. Jageneau, *personal communication.*)

In patients with pregrangrene (27), Bürger's disease (45), and Suddeck's atrophy (39), the injection of ketanserin causes a rapid rise in blood flow and a marked reduction of pain.

Ketanserin was also studied during an acute thrombotic episode such as acute hemorrhoidal thrombosis or acute peripheral thrombophlebitis. Three double-blind placebo-controlled studies have shown that ketanserin relieves pain and tension within minutes after the intravenous injection or within 2 hr after oral treatment (16,18,48). The effect on pain in patients with acute peripheral thrombophlebitis is shown in Fig. 6. Ketanserin does not influence the organization or the disorganization of the thrombus. It thus acts symptomatically, probably by relieving vasospasm around the thrombus.

Effects on Blood Gases

During pharmacokinetic studies with ketanserin it had been observed that the venous blood of resting healthy volunteers turned red like arterial blood within minutes after the injection of ketanserin or within 1 or 2 hr after oral treatment. Ketanserin causes a rise in venous P_{O_2} and a reduction in venous P_{CO_2} (Fig. 7) (10). The kinetics of blood gas changes parallel the kinetics of ketanserin blood levels. Blood gas changes are not seen after exercise (A. Jageneau, *personal communication*).

To investigate whether the increase in venous P_{O_2} is due to reduced oxygen extraction in the exchange capillary vessels, exercise tests were performed in healthy volunteers and in stress-prone pigs. Immediately after exercise on an ergometer,

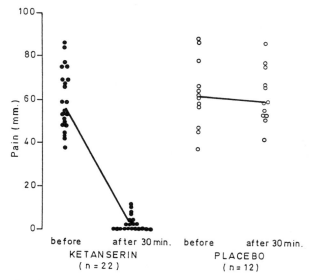

FIG. 6. Effect of a single intravenous injection of 10 mg ketanserin or placebo on pain in patients with acute peripheral thrombophlebitis, as evaluated on a visual analog scale. (From ref. 18.)

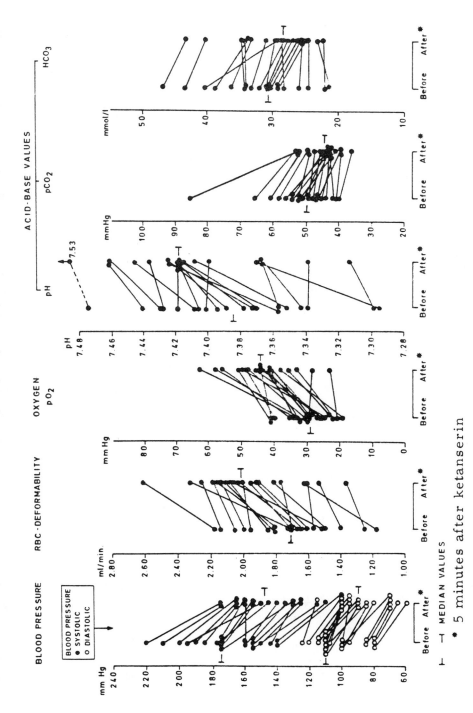

FIG. 7. Effects of a single intravenous injection of 10 mg ketanserin on arterial blood pressure, venous blood gases, and venous red blood cell deformability in 20 patients with essential hypertension or emphysema. (From ref. 10.)

venous P_{O_2} and venous lactic acid were similar in volunteers pretreated with ketanserin, as compared to the control values in the same volunteers (34). In pigs,
ketanserin treatment prevented exercise-induced acidosis and shortened the lactic
acid washout period (33).

These data suggest that oxygen extraction in the muscle is adequate after ketanserin treatment. The rise in venous P_{O_2} might be due to increased capillary perfusion:
Because tissue oxygen demand remains constant during rest, the increased capillary
supply of oxygen is not utilized and larger amounts of oxygen pass into the venous
circulation. During and after exercise, however, increased capillary perfusion may
result in improved oxygenation and removal of metabolic breakdown products. The
protective effect of ketanserin against halothane-induced malignant hyperthermia
in pigs might be partially due to a similar mechanism (L. Ooms and F. Verheyen,
this volume).

In patients with congestive heart failure, treatment with ketanserin resulted in an
improved venous oxygen saturation (17).

In patients with essential hypertension, blood gas changes after ketanserin treatment were accompanied by an increase in red blood cell deformability (Fig. 7)
(10).

Effects on Platelets

David and Demoulin studied *in vivo* platelet activation in 6 patients with refractory
heart failure before and 15 min after the intravenous injection of 10 mg ketanserin.
The platelet aggregation index, which was abnormal in 5 of 6 patients before
treatment, improved in all, indicating that the number of circulating aggregates had
decreased after ketanserin treatment (15; J. L. David, *personal communication*).

POSSIBLE SOURCES OF 5-HYDROXYTRYPTAMINE

The enterochromaffin cells of the gut are the major source of 5-hydroxytryp-
tamine. Under normal circumstances, the hepatic and pulmonary beds avidly remove
5-hydroxytryptamine from the circulation, allowing less than 1% of portal blood
5-hydroxytryptamine to pass (46). Free 5-hydroxytryptamine is picked up by platelets and transported throughout the body (46). 5-Hydroxytryptamine is released
from platelets during platelet aggregation (56).

5-Hydroxytryptamine-induced pathology may be expected: (a) when the protective mechanisms of metabolism and uptake are overwhelmed or altered; (b) when
there is excessive release of 5-hydroxytryptamine from platelets; and (c) when the
susceptibility of blood vessels to 5-hydroxytryptamine increases.

The Protective Mechanisms are Overwhelmed or Altered

The protective mechanisms of metabolism and uptake are overwhelmed or altered
in at least two conditions, carcinoid syndrome and septic shock. In patients with
carcinoid syndrome, massive amounts of 5-hydroxytryptamine are released from

enterochromaffin cell tumors in the intestine or in metastases. The patients have vascular, bronchial, and intestinal pathology. Ketanserin reduces the symptoms in these patients (G. Stage, *personal communication*). During septic shock, large amounts of 5-hydroxytryptamine enter the pulmonary circulation, apparently because the Küpfer cells in the liver inadequately remove 5-hydroxytryptamine from the portal system (42). Ketanserin reduces pulmonary hypertension during endotoxemic shock in dogs (30,44) and has been beneficial in patients with septic shock (14,32).

Excessive Release of 5-Hydroxytryptamine from Platelets

There is growing evidence that platelet aggregation and platelet release reaction are increased in many cardiovascular diseases, e.g., Raynaud's disease (54), septic shock (8), eclampsia (21,22), after vascular surgery (4,53). In acute thrombosis, aggregating platelets release large amounts of 5-hydroxytryptamine and other vasoactive substances (53,56). In all these diseases, ketanserin relieves vasoconstriction. An involvement of 5-hydroxytryptamine from platelets in the pathogenesis of these diseases may thus be postulated.

In patients with essential hypertension, the adhesiveness of platelets to glass is increased (5), beta-thromboglobulin levels in plasma are increased (31), and the 5-hydroxytryptamine content of platelets and the 5-hydroxytryptamine uptake by platelets are reduced (2). With increasing age, the 5-hydroxytryptamine content of platelets decreases (41), platelet release reaction increases and platelet survival shortens (55). The susceptibility of blood vessels to 5-hydroxytryptamine is increased in hypertensive and aging rats (6,13). Ketanserin reduces blood pressure in patients with essential hypertension (12,51). It is conceivable that an increased release of 5-hydroxytryptamine from platelets or an increased susceptibility of blood

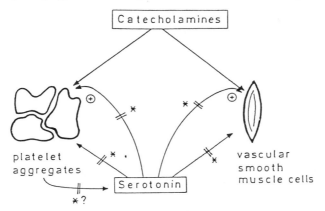

FIG. 8. Possible interaction between 5-hydroxytryptamine and catecholamines on platelet function and vascular contraction, and *(asterisk)* site of action of ketanserin (15). *Arrow:* direct effect of 5-hydroxytryptamine (serotonin). *Arrow with plus sign:* amplification of catecholamines by 5-hydroxytryptamine (serotonin).

vessels to 5-hydroxytryptamine, or both, contribute to the onset or the maintenance of essential hypertension (P. M. Vanhoutte, *this volume*).

CONCLUSIONS

The clinical effects of ketanserin are compatible with serotonergic antagonism. The possible interaction between 5-hydroxytryptamine and catecholamines on platelet function and vascular contraction are shown schematically in Fig. 8. Blockade of 5-hydroxytryptamine probably interrupts a vicious circle of platelet aggregation and 5-hydroxytryptamine release.

Whether all the effects of ketanserin are solely due to blockade of 5-hydroxytryptamine or whether other, yet unknown mechanisms interfere also, remains to be established.

REFERENCES

1. Barnard, E. A., and Barnard, P. J. (1979): Use of genetically dystrophic animals in hemotherapy trials and application of serotonin antagonists as antidystrophic drugs. *Ann. NY Acad. Sci.*, 317:374–399.
2. Bhargava, K. P., Raina, N., Misra, N., Shanker, K., and Vrat, S. (1979): Uptake of serotonin by human platelets and its relevance to CNS involvement in hypertension. *Life Sci.*, 25:195–200.
3. Cantalamessa, F., and de Caro, G. (1982): Ketanserin (R 41468), a new selective 5-HT$_2$ receptor blocking agent, inhibits the antidiuretic effect of serotonin (5-HT) in Wistar rats (*in manuscript*).
4. Cella, G., Schivazappa, L., Casonato, A., Molaro, L. G., Girolami, A., Westwick, J., Lane, D. A., and Kakkar, V. V. (1980): *In vivo* platelet release reaction in patients with heart valve prosthesis. *Haemostasis*, 9:263–275.
5. Coccheri, S., and Fiorentini, P. (1971): Platelet adhesiveness and aggregation in hypertensive patients. In: *Round-the-Table Conference on Normal and Modified Platelet Aggregation*, edited by J. Vermylen, G. de Gaetano, and M. Verstraete, Suppl. 525, pp. 273–275. Acta Medica Sandinavica.
6. Collis, M. G., and Vanhoutte, P. M. (1977): Vascular reactivity of isolated perfused kidneys from male and female spontaneously hypertensive rats. *Circ. Res.*, 41:759–767.
7. Colpaert, F. C., Niemegeers, C. J. E., and Janssen, P. A. J. (1982): A drug discrimination analysis of lysergic acid diethylamide: *In vivo* agonist and antagonist effects of purported 5-hydroxytryptamine antagonists and of R 47465, and LSD-antagonist. *J. Pharmacol. Exp. Ther. (in press)*.
8. Corrigan, J. J., Ray, W. L., and May, N. (1968): Changes in the blood coagulation system associated with septicemia. *New Engl. J. Med.*, 279:851–856.
9. De Clerck, F., and David, J. L. (1981): Pharmacological control of platelet and red blood cell function in the microcirculation. *J. Cardiovasc. Pharmacol.*, 3:1388–1412.
10. De Crée, J., Geukens, H., De Cock, W., Leempoels, J., and Verhaegen, H. (1980): The effect of an intravenous administration of R 41468 on blood gases and red blood cell deformability. Clinical Research Report on ketanserin, No. 32 (*unpublished*).
11. De Crée, J., Leempoels, J., De Cock, W., Geukens, H., and Verhaegen, H. (1981): The antihypertensive effects of a pure and selective serotonin-receptor blocking agent (R 41468) in elderly patients. *Angiology*, 32:137–144.
12. De Crée, J., Verhaegen, H., and Symoens, J. (1981): Acute blood-pressure-lowering effect of ketanserin. *Lancet*, 1:1161–1162.
13. De Mey, Ch., and Vanhoutte, P. M. (1981): Effect of age and spontaneous hypertension on the tachyphylaxis to 5-hydroxytryptamine and angiotensin II in the isolated rat kidney. *Hypertension*, 3:718–724.
14. Demeyere, R. (1981): Experience with ketanserin (R 41468) in two patients with septic shock. Case reports. Clinical Research Report on ketanserin, No. 45 (*unpublished*).
15. Demoulin, J.-C., Bertholet, M., Soumagne, D., David, J.-L., and Kulbertus, H. E. (1981): 5-HT$_2$ receptor blockade in the treatment of heart failure. A preliminary study. *Lancet*, 1:1186–1188.

16. Depuydt, L., Goethals, C., Gysen, J., Jacques, N., Lambrecht, R., Platteau, K., Sandra, M., Schiettekatte, L., and Verschueren, R. (1979): R 41468 in the treatment of acute external haemorrhoidal episodes. A double blind placebo-controlled multicenter study. Clincal Research Report on ketanserin, No. 4 *(unpublished)*.

17. Derbaudrenghien, J. P., and Lejeune, Ph.O. (1981): Treatment of congestive heart failure with R 41468. Case report *(in manuscript)*.

18. De Roose, J. (1981): Ketanserin (R 41468) in superficial thrombophlebitis. A double-blind placebo-controlled cross-over study *(in manuscript)*.

19. Di Perri, T., Laghi Pasini, F., Auteri, A., Pecchi, S., and Cappelli, R. (1981): Serotonergic mechanisms in vascular disorders. A clinical and pharmacological approach *(in manuscript)*.

20. Douglas, W. W. (1980): Histamine and 5-hydroxytryptamine (serotonin) and their antagonists. In: *The Pharmacological Basis of Therapeutics*, 6th ed., Chapter 26, edited by A. Goodman Gilman, L. S. Goodman, and A. Gilman, pp. 638–639. Mac Millan, New York.

21. Essman, W. B. (1978): *Serotonin in Health and Disease. Volume II: Physiological Regulation and Pharmacological Action*, p. 88. SP Medical and Scientific Books Division, Spectrum Publications, New York.

22. Henderson, A. H., Pugsley, D. J., and Thomas, D. P. (1970): Fibrin degradation products in pre-eclamptic toxaemia and eclampsia. *Br. Med. J.*, 3:545–547.

23. Heykants, J., Woestenborghs, R., Scheijgrond, H., and Symoens, J. (1981): Preliminary study of the pharmacokinetics of seroquinaline in healthy subjects following intravenous, intramuscular and oral administration. Clinical Research Report on ketanserin, No. 33 *(unpublished)*.

24. Jageneau, A. H. M., Hoerig, C., Loots, W., and Symoens, J. (1980): Plethysmographic registration of volume changes in a hand vein. Effects of serotonin and of a specific antagonist. *Angiology*, 31:828–832.

25. Kalenda, Z. (1980): The use of an anti-serotonin R 41468 in the treatment of complications following neurosurgery. (Abstract.) *7th World Congress of Anaesthesiologists*, Hamburg.

26. Kincius, C. A., and Pearson, J. W. (1981): The effect of serotonin antagonist R 41468 upon the blood pressure of the puerperal pre-eclamptic patient. (Abstract.) *Workshop "Stress and Serotonin in Animals and Man"*, Beerse, Belgium.

27. Kunnen, J. (1981): Standard Case Reports Nos. 11, 12 *(unpublished)*.

28. Leysen, J. E., Awouters, F., Kennis, L., Laduron, P. M., Vandenberk, J., and Janssen, P. A. J. (1981): Receptor binding profile of R 41468, a novel antagonist at 5-HT$_2$ receptors. *Life Sci.*, 28:1015–1022.

29. MacCanon, D. M., and Horvath, S. M. (1954): Hemodynamic effects of serotonin (5-hydroxytryptamine) injected into the pulmonary artery of anesthetized dogs. *Fed. Proc.*, 13:92–93.

30. Makabali, G. L., Mandal, A. K., and Morris, J. A. (1981): Endotoxemic shock: An implied role for serotonin *(in manuscript)*.

31. Mehta, J., and Mehta, P. (1981): Platelet function in hypertension and effect of therapy. *Am. J. Cardiol.*, 47:331–334.

32. Miranda, D. (1981): Standard Case Reports Nos. 1, 2, 21, 37, 40 *(unpublished)*.

33. Ooms, L. (1981): Exercise-induced myopathies and 5-HT$_2$ receptor blockers. (Abstract.) *Workshop "Stress and Serotonin in Animals and Man"*, Beerse, Belgium.

34. Pannier, J. L. (1981): Influence of ketanserin on performance. Clinical Research Report on ketanserin, No. 48 *(unpublished)*.

35. Rowley, D. A., and Benditt, E. P. (1956): 5-Hydroxytryptamine and histamine as mediators of vascular injury produced by agents which damage mast cells in rats. *J. Exp. Med.*, 103:399–411.

36. Rudolph, A. M., and Paul, M. H. (1957): Pulmonary and systemic vascular response to continuous infusion of 5-hydroxytryptamine (serotonin) in the dog. *Am. J. Physiol.*, 189:263–268.

37. Safar, M. (1981): Étude du R 41468 par voie intraveneuse chez l'hypertendu. Clinical Research Report on ketanserin, No. 38 *(unpublished)*.

38. Safar, M. (1981): Effect of a single oral dose of 40 mg or 160 mg on blood pressure and heart rate in patients with essential hypertension. Clinical Research Report on ketanserin, No. 46 *(unpublished)*.

39. Schoen, A. (1981): Standard Case Report No. 30 *(unpublished)*.

40. Shepherd, J. T., and Vanhoutte, P. M. (1979): *The Human Cardiovascular System. Facts and Concepts*, edited by J. T. Shepherd and P. M. Vanhoutte. Raven Press, New York.

41. Shuttleworth, R. D., and O'Brien, J. R. (1981): Intraplatelet serotonin and plasma 5-hydroxyindoles in health and disease. *Blood*, 57:505–509.

42. Sibbald, W., Peters, S., and Lindsay, R. M. (1980): Serotonin and pulmonary hypertension in human septic ARDS. *Crit. Care Med.*, 8:490–494.
43. Smirk, F. H. (1973): Experimental genetic hypertension. Part III. Genetics, epidemiology, and environmental factors in essential hypertension. In: *Hypertension: Mechanisms and Management*, edited by G. Onesti, K. Eun Kim, and J. H. Moyer, pp. 59–65. Grune & Stratton, New York.
44. Stanley, T. H. (1981): The cardiovascular and pulmonary effects of serotonin antagonism before and during endotoxic shock. (Abstract.) *Workshop "Stress and Serotonin in Animals and Man"*, Beerse, Belgium.
45. Tamsma, T. (1981): Standard Case Report No. 8 *(unpublished)*.
46. Thompson, J. H. (1971): Serotonin and the alimentary tract. *Res. Commun. Chem. Pathol. Pharmacol.*, 2:687–781.
47. Vaes, L. (1981): Treatment of a recurrent acute pulmonary oedema with R 41468. Case report. Clinical Research Report on ketanserin, No. 35 *(unpublished)*.
48. Van Herendael, B., De Crée, J., Verbruggen, F., and Verhaegen, H. (1980): The therapeutic effects of R 41468 in women with an acute outbreak of external haemorrhoids after delivery. A double-blind placebo-controlled study. Clinical Research Report on ketanserin, No. 23 *(unpublished)*.
49. Van Nueten, J. M., Janssen, P. A. J., Van Beek, J., Xhonneux, R., Verbeuren, T. J., and Vanhoutte, P. M. (1981): Vascular effects of R 41468, a novel antagonist of 5-HT$_2$ serotonergic receptors. *J. Pharmacol. Exp. Ther.*, 218:217–230.
50. Van Nueten, J. M., Janssen, P. A. J., De Ridder, W., and Vanhoutte, P. M. (1982): Interaction between 5-hydroxytryptamine and other vasoconstrictor substances in the isolated femoral artery of the rabbit; effect of ketanserin (R 41468). *Eur. J. Pharmacol.*, 77:281–287.
51. Wenting, G. J., Man in 't Veld, A. J., Woittiez, A. J., Boonsma, F., and Schalekamp, M. A. D. H. (1981): Treatment of hypertension with ketanserin, a new selective 5-HT$_2$ receptor antagonist. *Br. Med. J.*, 284:537–539.
52. Wilhelmi, G. (1957): Über die ulcerogene Wirkung von 5-Hydroxytryptamin aus Rattenmagen und deren Beëinflussung durch verschiedene Pharmaca. *Helv. Physiol. Pharmacol. Acta*, 15:83–84.
53. Yamazaki, H., Motomiya, T., Watanabe, C., Miyagawa, N., Yahara, Y., Okawa, Y., and Onozawa, Y. (1980): Consumption of larger platelets with decrease in adenine nucleotide content in thrombosis, disseminated intravascular coagulation, and postoperative state. *Thromb. Res.*, 18:77–88.
54. Zahavi, J., Hamilton, W. A. P., O'Reilly, M. J. G., Leyton, J., Cotton, L. T., and Kakkar, V. V. (1980): Plasma exchange and platelet function in Raynaud's phenomenon. *Thromb. Res.*, 19:85–93.
55. Zahavi, J., Jones, N. A. G., Leyton, J., Dubiel, M., and Kakkar, V. V. (1980): Enhanced *in vivo* platelet "release reaction" in old healthy individuals. *Thromb. Res.*, 17:329–336.
56. Zucker, M. B. (1975): The platelet release reactions. In: *Platelets, Drugs and Thrombosis*, edited by J. Hirsch, J. F. Cade, A. S. Gallus, and E. Schönbaum, pp. 27–34. S. Karger, Basel.

Copies of all unpublished reports can be obtained on request from the Documentation Department, Janssen Pharmaceutica, B-2340 Beerse, Belgium.

5-Hydroxytryptamine in Peripheral Reactions,
edited by Fred De Clerck and Paul M.
Vanhoutte. Raven Press, New York © 1982.

Hypotheses on the Release of Biologically Active Humoral Mediators Induced by Ketanserin (R 41 468): A Platelet Study

T. Di Perri, F. Laghi Pasini, A. Vittoria, and L. Ceccatelli

*Department of Internal Medicine, School of Medicine, University of Siena,
I-53100 Siena, Italy*

Ketanserin (R 41 468), a specific inhibitor of serotonergic 5-HT$_2$ receptors in blood vessels, platelets, and bronchi, is clinically useful in conditions where 5-hydroxytryptamine is a possible cause of pathology, in particular, in several circulatory disorders (2,3). Thus, ketanserin increases the leg resting blood flow in patients with peripheral obliterative arterial disease as well as in normal subjects (3). The cold-induced vasospastic reaction of patients with Raynaud's disease was completely reversed or prevented by the infusion of the drug (2,3). In patients suffering from acute cerebrovascular disease associated with a hypertensive reaction, as well as in essential hypertensive subjects, ketanserin rapidly normalizes arterial blood pressure (2,3). The drug-induced rapid decrease in peripheral resistance is not associated with a change in heart rate, which excludes an induction of the baroreceptor reflex. The addition of the drug either to water or to osmotic infusion in normal subjects is followed by several changes in renal function (T. Di Perri et al., *this volume*). The observation of the complex pharmacological effect of ketanserin on hemodynamics and on renal function led us to consider its similarity with the activity of different types of prostaglandins (5). Particularly, prostacyclin (PGI$_2$) infusion in man has been shown to induce a marked vasodilation in different vascular districts and to lower pulmonary arterial pressure and systemic diastolic blood pressure. Prostacyclin and prostaglandins, such as PGA$_1$, have a profound activity on the renal circulation resembling that of ketanserin (1). Hence, we have investigated the possibility that ketanserin might act not only as a specific serotonergic receptor antagonist, but also may release prostacyclin-like substances. The selection of our experimental model was based on the knowledge that prostacyclin possesses marked platelet antiaggregating properties and on the assumption that, in man, the induction of prostacyclin liberation augments the antiaggregating activity of the plasma. Neri Serneri et al. (4) showed that venous stasis is followed by the liberation of prostacyclin. We have tried to confirm the inducing effect of venous stasis on prostacyclin release and have studied the possible interference of ketanserin with the metabolism and release of prostaglandin-like substances in normal volunteers.

MATERIALS AND METHODS

Experiments were performed in two groups of healthy subjects: In the first group the action of venous stasis on the liberation of a plasmatic antiaggregating factor at the level of the platelet was studied. The effect of the infusion of ketanserin on the possible liberation of antiaggregating substances was observed in the second group.

Group I consisted of 8 volunteers (7 male, 1 female, mean age 35 years, range 25–47 years). None of them had taken drugs active on platelet function or on prostaglandin synthesis for 3 weeks before the test. Venous stasis was performed by means of sphingomanometric occlusion (50 mm Hg for 10 min) and citrated blood (3.8% trisodium citrate/blood in the ratio of 1:9) was collected, either at room temperature or at 4°C, before the test, after 10 min of venous stasis, and 30 min after recovery. The release of antiaggregating substances was tested in a standardized platelet aggregation system with normally functioning platelets. Group II consisted of 18 healthy volunteers (11 male, 7 female, mean age 32 years, range 24–42 years). None of them had taken drugs known to be active on platelet function for 3 weeks before the test. They received 10 mg of ketanserin intravenously, given in 2 min. Citrated plasma of the treated subjects was obtained at room temperature or at 4°C before, 3 min and 60 min after drug infusion, and tested for antiaggregating activity.

The aggregating system consisted of platelet-rich plasma from normal untreated subjects. Platelet-rich plasma was prepared from citrated blood by centrifugation at 100 g for 15 min and platelet-poor plasma by centrifugation at 1,440 g for 15 min. The platelet concentration in platelet-rich plasma was adjusted to 4×10^8/ml. Adenosine-5′-diphosphate-induced (ADP, Biochemia) platelet aggregation was studied with a turbidimetric method in an aggregometer Elvi 840 connected with a continuous recording system. Platelet-poor plasma was used for the 100% transmission setting of the instrument; 0.1 ml of platelet-poor plasma obtained from subjects to be tested for antiaggregating activity was incubated with 0.5 ml platelet-rich plasma at room temperature for 3, 5, and 10 min before the addition of the aggregating substance. The aggregation was performed at 37°C. In the basal (controls platelet-rich plasma + plasma before drug infusion or venous stasis at room temperature or at 4°C) the minimal dose of ADP able to induce an irreversible aggregation was determined. The same dose was utilized in the successive aggregation systems (platelet-rich plasma + plasma obtained after venous stasis and recovery, or 3 min and 60 min after drug infusion, at room temperature or at 4°C) and maximal percentage of change in the optical density was calculated.

In order to evaluate the effect of prostaglandin synthesis inhibition on the possible ketanserin-induced release of antiaggregating activity, the test with drug infusion was repeated after indomethacin pretreatment (200 mg/day per os for 3 days and 50 mg intravenously 30 min before test). The results were analyzed statistically with Student's t-test for paired observations.

RESULTS

The results are shown in Figs. 1 to 4. After 10 min venous stasis, a statistically significant release of antiaggregating activity was observed in plasma stored at 4°C, but not at room temperature. This activity rapidly disappeared after recovery from the venous stasis.

The infusion of 10 mg of ketanserin intravenously did not induce release of antiaggregating activity, if the entire population of treated subjects is considered. The statistical analysis did not show a significant activity in plasma stored at either room temperature or at 4°C. However, a more careful evaluation of the results

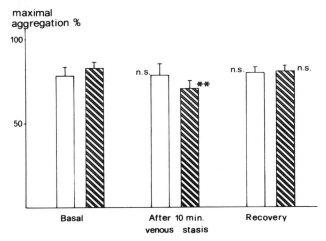

FIG. 1. Effect of venous stasis on the release in plasma of platelet antiaggregating activity ($n = 8$). **p < 0.01 (Student's *t*-test). *Open bar* = 20°C, *hatched bar* = 4°C.

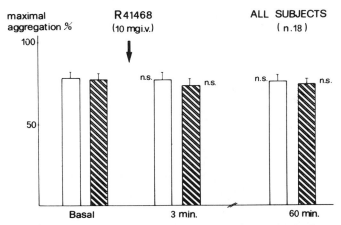

FIG. 2. Effect of an i.v. infusion of ketanserin (10 mg) on the release in plasma of platelet antiaggregating activity by R 41 468 in 18 healthy volunteers. No significant effect was present. Incubation period 10 min. *Open bar* = 20°C; *hatched bar* = 4°C.

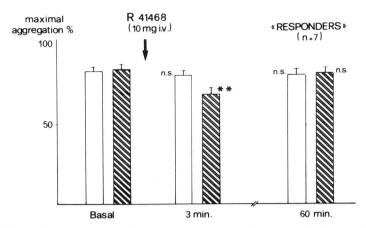

FIG. 3. Effect of an i.v. infusion of ketanserin (10 mg) on the release in plasma of platelet antiaggregating activity by R 41 468 in 7 "responders" subjects. A significant inhibitory effect on platelet aggregation was present in plasma collected 3 min after drug infusion and stored at 4°C. Incubation period 10 min. **p < 0.01 Student's t-test. *Open bar* = 20°C, *hatched bar* = 4°C.

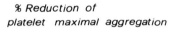

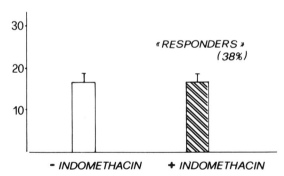

FIG. 4. Effect of indomethacin on the release in plasma of platelet antiaggregating activity induced by ketanserin in "responders" subjects. Indomethacin did not influence the ketanserin-induced release of antiaggregating activity in "responders."

allowed to define a subpopulation of 7 treated volunteers ("responders") in whom the infusion of the drug was followed by the appearance of antiaggregating activity, present at 4°C and rapidly destroyed at room temperature. The specific activity was present 3 min after ketanserin infusion but did not persist at the 60th min. The necessary incubation period of plasma with platelet-rich plasma for expressing the antiaggregating activity was 10 min. The pretreatment with indomethacin of "responders" subjects did not modify the release of the antiaggregating activity. No changes were observed in the "nonresponders" group with indomethacin.

DISCUSSION

As reported by others (4), venous stasis was able to induce the release of an endogenous antiaggregating activity. This effect rapidly disappeared at room temperature and was relatively stable at 4°C, thus confirming that the involved substance(s) could be related to prostacyclin. These results confirm the possibility to induce *in vivo* the release of endogenous prostacyclin-like activity. As regards the pharmacological study, our findings showed that in 7 out of 18 normal volunteers (38%), the intravenous administration of 10 mg of ketanserin induced the appearance of a plasmatic antiaggregating activity, as shown by a decrease of the maximal extent of platelet aggregation induced by ADP. This effect was evident 3 min after drug infusion in the plasma stored at 4°C but not at room temperature, which excludes a direct effect of the drug on the aggregating system. In the "nonresponders," no antiaggregating activity appeared; however, in all tested subjects a similar increase of muscular blood flow was observed, demonstrating the pharmacological activity of the infused compound. In order to evaluate the effect of prostaglandin synthesis inhibition on ketanserin-induced release of antiaggregating activity, the test was repeated after indomethacin treatment. In the "responders," as well as in the "nonresponders" group, no changes were observed after prostacyclin synthesis inhibition. Thus, if ketanserin induces the release of an endogenous antiaggregatory substance, it is unlikely that prostacyclin is involved.

On the whole, the present data do not sufficiently support the working hypothesis that part of the effect of ketanserin is humoral in nature. However, the limited number of subjects and the use of a single dose of the drug may not permit final conclusions in that regard. Likewise, more sophisticated chemical and/or biological techniques may be requested to obtain conclusive results. In any case, the eventual appearance of a thermolabile plasmatic factor with antiaggregating properties seems to be dissociated from the vasodilator activity of ketanserin, thus confirming the direct pharmacological effect of the drug on vascular smooth muscle cells.

REFERENCES

1. Di Perri, T., Forconi, S., Puccetti, F., Vittoria, A., and Guerrini, M. (1980): Effects of prostaglandin A_1 on renal handling of salt and water in congestive heart failure. *J. Cardiovasc. Pharmacol.*, 2:215–227.
2. Janssen Pharmaceutica (1980): R 41 468: The first pure and selective serotonin S_2 receptor blocking agent. Investigational New Drug Brochure.
3. Laghi Pasini, F., Auteri, A., Pecchi,, S., Cappelli, R., and Di Perri, T. (1982): Effect of a new antiserotonergic drug (R 41 468) in clinical conditions associated with circulatory disorders. *Proceedings of the Second Workshop on Peripheral Hemodynamics*, Siena, Italy *(in press)*.
4. Neri Serneri, G. G., Masotti, G., Poggesi, L., and Galanti, C. (1978): Release of PgI_2 in humans after local blood flow changes (post-ischemic hyperemia and venous stasis). *Proceedings of 5° International Congress on Thromboembolism*, p. 249. Bologna, Italy.
5. Van Nueten, J. M., Janssen, P. A. J., Van Beek, J., Verbeuren, T. J., and Vanhoutte, P. M. (1981): Vascular effects of ketanserin (R 41 468), a novel antagonist of 5-HT$_2$ serotonergic receptors. *J. Pharmacol. Exp. Ther.*, 218:217–230.

5-Hydroxytryptamine in Peripheral Reactions,
edited by Fred De Clerck and Paul M.
Vanhoutte. Raven Press, New York © 1982.

Action of Ketanserin (R 41 468) on Maximal Water and Osmotic Diuresis in Normal Subjects

T. Di Perri, F. Laghi Pasini, A. Vittoria, and G. Martelli

Department of Internal Medicine, School of Medicine, University of Siena,
I-53100 Siena, Italy

Ketanserin (R 41 468) increases muscular blood flow in normal subjects and patients with peripheral obliterative arterial disease, prevents cold-induced Raynaud's phenomenon, and lowers arterial blood pressure in hypertensive patients without changing heart rate (3; J. Symoens, *this volume*). The molecular mechanism of action of the drug is not fully understood but, at present, the most likely working hypothesis is that it possesses specific inhibitory properties of $5-HT_2$ serotonergic receptors. The decrease in peripheral resistance in skeletal muscle after acute infusion of the drug is accompanied by an increase in blood flow and complex metabolic changes like an increase of the venous Po_2 (J. Symoens, *this volume*).

The effect of the drug on renal function in man is not known. Both water and osmotic maximal diuresis enhance ionic and water transtubular transport in a specific way, leading to a diuretic response that is quantitatively correlated with the production of free water during water diuresis, and with the reabsorption of free water during osmotic diuresis (1,2).

The study of these two types of diuresis allows us not only to explore the diluting and concentrating activity of the kidney but also to test the action of drugs on the modification of kidney function caused by maximal diuresis. The aim of this study was to investigate the acute effect of ketanserin in normal man by infusing it during the induction of maximal diuresis.

MATERIALS AND METHODS

Six healthy volunteers (4 males, 2 females; mean age 38 years, range 25–46) were selected for the study. The subjects were divided in two groups. For each group of 3 subjects a different experimental procedure was used: one consisting of water loading and the other of water restriction according to a standardized protocol (1,2).

In the water-loaded group, the basal clearance period was 60 min. Successively, an initial water load of 10 ml/kg body weight in 5 min was given per os, followed

TABLE 1. Water load and ketanserin in normal subjects

	B	I	II	III	IV	F	P
U V ml/m'	0.38 ± 0.068	8.44 ± 1.994	10.33 ± 2.07	13.49 ± 2.41	16.33 ± 0.997	7.99	0.04
U Na mEq/m'	0.086 ± 0.028	0.303 ± 0.004	0.906 ± 0.211	1.699 ± 0.684	1.266 ± 0.268	2.71	0.09
U K mEq/m'	0.011 ± 0.002	0.044 ± 0.017	0.042 ± 0.016	0.038 ± 0.011	0.035 ± 0.013	0.7	0.5
U Cl mEq/m'	0.056 ± 0.026	0.317 ± 0.002	0.992 ± 0.232	1.743 ± 0.698	1.354 ± 0.262	2.99	0.07
U Ca mEq/m'	0.003 ± 0.001	0.022 ± 0.006	0.020 ± 0.003	0.031 ± 0.003	0.036 ± 0.006	7.24	0.005
U Mg mEq/m'	0.002 ± 0.001	0.024 ± 0.010	0.018 ± 0.005	0.036 ± 0.010	0.044 ± 0.017	1.51	0.2
U P mg/m'	0.296 ± 0.058	0.563 ± 0.069	0.490 ± 0.119	0.542 ± 0.117	0.589 ± 0.171	0.8	0.5
U Au mg/m'	0.485 ± 0.035	0.832 ± 0.158	0.528 ± 0.027	0.674 ± 0.087	0.725 ± 0.145	1.36	0.3
C Cr ml/m'	107.7 ± 0.781	125.0 ± 2.69	125.5 ± 9.79	127.6 ± 3.36	119.1 ± 9.66	1.79	0.2
C Osm ml/m'	1.141 ± 0.058	4.254 ± 0.584	2.182 ± 0.189	2.738 ± 0.233	3.273 ± 0.304	11.31	0.001
C H₂O ml/m'	0.241 ± 0.441	5.820 ± 1.71	8.146 ± 1.79	10.76 ± 2.21	13.05 ± 0.791	8.22	0.003
C Na + C H₂O	0.680 ± 0.171	6.480 ± 1.419	11.93 ± 1.610	18.31 ± 6.12	18.61 ± 1.158	5.04	0.01
100 GFR							

Columns refer to clearance periods: B, basal (60 min); I, dextrose (60 min); II, dextrose (30 min); III, dextrose + ketanserin (30 min); IV, dextrose + ketanserin (30 min). F and P values obtained with analysis of variance.

Abbreviations: UV, urinary volume; UNa, urinary sodium; UK, urinary potassium; UCl, urinary chloride; UCa, urinary calcium; UMg, urinary magnesium; UP, urinary phosphate; UAu, urinary uric acid; CCr, creatinine clearance; COsm, osmolar clearance; CH₂O, positive free-water clearance; CNa, sodium clearance; GFR, glomerular filtration rate; CNa + CH₂O/100 GFR, delivery of filtrate from the proximal tubule.

TABLE 2. *Osmotic load and ketanserin in normal subjects*

	B	I	II	III	IV	F	P
U V ml/m'	0.67 ± 0.112	5.21 ± 1.03	14.16 ± 2.048	18.16 ± 3.48	19.81 ± 2.420	5.92	0.03
U Na mEq/m'	0.073 ± 0.002	0.500 ± 0.041	1.154 ± 0.202	1.429 ± 0.271	1.569 ± 0.219	6.0	0.03
U K mEq/m'	0.017 ± 0.003	0.079 ± 0.016	0.118 ± 0.008	0.112 ± 0.019	0.135 ± 0.018	5.3	0.04
U Cl mEq/m'	0.076 ± 0.008	0.403 ± 0.046	0.922 ± 0.131	1.224 ± 0.230	1.355 ± 0.137	8.58	0.01
U Ca mEq/m'	0.004 ± 0.001	0.015 ± 0.021	0.023 ± 0.006	0.034 ± 0.007	0.042 ± 0.011	2.417	0.1
U Mg mEq/m'	0.004 ± 0.001	0.010 ± 0.001	0.012 ± 0.026	0.013 ± 0.006	0.012 ± 0.005	0.6	0.6
U P mg/m'	0.418 ± 0.010	0.389 ± 0.013	0.652 ± 0.151	0.656 ± 0.178	0.626 ± 0.108	0.5	0.6
U Au mg/m'	0.655 ± 0.016	0.982 ± 0.031	1.191 ± 0.068	1.211 ± 0.113	1.249 ± 0.074	5.4	0.04
C Cr ml/m'	109.6 ± 0.920	128.3 ± 3.4	126.9 ± 8.2	106.7 ± 5.9	109.8 ± 5.4	1.9	0.2
C Osm ml/m'	1.570 ± 0.082	9.0 ± 0.895	20.63 ± 3.112	23.17 ± 3.420	25.07 ± 2.58	8.85	0.01
T CH$_2$O ml/m'	0.895 ± 0.038	3.791 ± 0.072	6.470 ± 0.161	5.0 ± 0.164	5.264 ± 0.070	175.9	0.0002

Columns refer to clearance periods: B, basal (60 min); I, mannitol (60 min); II, mannitol (30 min); III, mannitol + ketanserin (30 min); IV, mannitol + ketanserin (30 min). F and P values obtained with analysis of variance.

Abbreviations: UV, urinary volume; UNa, urinary sodium; UK, urinary potassium; UCl, urinary chloride; UCa, urinary calcium; UMg, urinary magnesium; UP, urinary phosphate; UAu, urinary uric acid; CCr, creatinine clearance; COsm, osmolar clearance; TcH$_2$O, negative free-water clearance.

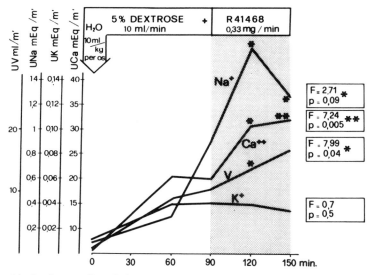

FIG. 1. Maximal water diuresis in normal subjects ($n = 3$). Effect of ketanserin on UV, UNa, UK, and UCa. (See Table 1 for definition of abbreviations.)

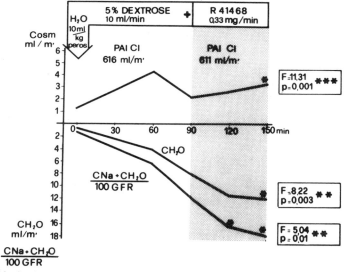

FIG. 2. Maximal water diuresis in normal subjects ($n = 3$). Effect of ketanserin on osmotic clearance (COsm) and fluid reaching the distal tubule.

by an infusion of 5% dextrose in water at the rate of 10 ml/min. After two clearance periods, the first of 60 and the second of 30 min, ketanserin was added to the dextrose solution in an amount sufficient to ensure an infusion of 0.33 mg/min for 60 min, divided into two successive clearance periods of 30 min.

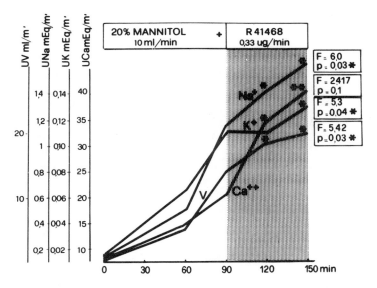

FIG. 3. Maximal osmotic diuresis in normal subjects ($n = 3$). Effect of ketanserin on UV, UNa, UK, and UCa. (See Table 1 for definition of abbreviations.)

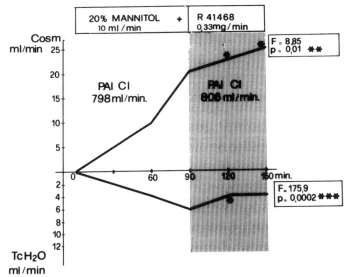

FIG. 4. Maximal osmotic diuresis in normal ($n = 3$). Effect of ketanserin on osmotic clearance (COsm) and negative free-water clearance (TcH$_2$O).

In the water-restricted group, the volunteers were deprived of water overnight. After 60 min of basal clearance, an infusion of 20% mannitol in water was started at the rate of 10 ml/min, during two successive periods of clearance of 60 and 30 min. At the end of the second period, ketanserin was added to the mannitol solution in an amount sufficient to ensure an infusion of 0.33 mg/min, prolonging the infusion for 60 min divided into two 30 min clearance periods. Urine was collected with a bladder catheter. Blood samples were collected in heparinized tubes before and after the initial dextrose or mannitol load and after the infusion of ketanserin.

The determination of sodium, potassium, calcium, and magnesium was made by atomic spectrophotometry (Shandon Southern A 3300). Chloride was measured by the method of Schales and Schales (4). Phosphate was measured by a colorimetric method (Phosphor B test, Wako Chemicals), uric acid by colorimetry (Urimeter Sclavo). Creatinine was measured by the kinetic colorimetric method (Sclavo). Paraaminohippurate (PAH) was measured by a colorimetric method in the presence of N-(1-naphthyl)ethylenediamine dihydrochloride (5). Osmolality was measured by the freezing point depression method in a semiautomatic osmometer (Knauser). We determined urinary volume per min, sodium (UNa), potassium (UK), calcium (UCa), magnesium (UMg), chloride (UCl) per min of output and urinary osmolality. In plasma the osmolality and the concentration of sodium (PNa) and all the other electrolytes considered were measured. We calculate the osmolar clearance, glomerular filtration rate (GFR), determined from endogenous creatinine clearance and renal plasmatic flow by means of the PAH clearance. Positive free-water clearance (CH_2O) in the water-load protocol and negative free-water clearance (TcH_2O) in the water-deprivation protocol were calculated and expressed in ml/min. In the water-loaded group, the delivery of filtrate from the proximal tubule was calculated using the formula: $CNa + CH_2O/100$ ml GFR (in ml/min), where CNa is the sodium clearance.

The data are expressed as means $\pm$ the standard error of the mean, for each group of values. All data were statistically evaluated by means of the analysis of variance (one way) and the mean values obtained at the end of each of the two clearance periods with ketanserin were tested for significance with Student's t-test for paired variables (t_1 at 120th min and t_2 at 150th min), in comparison with values obtained at the end of the simple dextrose or mannitol infusion.

RESULTS

Findings for water-loaded and water-deprived normal subjects, during the simple dextrose or mannitol infusion, are shown in the figures and tables and described in detail elsewhere (1). Statistical analysis showed significant modifications of UV, UCl, UCa, COsm, CH_2O and $CNa + CH_2/100$ ml GFR in maximal water diuresis and of UV, UNa, UK, UCl, UAu, COsm, and TcH_2O in osmotic diuresis (Tables 1 and 2).

When ketanserin was added to the dextrose infusion, remarkable modifications of the renal function were observed. A rapid and marked increase in urine volume ($t_1 = 6.16$) and output of sodium ($t_1 = 4.88$; $t_2 = 4.50$) as well as calcium ($t_1 = 4.35$; $t_2 = 7.33$) was registered in comparison with the findings recorded immediately before the addition of the drug. No variations in potassium excretion were observed. Moreoever there was a significant increase in the amount of osmotic clearance ($t_2 = 44.76$) and of free-water clearance ($t_2 = 4.92$) and, at the same time, a progressive and marked increase in the filtrate fluid entering the distal tubule ($-t_1 = 5.14$; $t_2 = 5.34$). The changes in glomerular filtration in renal plasmatic flow (PAH clearance) were not statistically significant (Figs. 1 and 2).

In the water-restricted subjects, the addition of ketanserin to the hypertonic mannitol infusion was followed immediately by an important and progressive increase in urinary volume ($t_1 = 5.28$; $t_2 = 4.90$) and excretion of sodium ($t_1 = 4.96$; $t_2 = 5.29$), potassium ($t_2 = 4.62$) and calcium ($t_1 = 5.11$; $t_2 = 4.43$); free-water reabsorption significantly decreased at the end of the first clearance period in comparison with the findings recorded immediately before the addition of the drug ($t_1 = 4.44$). No statistically important changes in the endogenous creatinine clearance and renal plasmatic flow were observed (Figs. 3 and 4).

DISCUSSION

In normal volunteers the infusion of ketanserin either during the water load (to study maximal water diuresis) or during the mannitol load in the dehydrated subjects (to study maximal osmotic diuresis) was followed by significant quantitative and qualitative changes. Ketanserin, when added either to water or to mannitol infusion, had a diuretic effect since it induced a marked increase of urine volume, and a saluretic effect since it induced an increase of sodium excretion. These changes were of rapid onset after the start of the drug infusion and were not associated with significant modifications of renal blood flow or glomerular filtration rate. These findings suggest that the mode of action of ketanserin is to interfere with the transcellular transport of ions and water at the tubular level. That ketanserin selectively inhibits salt reabsorption in the proximal tubule is suggested, in water-loaded subjects, by the larger amount of filtrate entering the distal tubule and the increase of free-water clearance. The latter finding appeared to depend strongly upon the amount of saline output to the diluting segment of the loop of Henle which, in turn, is determined by the inhibition of salt reabsorption in the proximal tubule. The increase of calcium excretion fits with this interpretation since the proximal tubule is the main site of its reabsorption. On the basis of these findings an increase of potassium excretion would be expected as a functional change which normally follows an increase in sodium output to the distal convoluted tubule; but it was not seen so. Therefore, a secondary site of action of the drug at this level must be admitted. In the dehydrated subjects submitted to osmotic load, the addition of ketanserin was not followed by an increase of free-water reabsorption as a functional consequence of the inhibition of saline reabsorption in the proximal tubule. This finding is not easy to explain without admitting that the drug specifically inhibits the tubular reabsorption of water. In conclusion, a marked diuretic and saluretic activity of ketanserin was observed in normal subjects undergoing maximal diuresis. We do not know, at present, whether ketanserin alone shows a similar activity in the nonstimulated subject but, certainly, it significantly interferes with kidney functions when a maximal diuresis is induced. The observed changes after ketanserin infusion are comparable to that observed with the infusion of PGA_1, using the same model of investigation (2). Both drugs act on proximal sodium reabsorption stimulating free-water clearance production, but did not modify free-water reabsorption. However, PGA_1 simultaneously augments renal blood flow and potassium excretion, an effect which was not observed for ketanserin, illustrating the differences in the mechanism of action of these two drugs on the human kidney.

REFERENCES

1. Di Perri, T., Forconi, S., Rubegni, M., Puccetti, J., and Vittoria, A. (1967): Su alcuni aspetti della funzione renale nello scompenso di cuore. *Boll. Soc. Ital. Cardiol.*, 13:46–57.
2. Di Perri, T., Forconi, S., Puccetti, F., Vittoria, A., and Guerrini, M. (1980): Effects of prostaglandin A_1 on renal handling of salt and water in congestive heart failure. *J. Cardiovasc. Pharmacol.*, 2:215–227.
3. Laghi Pasini, F., Auteri, A., Pecchi, S., Cappelli, R., and Di Perri, T. (1982): Effect of a new antiserotonergic drug (R 41 468) in clinical conditions associated with circulatory disorders. *Proceedings of the Second Workshop on Peripheral Hemodynamics*, Siena, Italy *(in press)*.
4. Schales, O., and Schales, S. S. (1941): A simple and accurate method for the determination of chloride in biological fluids. *J. Biol. Chem.*, 140:879–884.
5. Smith, H. W., Finkelstein, N., Aliminosa, L., and Smith, W. W. (1945): The renal clearances of substituted hippuric acid derivatives and other aromatic acids in dog and man. *J. Clin. Invest.*, 24:388–395.

Subject Index

Subject Index